Mohrman and Heller's
Cardiovascular Physiology

Notice

Medicine is an ever-changing science. As new research and clinical experience broaden our knowledge, changes in treatment and drug therapy are required. The authors and the publisher of this work have checked with sources believed to be reliable in their efforts to provide information that is complete and generally in accord with the standards accepted at the time of publication. However, in view of the possibility of human error or changes in medical sciences, neither the authors nor the publisher nor any other party who has been involved in the preparation or publication of this work warrants that the information contained herein is in every respect accurate or complete, and they disclaim all responsibility for any errors or omissions or for the results obtained from use of the information contained in this work. Readers are encouraged to confirm the information contained herein with other sources. For example, and in particular, readers are advised to check the product information sheet included in the package of each drug they plan to administer to be certain that the information contained in this work is accurate and that changes have not been made in the recommended dose or in the contraindications for administration. This recommendation is of particular importance in connection with new or infrequently used drugs.

a LANGE medical book

Mohrman and Heller's Cardiovascular Physiology

10th edition

David M. Harris, PhD
Associate Professor of Physiology
Department of Medical Education
University of Central Florida College of Medicine
Orlando, Florida

New York   Chicago   San Francisco   Athens   London   Madrid
Mexico City   Milan   New Delhi   Singapore   Sydney   Toronto

ISBN 978-1-264-61761-6
MHID 1-264-61761-5
ISSN 1541-9002

This book was set in Adobe Garamond Pro by MPS Limited.
The editors were Sydney Keen Vitale and Kim J. Davis.
The production supervisor was Catherine H. Saggese.
The text was designed by Eve Siegel.
Project management was provided by Pradhiba Kannaiyan, MPS Limited.
This book is printed on acid-free paper.

McGraw-Hill Education books are available at special quantity discounts to use as premiums and sales promotions or for use in corporate training programs. To contact a representative, please visit the Contact Us pages at www.mhprofessional.com.

Contents

Preface

It is an honor to serve as a primary author of such a well-written text that appropriately clarifies the concepts of cardiovascular physiology. I have nothing but gratitude to the founding authors, Drs. Mohrman and Heller, for their focus on learners not getting "lost in the forest for the trees." I vividly remember using this textbook during my graduate education in the late 1990s and early 2000s at Temple University as I developed my love for cardiovascular physiology. Thank you to them for helping me to share the passion with future learners.

The cardiovascular system is simple in a conceptual nature as its function is to establish a pressure gradient to ensure perfusion throughout the body and ultimately the brain. On the other side, the cardiovascular system is complex in design as it consists of multiple components that students learn separately until they eventually discover that the variables are dependent on each other. Despite the cardiovascular system being challenging, certain concepts transcend across the system (Ohm's Law) and as students learn them, they are able to better understand pathologies and disease states of the cardiovascular system and the related clinical signs and symptoms.

The tenth edition focuses on ensuring that mechanisms are the most up-to-date. Additionally, questions have been updated and clarified to help learners gauge their understanding.

Foremost, I thank my wife Renata and my two daughters, Isabella and Alicia, for their support and loving me even on my "worst" days. I would also like to thank my mentors, colleagues, and learners for what they have taught me over the years through various conversations and sessions.

David M. Harris, PhD

Overview of the Cardiovascular System

1

OBJECTIVES

The student understands the homeostatic role of the cardiovascular system, the basic principles of cardiovascular transport, and the basic structure and function of the components of the system:

▶ *Defines homeostasis.*

▶ *Identifies the major body fluid compartments and states the approximate volume of each.*

▶ *Lists 3 conditions provided by the cardiovascular system that are essential for regulating the composition of interstitial fluid (i.e., the internal environment).*

▶ *Predicts the relative changes in flow through a tube caused by changes in tube length, tube radius, fluid viscosity, and pressure difference.*

▶ *Uses the Fick principle to describe convective transport of substances through the CV system and to calculate a tissue's rate of utilization (or production) of a substance.*

▶ *Identifies the chambers and valves of the heart and describes the pathway of blood flow through the heart.*

▶ *Defines cardiac output and identifies its 2 determinants.*

▶ *Describes the site of initiation and pathway of action potential propagation in the heart.*

▶ *States the relationship between ventricular filling and cardiac output (the Starling law of the heart) and describes its importance in the control of cardiac output.*

▶ *Identifies the distribution of sympathetic and parasympathetic nerves in the heart and lists the basic effects of these nerves on the heart.*

▶ *Lists the 5 factors essential to proper ventricular pumping action.*

▶ *Lists the major different types of vessels in a vascular bed and describes the morphological differences among them.*

▶ *Describes the basics and functions of the different vessel types.*

▶ *Identifies the major mechanisms in vascular resistance control and blood flow distribution.*

▶ *Describes the basic composition of the fluid and cellular portions of blood.*

1

EVOLUTION AND HOMEOSTATIC ROLE
OF THE CARDIOVASCULAR SYSTEM

All living organisms require outside energy sources to survive. Indeed, Darwin deduced his evolutionary concepts largely from observations of external adaptations that evolved in different organisms to exploit unique sources of "food" energy. Clearly, one strong evolutionary force has been to maximize the ability to obtain outside energy.

In the big picture of "survival of the fittest," equally important to obtaining outside energy is making efficient use of it once it is obtained. Therefore, we contend that developing energy-efficient mechanisms to accomplish all internal tasks necessary for successful life has also been a strong evolutionary force and probably applies to all "internal" processes.

In this text, we focus on how the design and operation of the human cardiovascular system has evolved to accomplish its essential tasks with a minimum of energy expenditure.

A 19th-century French physiologist, Claude Bernard (1813–1878), first recognized that all higher organisms actively and constantly strive to prevent the external environment from upsetting the conditions necessary for life within the organism. Thus, the temperature, oxygen concentration, pH, ionic composition, osmolarity, and many other important variables of our *internal environment* are closely controlled. This process of maintaining the "constancy" of our internal environment has come to be known as *homeostasis*. To aid in this task, an elaborate material transport network, the cardiovascular system, has evolved.

Three compartments of watery fluids, known collectively as the *total body water*, account for approximately 60% of body weight in a normal adult. This water is distributed among the *intracellular, interstitial*, and *plasma* compartments, as indicated in Figure 1–1. Note that about two-thirds of our body water is contained within cells (intracellular) and communicates with the interstitial fluid across the plasma membranes of cells. The fluid outside of the cells (i.e., extracellular fluid) consists of interstitial and plasma volumes. Only a small amount of this fluid, the *plasma volume*, circulates within the cardiovascular system because blood also contains suspended blood cells that collectively occupy approximately 40% of its volume. However, it is the circulating plasma that directly interacts with the interstitial fluid of body organs across the walls of the capillary vessels.

The interstitial fluid is the immediate environment of individual cells. (It is the "internal environment" referred to by Bernard.) These cells must draw their nutrients from and release their products into the interstitial fluid. The interstitial fluid cannot, however, be considered a large reservoir for nutrients or a large sink for metabolic products because its volume is less than half that of the cells that it serves. The well-being of individual cells, therefore, depends heavily on the homeostatic mechanisms that regulate the composition of the interstitial fluid. This task is accomplished by continuously exposing the interstitial fluid to "fresh" circulating plasma fluid.

As blood passes through capillaries, solutes exchange between plasma and interstitial fluid by the process of *diffusion*. The net result of transcapillary diffusion is

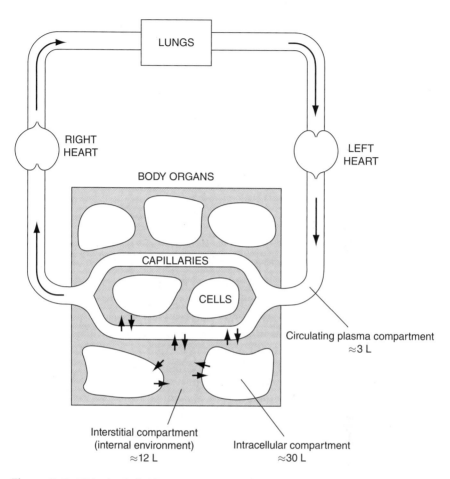

Figure 1–1. Major body fluid compartments with average volumes indicated for a normal 70-kg adult human. Total body water is approximately 60% of body weight.

always that the interstitial fluid tends to take on the composition of the incoming blood. If, for example, potassium ion concentration in the interstitium of a particular skeletal muscle was higher than that in the plasma entering the muscle, then potassium would diffuse into the blood as it passes through the muscle's capillaries. Because this removes potassium from the interstitial fluid, its potassium ion concentration would decrease. It would stop decreasing when the net movement of potassium into capillaries no longer occurs, that is, when the concentration of the interstitial fluid reaches that of incoming plasma.

Three conditions are essential for this circulatory mechanism to effectively control the composition of the interstitial fluid: (1) there must be adequate blood flow through the tissue capillaries; (2) the chemical composition of the incoming (or arterial) blood must be controlled to be that which is optimal in the interstitial fluid; and (3) diffusion distances between plasma and tissue cells must be short. Figure 1–1 shows how the cardiovascular transport system operates to accomplish these tasks. Diffusional transport within tissues occurs over extremely small distances because no cell in the body is located farther than approximately 10 μm from a capillary. Over such microscopic distances, diffusion is a very rapid process that can move huge quantities of material. Diffusion, however, is a very poor mechanism for moving substances from the capillaries of an organ, such as the lungs, to the capillaries of another organ that may be 1 m or more distant. Consequently, substances are transported between organs by the process of *convection*, by which the substances easily move along with blood flow because they are either dissolved or contained within blood. The relative distances involved in cardiovascular transport are not well illustrated in Figure 1–1. If the figure was drawn to scale, with 1 inch representing the distance from capillaries to cells within a calf muscle, then the capillaries in the lungs would have to be located about 15 miles away!

OVERALL DESIGN OF THE CARDIOVASCULAR SYSTEM

The overall functional arrangement of the cardiovascular system is illustrated in Figure 1–2. Because a functional rather than an anatomical viewpoint is expressed in this figure, the role of heart appears in 3 places: as the right heart pump, as the left heart pump, and as the heart muscle tissue. It is common practice to view the cardiovascular system as (1) the *pulmonary circulation*, composed of the right heart pump and the lungs, and (2) the *systemic circulation*, in which the left heart pump supplies blood to the systemic organs (all structures except the gas exchange portion of the lungs). The pulmonary and systemic circulations are *arranged in series*, that is, one after the other. Consequently, both the right and left hearts must pump an identical volume of blood per minute. This amount is called the *cardiac output*.

As indicated in Figure 1–2, most *systemic* organs are functionally *arranged in parallel* (i.e., side by side) within the cardiovascular system. There are 2 important consequences of this parallel arrangement. First, nearly all systemic organs receive blood of identical composition—that which has just left the lungs and is known as *arterial blood*. Second, the flow through any one of the systemic organs can be controlled independently of the flow through the other organs. Thus, for example, the cardiovascular response to whole-body exercise can involve increased blood flow through some organs, decreased blood flow through others, and unchanged blood flow through yet others.

Many of the organs in the body help perform the task of continually reconditioning the blood circulating in the cardiovascular system. Key roles are played by organs, such as the lungs, that communicate with the external environment. As is evident from the arrangement shown in Figure 1–2, any blood that has just passed through a systemic organ returns to the right heart and is pumped through the lungs, where oxygen and carbon dioxide are exchanged. Thus, the blood's gas composition is always reconditioned immediately after leaving a systemic organ.

Like the lungs, many of the systemic organs also serve to recondition the composition of blood, although the flow circuitry precludes their doing so each time

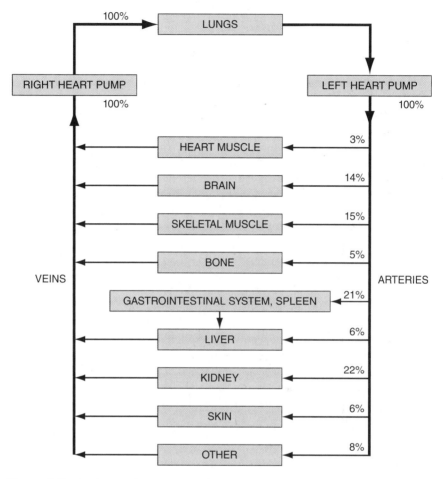

Figure 1–2. Cardiovascular circuitry, indicating the percentage distribution of cardiac output to various organ systems in a resting individual.

the blood completes a single circuit. The kidneys, for example, continually adjust the electrolyte composition of the blood passing through them. Because the blood conditioned by the kidneys mixes freely with all the circulating blood and because electrolytes and water freely pass through most capillary walls, the kidneys control the electrolyte balance of the entire internal environment. To achieve this, it is necessary that a given unit of blood pass often through the kidneys. In fact, the kidneys normally receive about one-fifth of the cardiac output under resting conditions. This greatly exceeds the amount of flow that is necessary to supply the nutrient needs of the renal tissue. This situation is common to organs that have a blood-conditioning function.

Blood-conditioning organs can also withstand, at least temporarily, severe reduction of blood flow. Skin, for example, can easily tolerate a large reduction in blood flow when it is necessary to conserve body heat. Most of the large abdominal organs also fall into this category. The reason is simply that because of their blood-conditioning functions, their normal blood flow is far more than that necessary to maintain their basal metabolic needs.

The brain, heart muscle, and skeletal muscles typify organs in which blood flows solely to supply the metabolic needs of the tissue. They do not recondition the blood for the benefit of any other organ. Normally, the blood flow to the brain and the heart muscle is only slightly greater than that required for their metabolism; hence, they do not tolerate blood flow interruptions well. Unconsciousness can occur within a few seconds after the stoppage of cerebral flow, and permanent brain damage can occur in as little as 4 minutes without flow. Similarly, the heart muscle (*myocardium*) normally consumes approximately 75% of the oxygen supplied to it, and the heart's pumping ability begins to deteriorate within beats of a coronary flow interruption. As we shall see later, the task of providing adequate blood flow to the brain and the heart muscle receives a high priority in the overall operation of the cardiovascular system.

Cardiac muscle must do physical work to move blood through the circulatory system. Note in Figure 1–2 that the cardiac muscle itself requires only about 3% of all the blood it is pumping to sustain its own operation. The clear implication is that the heart has evolved into a very efficient pump.

Within any given tissue, the blood flow required to maintain local homeostasis is directly related to its current cellular metabolic rate. Under the challenges of daily life, metabolic activity of many individual organs can change dramatically from situation to situation. For example, metabolic rate of maximally active skeletal muscle can be 50 times that of its inactive (resting) rate. Thus, it is essential for the cardiovascular system to rapidly adapt to ever-changing needs in the body. As far as the heart is concerned, the bottom line is how much blood flow it must produce in different situations, regardless of where that total flow is directed. Cardiac output in a resting human adult is about 5 to 6 L/min (80 gallons/h, 2000 gallons/day!) and can increase to 3 to 4 times that amount during maximal exercise. Presumably, the cardiovascular system has evolved to efficiently operate over that range.

THE BASIC PHYSICS OF BLOOD FLOW

One of the most important keys to comprehending how the cardiovascular system operates is to have a thorough understanding of the relationship among the physical factors that determine the rate of fluid flow through a tubular vessel.

The tube depicted in Figure 1–3 might represent a segment of any vessel in the body. It has a certain length (L) and a certain internal radius (r) through which blood flows. Fluid flows through the tube only when the pressures in the fluid at the inlet and outlet ends (P_i and P_o) are unequal, that is, when there is a pressure difference (ΔP) between the ends. Pressure differences supply the driving force for flow. Because friction develops between the moving fluid and the stationary walls of a tube, vessels tend to resist fluid movement

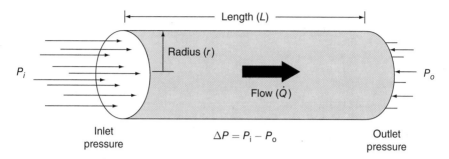

Figure 1–3. Factors influencing fluid flow through a tube.

through them. This *vascular resistance* is a measure of how difficult it is to make fluid flow through the tube, that is, how much of a pressure difference it takes to cause a certain flow. The all-important relationship among flow, pressure difference, and resistance is described by the *basic flow equation* as follows:

$$\text{Flow} = \frac{\text{Pressure difference}}{\text{Resistance}}$$

or

$$\dot{Q} = \frac{\Delta P}{R}$$

where $\dot{Q}$ = flow rate (volume/time), ΔP = pressure difference (mm Hg[1]), and R = resistance to flow (mm Hg × time/volume).

The basic flow equation may be applied not only to a single tube but also to complex networks of tubes, for example, the vascular bed of an organ or the entire systemic system. The flow through the brain, for example, is determined by the difference in pressure between cerebral arteries and veins divided by the overall resistance to flow through the vessels in the cerebral vascular bed. It should be evident from the basic flow equation that there are only 2 ways in which blood flow through any organ can be changed: (1) by changing the pressure difference across its vascular bed or (2) by changing its vascular resistance. Most often, it is changes in an organ's vascular resistance that cause the flow through the organ to change.

From the work of the French physician Jean Leonard Marie Poiseuille (1799–1869), who performed experiments on fluid flow through small glass capillary tubes, it is known that the resistance to flow through a cylindrical tube depends

---

[1] Although pressure is most correctly expressed in units of force per unit area, it is customary to express pressures within the cardiovascular system in millimeters of mercury. For example, mean arterial pressure may be said to be 100 mm Hg because it is same as the pressure existing at the bottom of a mercury column 100 mm high. All cardiovascular pressures are expressed relative to atmospheric pressure, which is approximately 760 mm Hg.

on several factors, including the radius and length of the tube and the viscosity of the fluid flowing through it. These factors influence resistance to flow as follows:

$$R = \frac{8L\eta}{\pi r^4}$$

where r = inside radius of the tube, L = tube length, and η = fluid viscosity.

Note especially that the internal radius of the tube is raised to the fourth power in this equation. Thus, even small changes in the internal radius of a tube have a huge influence on its resistance to flow. For example, halving the inside radius of a tube will increase its resistance to flow by 16-fold.

The preceding 2 equations may be combined into one expression known as the *Poiseuille equation*, which includes all the terms that influence flow through a cylindrical vessel:

$$\dot{Q} = \Delta P \frac{\pi r^4}{8L\eta}$$

Again, note that flow occurs only when a pressure difference exists. (If $\Delta P = 0$, then flow = 0.) It is not surprising then that arterial blood pressure is an extremely important and carefully regulated cardiovascular variable. Also note once again that for any given pressure difference, tube radius has a very large influence on the flow through a tube. It is logical, therefore, that organ blood flows are regulated primarily through changes in the radii of vessels within organs. Although vessel length and blood viscosity are factors that influence vascular resistance, they are not variables that can be easily manipulated for the purpose of moment-to-moment control of blood flow.

In regard to the overall cardiovascular system, as depicted in Figures 1–1 and 1–2, one can conclude that blood flows through the vessels within an organ only because a pressure difference exists between the blood in the arteries supplying the organ and the veins draining it. The primary job of the heart pump is to keep the pressure within arteries higher than that within veins. Normally, the average pressure in systemic arteries is approximately 100 mm Hg, and the average pressure in systemic veins is approximately 0 mm Hg.

Therefore, because the pressure difference (ΔP) is nearly identical across all systemic organs, cardiac output is distributed among the various systemic organs, primarily based on their individual resistances to flow. Because blood preferentially flows along paths of least resistance, organs with relatively low resistance naturally receive relatively high flow.

MATERIAL TRANSPORT BY BLOOD FLOW

Substances are carried between organs within the cardiovascular system by the process of *convective transport*, the simple process of being swept along with the flow of the blood in which they are contained. The rate at which a substance (X) is transported by this process depends solely on the concentration of the substance in the blood and the blood flow rate.

$$\text{Transport rate} = \text{Flow rate} \times \text{Concentration}$$

$$\dot{X} = \dot{Q} \times [X]$$

where $\dot{X}$ = rate of transport of X (mass/time), $\dot{Q}$ = blood flow rate (volume/time), and $[X]$ = concentration of X in blood (mass/volume).

It is evident from the preceding equation that only 2 methods are available for altering the rate at which a substance is carried to an organ: (1) a change in the blood flow rate through the organ or (2) a change in the arterial blood concentration of the substance. The preceding equation might be used, for example, to calculate how much oxygen is carried to a certain skeletal muscle each minute. Note, however, that this calculation would not indicate whether the muscle used the oxygen carried to it.

The Fick Principle

One can extend the convective transport principle to calculate the rate at which a substance is being removed from (or added to) the blood as it passes through an organ. To do so, one must simultaneously consider the rate at which the substance is entering the organ in the arterial blood *and* the rate at which the substance is leaving the organ in the venous blood. The basic logic is simple. For example, if something goes into an organ in arterial blood and does not come out on the other side in venous blood, it must have left the blood and entered the tissue within the organ. This concept is referred to as the *Fick principle* (Adolf Fick, a German physician, 1829–1901) and may be formally stated as follows:

$$\dot{X}_{tc} = \dot{Q} \times ([X]_a - [X]_v)$$

where $\dot{X}_{tc}$ = transcapillary efflux rate of X, $\dot{Q}$ = blood flow rate, and $[X]_{a,v}$ = arterial and venous concentrations of X.

The Fick principle is useful because it offers a practical method to deduce a tissue's *steady-state* rate of consumption (or production) of any substance. To understand why this is so, one further step in logic is necessary. Consider, for example, what possibly can happen to a substance that enters a tissue from the blood. It can either (1) increase the concentration of itself within the tissue or (2) be metabolized (i.e., converted into something else) within the tissue. A steady state implies a stable situation wherein nothing (including the substance's tissue concentration) is changing with time. Therefore, in the *steady state*, the rate of the substance's loss from blood within a tissue must equal its rate of metabolism within that tissue.

THE HEART

Pumping Action

The heart lies in the center of the thoracic cavity and is suspended by its attachments to the great vessels within a thin fibrous sac called the *pericardium.* A small amount of fluid in the sac lubricates the surface of the heart and allows it to move freely during contraction and relaxation. Blood flow through all organs is passive and occurs only because arterial pressure is kept higher than venous pressure by the pumping action of the heart. The right heart pump provides the energy necessary to move blood through the pulmonary vessels, and the left heart pump provides the energy to move blood through the systemic organs.

The pathway of blood flow through the chambers of the heart is indicated in Figure 1–4. Venous blood returns from the systemic organs to the right atrium via the superior and inferior venae cavae. This "venous" blood is deficient in oxygen because it has just passed through systemic organs that all extract oxygen from blood for their metabolism. It then passes through the *tricuspid valve* into the right ventricle, and from there it is pumped through the *pulmonic valve* into the pulmonary circulation via the pulmonary arteries. Within the capillaries of the lung, blood is "reoxygenated" by exposure to oxygen-rich inspired air. Oxygenated pulmonary venous blood flows in pulmonary veins to the left atrium and passes through the *mitral valve* into the left ventricle. From there it is pumped through the *aortic valve* into the aorta to be distributed to the systemic organs.

Although the gross anatomy of the right heart pump is somewhat different from that of the left heart pump, the pumping principles are identical. Each pump consists of a ventricle, which is a closed chamber surrounded by a muscular wall, as illustrated in Figure 1–5. The valves are structurally designed to allow flow in only one direction and *passively* open and close in

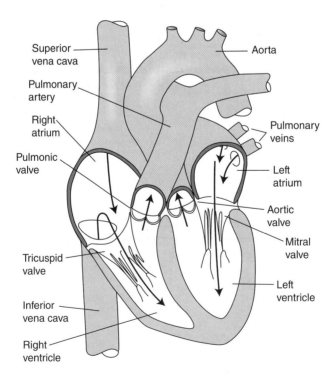

Figure 1–4. Pathway of blood flow through the heart.

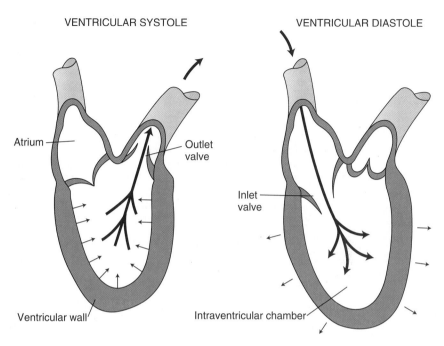

Figure 1–5. Ventricular pumping action.

response to the direction of the pressure differences across them. Ventricular pumping action occurs because the volume of the intraventricular chamber is cyclically changed by rhythmic and synchronized contraction and relaxation of the individual cardiac muscle cells that lie in a circumferential orientation within the ventricular wall.[2]

When the ventricular muscle cells contract, they generate a circumferential tension in the ventricular walls that causes the pressure within the chamber to increase. As soon as the ventricular pressure exceeds the pressure in the pulmonary artery (right pump) or aorta (left pump), blood is forced out of the chamber through the outlet valve, as shown in Figure 1–5. This phase of the cardiac cycle during which the ventricular muscle cells contract is called *systole.* Contraction of the ventricular muscle increases tension in the chordae tendineae, which prevents the atrioventricular (AV) valve from opening despite the large pressure difference between the ventricle and atrium. When the ventricular muscle cells relax, the pressure in the ventricle falls below that in the atrium, the AV valve opens, and the ventricle refills with blood, as shown on the right side in Figure 1–5. This portion of the cardiac cycle is called *diastole.* The outlet valve is closed during diastole

---

[2] The basic pumping principle of the heart has a very long evolutionary history. Eons before mammals evolved, bivalve mollusks were using the same principle to pump water through themselves to harvest food energy from microscopic organisms living in that water.

because arterial pressure is greater than intraventricular pressure. After the period of diastolic filling, the systolic phase of a new cardiac cycle is initiated.

⑤ The amount of blood pumped per minute from each ventricle (the *cardiac output*, CO) is determined by the volume of blood ejected per beat (the *stroke volume*, SV) and the number of heart beats per minute (the *heart rate*, HR) as follows:

$$CO = SV \times HR$$
$$volume/min = volume/beat \times beats/min$$

It should be evident from this relationship that *all* influences on cardiac output must act through changes in either the HR or the SV.

An important implication of the above is that the volume of blood that the ventricle pumps with each heartbeat (i.e., the SV) must equal the blood volume inside the ventricle at the end of diastole (*end-diastolic volume*, EDV) minus ventricular volume at the end of systole (*end-systolic volume*, ESV). That is,

$$SV = EDV - ESV$$

Thus, SV can only be changed by changes in EDV and/or ESV. The implication for the bigger picture is that cardiac output can *only* be changed by changes in HR, EDV, and/or ESV.

Cardiac Excitation

Efficient pumping action of the heart requires a precise coordination of the contraction of millions of individual cardiac muscle cells. Contraction of each cell is triggered when an electrical excitatory impulse (*action potential*) sweeps over its membrane. Proper coordination of the contractile activity of the individual cardiac muscle cells is achieved primarily by the conduction of action potentials from one cell to the next via gap junctions that connect all cells of the heart into a functional syncytium (i.e., acting as one synchronous unit). In addition, muscle cells in certain areas of the heart are specifically adapted to control the frequency of cardiac excitation, the pathway of conduction, and the rate of impulse propagation through various regions of the heart. The major components of this specialized excitation and conduction system are shown in Figure 1–6. These include the *sinoatrial node* (SA node), the *atrioventricular node* (AV node), the *bundle of His*, and the right and left *bundle branches* made up of specialized cells called *Purkinje fibers*.

The SA node contains specialized cells that normally function as the heart's pacemaker and initiate the action potential that is conducted through the heart. The AV node contains slowly conducting cells that normally function to create a slight delay between atrial contraction and ventricular contraction. The Purkinje fibers are specialized for rapid conduction and ensure that all ventricular cells contract at nearly the same instant. The overall message is that HR is normally controlled by the electrical activity of the SA nodal cells. The rest of the conduction

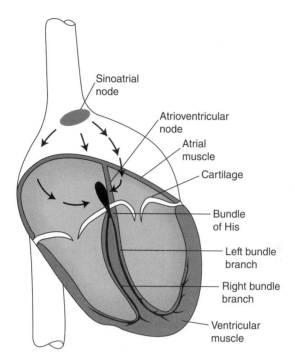

Figure 1–6. Electrical conduction system of the heart.

system ensures that all the rest of the cells in the heart follow along in proper lockstep for efficient pumping action.

Control of Cardiac Output

AUTONOMIC NEURAL INFLUENCES

Although the heart can inherently beat on its own, cardiac function can be influenced profoundly by neural inputs from both the sympathetic and parasympathetic divisions of the autonomic nervous system. These inputs allow us to modify cardiac pumping as is appropriate to meet changing homeostatic needs of the body. All portions of the heart are richly innervated by *adrenergic sympathetic fibers.* When active, these sympathetic nerves release *norepinephrine* (noradrenaline) on cardiac cells. Norepinephrine interacts with β_1-adrenergic receptors on cardiac muscle cells to increase the HR, increase the action potential conduction velocity, and increase the force of contraction and rates of contraction and relaxation. Overall, sympathetic activation acts to increase cardiac pumping.

Cholinergic parasympathetic nerve fibers travel to the heart via the vagus nerve and innervate the SA node, the AV node, and the atrial muscle. When active, these parasympathetic nerves release *acetylcholine* on cardiac muscle cells. Acetylcholine interacts with *muscarinic* receptors on cardiac muscle cells to decrease the HR

(SA node) and decrease the action potential conduction velocity (AV node). Parasympathetic nerves may also act to decrease the force of contraction of atrial (not ventricular) muscle cells. Overall, parasympathetic activation acts to decrease cardiac pumping.

DIASTOLIC FILLING: THE STARLING LAW OF THE HEART

One of the most fundamental causes of variations in SV was described by William Howell in 1884 and by Otto Frank in 1894 and formally stated by E. H. Starling in 1918. These investigators demonstrated that, with other factors being equal, if cardiac filling increases during diastole, the volume ejected during systole also increases. Consequently, and as illustrated in Figure 1–7, SV increases nearly in proportion to increases in EDV. This phenomenon is commonly referred to as the *Starling law of the heart*. In a subsequent chapter, we will describe how the Starling law is a direct consequence of the intrinsic mechanical properties of cardiac muscle cells. However, knowing the mechanisms behind the Starling law is not ultimately as important as appreciating its consequences. The primary consequence is that SV (and therefore cardiac output) is strongly influenced by cardiac filling during diastole. Therefore, we shall later pay particular attention to the factors that affect cardiac filling and how they participate in the normal regulation of cardiac output.

Requirements for Effective Operation

For effective and efficient ventricular pumping action, the heart must be functioning properly in 5 basic respects:

1. The contractions of individual cardiac muscle cells must occur at regular intervals and be synchronized (not *arrhythmic*).
2. The valves must open fully (not *stenotic*).

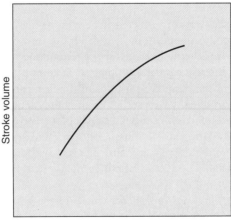

Figure 1–7. The Starling law of the heart.

3. The valves must not leak (not *insufficient* or *regurgitant*).
4. The muscle contractions must be forceful (not *failing*).
5. The ventricles must fill adequately during diastole.

In the subsequent chapters, we will study in detail how these requirements are met in the normal heart. Moreover, we will describe how failures in any of these respects lead to distinctly different, clinically relevant, pathologies and symptoms.

THE VASCULATURE

Blood that is ejected into the aorta by the left heart passes consecutively through many different types of vessels before it returns to the right heart. As illustrated in Figure 1–8, the major vessel classifications are *arteries, arterioles, capillaries, venules,* and *veins*. These consecutive vascular segments are distinguished from one another by differences in their physical dimensions, morphological characteristics,

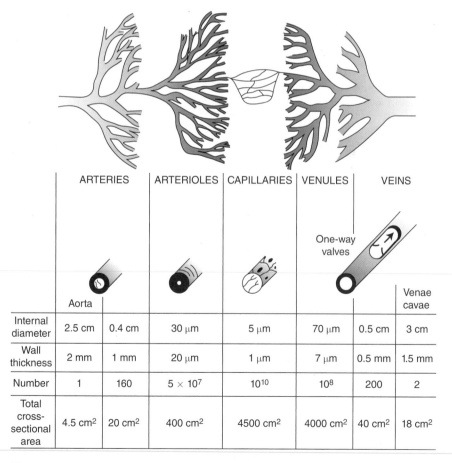

	ARTERIES	ARTERIOLES	CAPILLARIES	VENULES		VEINS	
	Aorta						Venae cavae
Internal diameter	2.5 cm	0.4 cm	30 μm	5 μm	70 μm	0.5 cm	3 cm
Wall thickness	2 mm	1 mm	20 μm	1 μm	7 μm	0.5 mm	1.5 mm
Number	1	160	5×10^7	10^{10}	10^8	200	2
Total cross-sectional area	4.5 cm^2	20 cm^2	400 cm^2	4500 cm^2	4000 cm^2	40 cm^2	18 cm^2

Figure 1–8. Structural characteristics of the peripheral vascular system.

and functions. One thing that all these vessels have in common is that they are lined with a contiguous single layer of endothelial cells. In fact, this is true for the entire circulatory system including the heart chambers and even the valve leaflets.

Vessel Characteristics

Some representative physical characteristics of these major vessel types are shown in Figure 1–8. It should be realized, however, that the vascular bed is a continuum and that the transition from one type of vascular segment to another does not occur abruptly. The total cross-sectional area through which blood flows at any level in the vascular system is equal to the sum of the cross-sectional areas of all the individual vessels arranged in parallel at that level. The number and total cross-sectional area values presented in Figure 1–8 are estimates for the entire systemic circulation.

Arteries are thick-walled vessels that contain, in addition to some smooth muscle, a large component of elastin and collagen fibers. Primarily because of the elastin fibers, which can stretch to twice their unloaded length, arteries can expand under increased pressure to accept and temporarily store some of the blood ejected by the heart during systole and then, by passive recoil, supply this blood to the organs downstream during diastole. The aorta is the largest artery and has an internal (luminal) diameter of approximately 25 mm. Arterial diameter decreases with each consecutive branching, and the smallest arteries have diameters of approximately 0.1 mm. The consecutive arterial branching pattern causes an exponential increase in arterial numbers. Thus, although individual vessels get progressively smaller, the total cross-sectional area available for blood flow within the arterial system increases to several fold greater than the aorta. Arteries are often referred to as *conduit* vessels because they have relatively low and unchanging resistance to flow.

Arterioles are smaller and structured differently than arteries. In proportion to lumen size, arterioles have much thicker walls with more smooth muscle and less elastic material than do arteries. Because arterioles are so muscular, their diameters can be actively changed to regulate the blood flow through peripheral organs. Despite their minute size, arterioles are so numerous that in parallel, their collective cross-sectional area is much larger than that at any level in arteries. Arterioles are often referred to as *resistance* vessels because of their high and changeable resistance, which regulates peripheral blood flow through individual organs.

Capillaries are the smallest vessels in the vasculature. In fact, red blood cells with diameters of 7 μm must deform to pass through them. The capillary wall consists of a single layer of endothelial cells that separates the blood from the interstitial fluid by only approximately 1 μm. Capillaries contain no smooth muscle and thus lack the ability to change their diameters actively. They are so numerous that the total collective cross-sectional area of all the capillaries in systemic organs is more than 1000 times that of the root of the aorta. Given that capillaries are approximately 0.5 mm in length, the total surface area available for exchange of material between blood and interstitial fluid can be calculated to exceed 100 m^2. For obvious reasons, capillaries are viewed as the *exchange* vessels of the cardiovascular system. In addition to the transcapillary diffusion of solutes that occurs across these vessel walls, there can sometimes be net movements of fluid (volume) into and/or out of capillaries. For example, tissue swelling (*edema*) is a result of net fluid movement from plasma into the interstitial space.

After leaving capillaries, blood is collected in venules and veins and returned to the heart. Venous vessels have very thin walls in proportion to their diameters. Their walls contain smooth muscle, and their diameters can actively change. Because of their thin walls, venous vessels are quite distensible. Therefore, their diameters change passively in response to small changes in transmural distending pressure (i.e., the difference between the internal and external pressures across the vessel wall). Venous vessels, especially the larger ones, also have one-way valves that prevent reverse flow. As will be discussed later, these valves are especially important in the cardiovascular system's operation during standing and during exercise. It turns out that peripheral venules and veins normally contain more than 50% of the total blood volume. Consequently, they are commonly thought of as the *capacitance* vessels. More importantly, *changes* in venous volume greatly influence cardiac filling and therefore cardiac pumping. Thus, peripheral veins play an extremely important role in controlling cardiac output.

Control of Blood Vessels

Blood flow through individual vascular beds is profoundly influenced by changes in the activity of sympathetic nerves innervating arterioles. These nerves release norepinephrine at their endings that interacts with α-*adrenergic* receptors on the smooth muscle cells to cause contraction and thus arteriolar constriction. The reduction in arteriolar diameter increases vascular resistance and decreases blood flow. These neural fibers provide the most important means of *reflex* control of vascular resistance and organ blood flow.

Arteriolar smooth muscle is also very responsive to changes in the local chemical conditions within an organ that accompany changes in the metabolic rate of the organ. For reasons to be discussed later, increased tissue metabolic rate leads to arteriolar dilation and increased tissue blood flow.

Venules and veins are also richly innervated by sympathetic nerves, and smooth muscle constricts when these nerves are activated. The mechanism is the same as that involved with arterioles. Thus, increased sympathetic nerve activity is accompanied by decreased venous volume. The importance of this phenomenon is that venous constriction tends to increase cardiac filling and therefore cardiac output via the Starling law of the heart.

To the best of our knowledge, there is no important neural or local metabolic control of either arterial or capillary vessel tone or diameter.

Overall Vascular Function

In essence, the bulk of the vascular system is simply the network of "pipes" necessary to route blood flow from the heart through capillary beds in organs throughout the body and then collect it again to return it to the heart. Because blood is a viscous fluid, there is an unavoidable energy loss (to heat via fluid friction) as it flows through any vessel. Thus, there is an energy cost to just distributing the blood throughout the body. This energy loss as blood moves through the vasculature is important because it determines how much work the heart must do to produce that flow in the first place.

There are many possible plumbing schemes (e.g., various combinations of vessels of different diameters, lengths, and branching patterns) that could accomplish the goal of distributing blood to capillary beds throughout the body. However, some would do so with less frictional energy loss than others. We contend that the vascular system has evolved to distribute the cardiac output with minimal energy loss in the process.

BLOOD

Blood is a complex fluid that serves as the medium for transporting substances between the tissues of the body and performs a host of other functions as well. Normally, approximately 40% of the volume of whole blood is occupied by blood cells that are suspended in the watery fluid, *plasma*, which accounts for the rest of the volume. The fraction of blood volume occupied by cells is termed as the *hematocrit*, a clinically important parameter.

Hematocrit = Cell volume/Total blood volume

One of the reasons that a person's hematocrit is clinically relevant is that the viscosity of blood increases dramatically with increases in its hematocrit. Recall that fluid viscosity is one physical factor that affects the flow through a tube. Other factors equal, the higher the blood viscosity, the more work the heart must do to produce any given flow through the vasculature.

Blood Cells

Blood contains 3 general types of "formed elements": red cells, white cells, and platelets (see Appendix A). All are formed in bone marrow from a common stem cell. Red cells are by far the most abundant. They are specialized to carry oxygen from the lungs to other tissues by binding oxygen to *hemoglobin*, an iron-containing heme protein contained within red blood cells. Because of the presence of hemoglobin, blood can transport 40 to 50 times the amount of oxygen that plasma alone could carry. In addition, the hydrogen ion buffering capacity of hemoglobin is vitally important to the blood's capacity to transport carbon dioxide.

A small, but important, fraction of the cells in blood is white cells or *leukocytes*. Leukocytes are involved in immune processes. Appendix A gives more information on the types and functions of leukocytes. Platelets are small cell fragments that are important in the blood-clotting process.

Plasma

Plasma is the liquid component of blood and, as indicated in Appendix B, is a complex solution of electrolytes and proteins. *Serum* is the fluid obtained from a blood sample after it has been allowed to clot. For all practical purposes, the composition of serum is identical to that of plasma except that it contains none of the clotting proteins.

Inorganic *electrolytes* (inorganic ions such as sodium, potassium, chloride, and bicarbonate) are the most concentrated solutes in plasma. Of these, sodium and chloride are by far the most abundant and, therefore, are primarily responsible for plasma's normal osmolarity of approximately 300 mOsm/L. To a first approximation, the "stock" of the plasma soup is a 150-mM solution of sodium chloride. Such a solution is called "isotonic saline" and has many clinical uses as a fluid that is compatible with cells.

Plasma normally contains many different *proteins*. Most plasma proteins can be classified as *albumins*, *globulins*, or *fibrinogen* based on different physical and chemical characteristics used to separate them. More than 100 distinct plasma proteins have been identified and each presumably serves some specific function. Many plasma proteins are involved in blood clotting or immune/defense reactions. Many others are important carrier proteins for a variety of substances, including fatty acids, iron, copper, vitamin D, and certain hormones.

Proteins do not readily cross capillary walls and, in general, their plasma concentrations are much higher than their concentrations in the interstitial fluid. As will be discussed, plasma proteins play an important osmotic role in transcapillary fluid movement and consequently in the distribution of extracellular volume between the plasma and interstitial compartments. *Albumin* plays an especially strong role in this regard simply because it is by far the most abundant of the plasma proteins.

Plasma also serves as the vehicle for transporting nutrients and waste products. Thus, a plasma sample contains many small organic molecules such as glucose, amino acids, urea, creatinine, and uric acid whose measured values are useful in clinical diagnosis.

PERSPECTIVES

In this first chapter, we have argued that maintaining bodily homeostasis is the bottom-line task of the cardiovascular system. To maintain homeostasis in any tissue in any given situation, that tissue must receive a blood flow through its capillaries that is matched to support the local current metabolic needs of that tissue. Adequate arterial pressure is necessary to produce tissue blood flow in the first place but arterial pressure is only one factor in achieving adequate tissue blood flow. Constant arterial pressure by itself does not ensure that there will be homeostasis throughout the body. What constant arterial pressure does do is allow an individual organ to control its own blood flow by varying the local resistance to blood flow according to its current metabolic needs. Moreover, this local control allows any organ to regulate its own flow without disturbing the flows through other organs. At this juncture, we would also like to draw the reader's attention to Appendix C, which is a shorthand compilation of many of the key cardiovascular relationships that we have and will encounter in due course.

KEY CONCEPTS

 The primary role of the cardiovascular system is to maintain homeostasis in the interstitial fluid.

 The physical law that governs cardiovascular operation is that flow through any segment is equal to pressure difference across that segment divided by its resistance to flow, that is, $\dot{Q} = \Delta P / R$.

 The rate of transport of a substance within the blood (X) is a function of its concentration in the blood [X] and the blood flow rate, that is, $\dot{X} = \dot{Q}[X]$.

 The heart pumps blood by rhythmically filling and ejecting blood from the ventricular chambers that are served by passive one-way inlet and outlet valves.

 Cardiac output (CO) is a function of the heart rate (HR) and stroke volume (SV), that is, $CO = HR \times SV$.

 Changes in heart rate and stroke volume (and therefore cardiac output) can be accomplished by alterations in ventricular filling and by alterations in autonomic nerve activity to the heart.

 Blood flow through individual organs is regulated by changes in the diameter of their arterioles.

 Changes in arteriolar diameter can be accomplished by alterations in sympathetic nerve activity and by variations in local conditions.

 Blood is a complex suspension of red cells, white cells, and platelets in plasma that is ideally suited to carry gases, salts, nutrients, and waste molecules throughout the system.

 STUDY QUESTIONS

1–1. Which organ in the body always receives the most blood flow?

1–2. Whenever blood flow to one organ increases, blood flow to other organs must decrease. True or false?

1–3. When a heart valve does not close properly, a sound called a "murmur" can often be detected as the valve leaks. Would you expect a leaky aortic valve to cause a systolic or diastolic murmur?

1–4. The primary effect of slowing action potential conduction through the AV node is to lower the heart rate. True or false?

1–5. Suppose the diameters of the vessels within an organ increase by 10%. Other factors equal, how would this affect the

　a. resistance to blood flow through the organ?

　b. blood flow through the organ?

1–6. The pressure in the aorta is normally about 100 mm Hg, whereas that in the pulmonary artery is normally about 15 mm Hg. A few of your fellow students offer the following alternative hypotheses about why pulmonary artery pressure is less:

　a. The right heart pumps less blood than the left heart.

　b. The right heart rate is slower than the left heart rate.

　c. The right ventricle is less muscular than the left ventricle.

　d. The pulmonary vascular bed has less resistance than the systemic bed.

　e. The stroke volume of the right heart is less than that of the left heart.

　Which of their suggestions is correct?

1–7. Usually, an individual who has lost a significant amount of blood is weak and may present with incoherence or dizziness. Why would blood loss contribute to these presentations?

1–8. What direct cardiovascular effects would you expect from an intravenous injection of a drug that stimulates α-adrenergic receptors but not β-adrenergic receptors?

1–9. Individuals with high arterial blood pressure (hypertension) are often treated with drugs that block β-adrenergic receptors. What is a rationale for such treatment?

1–10. The clinical laboratory reports a serum sodium ion value of 140 mEq/L in a blood sample you have taken from a patient. What does this suggest about the sodium ion concentration in plasma, in interstitial fluid, and in intracellular fluid?

1–11. Explain how it is that the water flow into your kitchen sink changes when you turn the handle on its faucet.

1–12. A common "side effect" of β-blocker therapy is decreased exercise tolerance. Why is this not surprising?

1–13. You need to determine the correct dose of an IV drug that distributes only within the extracellular space. Which of the following values would be the closest estimate of the extracellular fluid volume of a healthy young adult male weighing 100 kg (220 lb)?

　a. 3 L

　b. 5 L

　c. 8 L

　d. 10 L

　e. 20 L

1–14. Determine the rate of glucose uptake by an exercising skeletal muscle ($\dot{G}_m$) from the following data:

Arterial blood glucose concentration, $[G]_a = 50\ mg/100\ mL$

Muscle venous blood glucose concentration, $[G]_v = 30\ mg/100\ mL$

Muscle blood flow $\dot{Q} = 60\ mL / min$

1–15.   The Fick principle implies that doubling the flow through an organ will necessarily double the organ's rate of metabolism (or production) of a substance. True or False?

1–16.   Five requirements for normal cardiac pumping action are listed in this chapter. Recall that CO = HR × (EDV − ESV). Use this as a basis for explaining in detail why a lack of each of the requirements would adversely affect CO.

Characteristics of Cardiac Muscle Cells

2

OBJECTIVES

The student understands the ionic basis of the spontaneous electrical activity of cardiac muscle cells:

▶ Describes how membrane potentials are created across semipermeable membranes by transmembrane ion concentration differences.

▶ Defines equilibrium potential and knows its normal value for potassium and sodium ions.

▶ States how membrane potential reflects a membrane's relative permeability to various ions.

▶ Defines resting potential and action potential.

▶ Describes the characteristics of "fast" and "slow" response action potentials.

▶ Identifies the refractory periods of the cardiac cell electrical cycle.

▶ Defines threshold potential and describes the interaction between ion channel conditions and membrane potential during the depolarization phase of the action potential.

▶ Defines pacemaker potential and describes the basis for rhythmic electrical activity of cardiac cells.

▶ Names the important ion channels involved in the permeability alterations during the various phases of the cardiac cycle.

The student knows the normal process of cardiac electrical excitation:

▶ Describes gap junctions and their role in cardiac excitation.

▶ Describes the normal pathway of action potential conduction through the heart.

▶ Indicates the timing at which various areas of the heart are electrically excited and identifies the characteristic action potential shapes and conduction velocities in each major part of the conduction system.

▶ States the relationship between electrical events of cardiac excitation and the P, QRS, and T waves, the PR and QT intervals, and the ST segment of the electrocardiogram (ECG).

The student understands the factors that control the heart rate and action potential conduction in the heart:

▶ States how diastolic potentials of pacemaker cells can be altered to produce changes in the heart rate.

▶ Describes how cardiac sympathetic and parasympathetic nerves alter the heart rate and conduction of cardiac action potentials.

▶ Defines the terms chronotropic and dromotropic.

23

The student understands the contractile processes of cardiac muscle cells:
▶ *Lists the subcellular structures responsible for cardiac muscle cell contraction.*
▶ *Defines and describes the excitation–contraction process.*
▶ *Defines isometric, isotonic, and afterloaded contractions of the cardiac muscle.*
▶ *Identifies the influence of altered preload on the tension-producing and shortening capabilities of the cardiac muscle.*
▶ *Describes the influence of altered afterload on the shortening capabilities of the cardiac muscle.*
▶ *Defines the terms contractility and inotropic state and describes the influence of altered contractility on the tension-producing and shortening capabilities of the cardiac muscle.*
▶ *Describes the effect of altered sympathetic neural activity on the cardiac inotropic state.*
▶ *States the relationships between ventricular volume and muscle length, between intraventricular pressure and muscle tension and the law of Laplace.*

Cardiac muscle cells are responsible for providing the power to drive blood through the circulatory system. Coordination of their activity depends on an electrical stimulus that is regularly initiated at an appropriate rate and reliably conducted through the entire heart. Mechanical pumping action depends on a robust contraction of the muscle cells that results in repeating cycles of tension development, shortening, and relaxation. In addition, mechanisms to adjust the excitation and contraction characteristics must be available to meet the changing demands of the circulatory system. This chapter focuses on these electrical and mechanical properties of cardiac muscle cells that underlie normal heart function.

ELECTRICAL ACTIVITY OF CARDIAC MUSCLE CELLS

In all striated muscle cells, contraction is triggered by a rapid voltage change called an *action potential* that occurs on the cell membrane. Cardiac muscle cell action potentials differ sharply from those of skeletal muscle cells in 3 important ways that promote synchronous rhythmic excitation of the heart: (1) they can be self-generating; (2) they are conducted directly from cell to cell; and (3) they have long duration, which precludes fusion of individual twitch contractions. To understand these special electrical properties of the cardiac muscle and how cardiac function depends on them, the basic electrical properties of excitable cell membranes must first be examined.

Membrane Potentials

All cells have an electrical potential (voltage) across their membranes. Such *transmembrane potentials* are caused by a separation of electrical charges across the membrane itself. The only way that the transmembrane potential can change is for electrical charges to move across (i.e., current to flow through) the cell membrane.

There are 2 important corollaries to this statement: (1) the rate of change of transmembrane voltage is directly proportional to the net current across the membrane; and (2) transmembrane voltage is stable (i.e., unchanging) only when there is no net current across the membrane.

Unlike a wire, current across cell membranes is not carried by electrons but by the movement of ions through the cell membrane. The 3 ions that are the most important determinants of cardiac transmembrane potentials are sodium (Na^+) and calcium (Ca^{2+}), which are more concentrated in the extracellular fluid than they are inside cells, and potassium (K^+), which is more concentrated in intracellular than extracellular fluid. (See Appendix B for normal values of many constituents of adult human plasma.) In general, such ions are very insoluble in lipids. Consequently, they cannot pass into or out of a cell through the lipid bilayer of the membrane itself. Instead, these ions cross the membrane only via various protein structures that are embedded in and span across the lipid cell wall. There are 3 general types of such transmembrane protein structures that are involved in ion movement across the cell membrane: (1) ion *channels*; (2) ion *exchangers*; and (3) ion *pumps*.[1] All are very specific for ions. For example, a "sodium channel" is a transmembrane protein structure that allows only Na^+ ions to pass into or out of a cell according to the net electrochemical forces acting on Na^+ ions.

The subsequent discussion concentrates on ion channel operation because ion channels (as opposed to exchangers and pumps) are responsible for the resting membrane potential and for the rapid changes in membrane potential that constitute the cardiac cell action potential. Ion channels are under complex control and can be "opened," "closed," or "inactivated." The net result of the status of membrane channels for a particular ion is commonly referred to as the membrane's *permeability* to that ion. For example, "high permeability to sodium" implies that many of the Na^+ ion channels are in their open state at that instant. Precise timing of the status of ion channels accounts for the characteristic membrane potential changes that occur when cardiac cells are activated.

Figure 2–1 shows how ion concentration differences can generate an electrical potential across the cell membrane. Consider first, as shown at the top of this figure, a cell that (1) has K^+ more concentrated inside the cell than outside, (2) is permeable only to K^+ (i.e., only K^+ channels are open), and (3) has no initial transmembrane potential. Because of the concentration difference, K^+ ions (positive charges) will diffuse out of the cell. Meanwhile, negative charges, such as protein anions, cannot leave the cell because the membrane is impermeable to them. Thus, the K^+ efflux will make the cytoplasm at the inside surface of the cell membrane more electrically negative (deficient in positively charged ions) and at the same time make the interstitial fluid just outside the cell membrane

---

[1] "Channels" can be thought of as passive ion-specific holes in the membrane through which a particular ion will move according to the electrochemical forces acting on it. "Exchangers" are passive devices that couple the movement of 2 or more specific ions across the membrane according to the collective net electrochemical forces acting on all the ions involved. "Pumps" use the chemical energy of splitting ATP to move ions across the cell membrane against prevailing electrochemical forces.

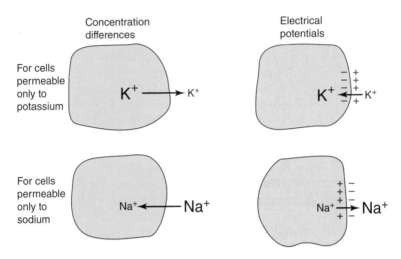

Figure 2-1. Electrochemical basis of membrane potentials.

more electrically positive (rich in positively charged ions). K^+ ion, being positively charged, is attracted to regions of electrical negativity. Therefore, when K^+ diffuses out of a cell, it creates an electrical potential across the membrane that tends to attract it back into the cell. There exists one membrane potential called the *potassium equilibrium potential* at which the electrical forces tending to pull K^+ into the cell exactly balance the concentration forces tending to drive K^+ out. When the membrane potential has this value, there is no *net* movement of K^+ across the membrane. With the normal concentrations of approximately 145 mM K^+ inside cells and 4 mM K^+ in the extracellular fluid, the K^+ equilibrium potential is roughly −90 mV (more negative inside than outside by nine-hundredths of a volt).[2] A membrane that is permeable only to K^+ will inherently and rapidly (essentially instantaneously) develop the potassium equilibrium potential. In addition, membrane potential changes require the movement of so few ions that concentration differences between the intracellular and extracellular fluid compartments are not significantly affected by the process.

As depicted in the bottom half of Figure 2–1, similar reasoning shows how a membrane permeable only to Na^+ would have the *sodium equilibrium potential* across it. The sodium equilibrium potential is approximately +70 mV, with a normal extracellular Na^+ concentration of 140 mM and an intracellular Na^+ concentration of 10 mM.

Real cell membranes, however, are never permeable to just Na^+ or just K^+. When a membrane is permeable to both ions, the membrane potential will lie somewhere between the Na^+ equilibrium potential and the K^+ equilibrium potential.

---

[2] The equilibrium potential (E_{eq}) for any ion (X^z) where z is the ion's charge is determined by its intracellular and extracellular concentrations as indicated in the Nernst equation:

$$E_{eq} = \frac{-61.5 \, mV}{z} \log_{10} \frac{[X^z] \text{inside}}{[X^z] \text{outside}}$$

Just what membrane potential will exist at any instant depends on the relative permeability of the membrane to Na^+ and K^+. The more permeable the membrane is to K^+ than to Na^+, the closer the membrane potential will be to -90 mV. Conversely, when the permeability to Na^+ is high relative to the permeability to K^+, the membrane potential will be closer to $+70$ mV.[3] A *stable* membrane potential that lies between the sodium and potassium equilibrium potentials implies that there is no *net* current across the membrane. This situation may well be the result of opposite but balanced sodium and potassium currents across the membrane.

Because of low or unchanging permeability or low concentration, roles played by ions other than Na^+ and K^+ in determining membrane potential are usually minor and often ignored. However, as discussed later, calcium ions (Ca^{2+}) do participate in the cardiac muscle action potential. Like Na^+, Ca^{2+} is more concentrated outside cells than inside. The equilibrium potential for Ca^{2+} is approximately $+100$ mV, and the cell membrane tends to become more positive on the inside when the membrane's permeability to Ca^{2+} rises.

Under resting conditions, most heart muscle cells have membrane potentials that are quite close to the potassium equilibrium potential. Thus, both electrical and concentration gradients favor the entry of Na^+ and Ca^{2+} into the resting cell. Left unchecked, this slow leak of Na^+ and Ca^{2+} into the cell and K^+ out of the cell would ultimately destroy the transmembrane potential. However, the very low permeability of the resting membrane to Na^+ and Ca^{2+} (in combination with a Na^+–Ca^{2+} exchanger and an energy-requiring sodium–potassium pump) prevents Na^+ and Ca^{2+} from gradually accumulating inside the resting cell.[4,5]

Cardiac Muscle Cell Action Potentials

 Action potentials of cells from different regions of the heart are not identical but have varying characteristics that are important to the overall process of cardiac excitation.

Some cells within a specialized conduction system can act as pacemakers and spontaneously initiate action potentials, whereas ordinary cardiac muscle cells do not (except under unusual conditions). Basic membrane electrical features of an ordinary cardiac muscle cell and a cardiac pacemaker-type cell are shown in Figure 2–2. Action potentials from these cell types are referred to as "fast-response" and "slow-response" action potentials, respectively.

---

[3] A quantitative description of how Na^+ and K^+ concentrations and the relative permeability (P_{Na}/P_K) to these ions affect membrane potential (E_m) is given by the following equation:

$$E_m = -61.5\,\mathrm{mV}\,\log_{10}\left(\frac{[K^+] + P_{Na}\,/\,P_K[Na^+]_i}{[K^+]_o + P_{Na}\,/\,P_K[Na^+]_o}\right)$$

[4] The sodium pump not only removes Na^+ from the cell but also pumps K^+ into the cell. Because more Na^+ is pumped out than K^+ is pumped in (3:2), the pump is said to be electrogenic. The resting membrane potential becomes slightly less negative than normal when the pump is abruptly inhibited.
[5] The steep sodium gradient promotes Na^+ entry into and Ca^{2+} removal from the cytoplasm via the Na^+–Ca^{2+} exchanger.

As shown in Figure 2–2A, fast-response action potentials are characterized by a rapid depolarization (phase 0) with a substantial overshoot (positive inside voltage), a rapid reversal of the overshoot potential (phase 1), a long plateau (phase 2), and a repolarization (phase 3) to a stable, high (i.e., large negative) resting membrane potential (phase 4). In comparison, the slow-response action potentials are characterized by a slower initial depolarization phase, a lower amplitude overshoot, a shorter and less stable plateau phase, and a repolarization to an unstable, slowly depolarizing "resting" potential (Figure 2–2B). The unstable resting potential seen in pacemaker cells with slow-response action potentials is variously referred to as *phase 4 depolarization, diastolic depolarization,* or

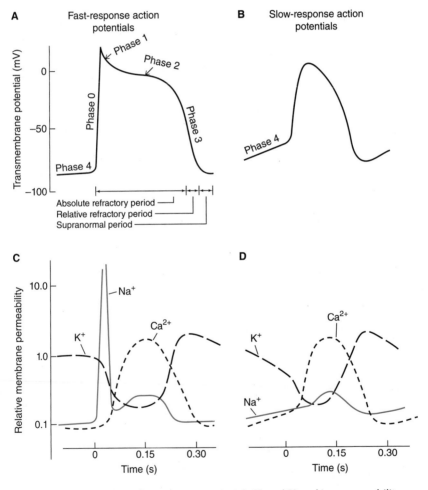

Figure 2–2. Time course of membrane potentials (A and B) and ion permeability changes (C and D) that occur during "fast-response" (left) and "slow-response" (right) action potentials.

pacemaker potential. Such cells are usually found in the sinoatrial (SA) and atrio-ventricular (AV) nodes.

As indicated at the bottom of Figure 2–2A, cells are in an absolute refractory state during most of the action potential (i.e., they cannot be stimulated to fire another action potential). Near the end of the action potential, the membrane is relatively refractory and can be re-excited only by a larger-than-normal stimulus. This long refractory state precludes summated or tetanic contractions from occurring in normal cardiac muscle. Immediately after the action potential, the membrane is transiently hyperexcitable and is said to be in a "vulnerable" or "supranormal" period. Similar alterations in membrane excitability occur during slow action potentials but are not well characterized at present.

 Recall that the membrane potential of any cell at any given instant depends on the relative permeability of the cell membrane to specific ions. As in all excitable cells, cardiac cell *action* potentials are the result of large, rapid, and transient changes in the ionic permeability of the cell membrane that are triggered by an initial small, localized depolarization and then propagated over the entire cell membrane. Figure 2–2C and 2–2D indicates the changes in the membrane's permeabilities to K^+, Na^+, and Ca^{2+} that produce the various phases of the fast- and slow-response action potentials.[6] Note that during the resting phase, the membranes of both types of cells are more permeable to K^+ than to Na^+ or Ca^{2+}. Therefore, the membrane potentials are close to the potassium equilibrium potential (of -90 mV) during this period.

In pacemaker-type cells, at least 3 mechanisms are thought to contribute to the slow depolarization of the membrane observed during the diastolic interval. First, there is a progressive decrease in the membrane's permeability to K^+ during the resting phase. Second, the permeability to Na^+ increases slowly. (This gradual increase in the Na^+/K^+ permeability ratio will cause the membrane potential to move slowly away from the K^+ equilibrium potential (-90 mV) in the direction of the Na^+ equilibrium potential.) Third, there is a slight increase in the permeability of the membrane to calcium ions late in diastole, which results in an inward movement of these positively charged ions and contributes to the diastolic depolarization. These permeability changes result in a specific current that occurs during diastole called the *i*-funny (i_f) current.

When the membrane potential depolarizes to a certain *threshold* potential in either type of cell, major rapid alterations in the permeability of the membrane to specific ions are triggered. Once initiated, these permeability changes cannot be stopped, and they proceed to completion.

The characteristic rapid rising phase of the fast-response action potential is a result of a sudden increase in Na^+ permeability. This produces what is referred

---

[6] The membrane's permeability to a particular ion is not synonymous with the transmembrane current of that ion. The transmembrane current of any ion is the product of the membrane's permeability to it times the electrochemical driving forces acting on it. For example, the resting membrane is quite permeable to K^+ but there is little net K^+ movement (current flow) because the resting membrane potential is very close to the potassium equilibrium potential.

to as the *fast inward current* of Na$^+$ and causes the membrane potential to move rapidly toward the sodium equilibrium potential. As indicated in Figure 2–2C, this period of very high sodium permeability (phase 0) is short-lived. A very brief increase in potassium permeability then occurs (not shown in Figure 2–2C) that allows a transient outward-going potassium current (i_{To}) and results in a small non-sustained repolarization after the peak of the action potential (phase 1). Development and maintenance of a prolonged depolarized *plateau* state (phase 2) is accomplished by the interactions of at least 2 separate processes: (1) a sustained reduction in K$^+$ permeability and (2) a slowly developed and sustained increase in the membrane's permeability to Ca^{2+}. In addition, under certain conditions, the electrogenic action of a Na$^+$–Ca^{2+} exchanger (in which 3 Na$^+$ ions move into the cell in exchange for a single Ca^{2+} ion moving out of the cell) may contribute to the maintenance of the plateau phase of the cardiac action potential.

The initial fast inward current is small (or even absent) in cells that have slow-response action potentials (Figure 2–2D). Therefore, the initial depolarization phase of these action potentials is somewhat slower than that of the fast-response action potentials and is primarily a result of an inward movement of Ca^{2+} ions. In both types of cells, the membrane is repolarized (during phase 3) to its original resting potential as the K$^+$ permeability increases to its high resting value and the Ca^{2+} and Na$^+$ permeabilities return to their low resting values. These late permeability changes produce what is referred to as the *delayed outward current*.

The overall smoothly graded permeability changes that produce action potentials are the net result of alterations in each of the many individual ion channels within the plasma membrane of a single cell.[7] These ion channels are generally made up of very long polypeptide chains that loop repeatedly across the cell membrane. These loops form a hollow conduction channel between the intracellular and extracellular fluids that are structurally quite specific for a particular ion. These channels can exist in 1 of 3 conformational states: *open, closed,* or *inactivated.* The status of the channels can be altered by configurational changes in certain subunits of the molecules within the channel (referred to as "gates" or plugs) so that when *open*, ions move down their electrochemical gradient either into or out of the cell (high permeability) and when *closed* or *inactivated*, no ions can move (low permeability).

The specific mechanisms that control the operation of these channels during the action potential are not fully understood. Certain types of channels are called *voltage-gated channels* (or voltage-operated channels) because their probability of being open varies with membrane potential. Another type of channels, called *ligand-gated channels* (or receptor-operated channels), are activated by certain neurotransmitters or other specific signal molecules. Table 2–1 lists a few of the important currents and channel types involved in cardiac cell electrical activity.

---

[7] The experimental technique of *patch clamping* has made it possible to study the operation of individual ion channels. The patch clamp data indicate that a single channel is either open or closed at any instant in time; there are no graded states of partial opening. What is graded is the percentage of time that a given channel spends in the open state, and the total number of channels that are currently in an open state.

Table 2–1. Characteristics of Important Cardiac Ion Channels in Order of Their Participation in an Action Potential

Current	Channel	Gating mechanism	Functional role
i_{K1}	K⁺ channel (inward rectifier), K_{ir}	Voltage	Maintains high K⁺ permeability during phase 4 Its decay contributes to diastolic depolarization Its suppression during phases 0-2 contributes to plateau
i_{Na}	Na⁺ channel (fast) Nav 1.5	Voltage	Accounts for phase 0 of action potential Inactivation may contribute to phase 1 of action potential
i_{To}	K⁺ channel (transient outward), K_{to}	Voltage	Contributes to phase 1 of action potential
i_{Ca}	Ca²⁺ channel (slow inward, L channels) Cav 1.2	Both	Contributes to phase 2 of action potential Inactivation may contribute to phase 3 of action potential Is enhanced by sympathetic stimulation and β-adrenergic agents
i_{K}	K⁺ channels (delayed rectifier), K_s, K_r, K_{ur}	Voltage	Causes phase 3 of action potential Is enhanced by increased intracellular Ca²⁺
i_{KATP}	K⁺ channel (ATP-sensitive)	Ligand	Increases K⁺ permeability when [ATP] is low
i_{KACh}	K⁺ channel (acetylcholine-activated)	Ligand	Responsible for effects of vagal stimulation Decreases diastolic depolarization (and the heart rate) Hyperpolarizes resting membrane potential Shortens phase 2 of the action potential
i_f ("funny")	Na⁺, Ca²⁺, K⁺ (pacemaker current via HCN channel)	Both	Is activated by hyperpolarization and cyclic nucleotides and contributes to the diastolic depolarization Is enhanced by sympathetic stimulation and β-adrenergic agents Is suppressed by vagal stimulation

The number of well-described ion channels in cardiac muscle is rapidly increasing and abnormalities in these channels (channelopathies) are now known to be responsible for a variety of excitation abnormalities. Our oversimplified description of channel function below is an effort to provide some basic understanding without the many complicating features of the electrical excitation process.

Some of the voltage-gated channels respond to a sudden-onset, sustained change in membrane potential by only a brief period of activation. However, changes in membrane potential of slower onset, but of the same magnitude, may fail to activate these channels at all. To explain such behavior, it is postulated that a given channel has 2 independently operating "gates"—an *activation gate* and an *inactivation gate*—both of which must be open for the channel to be open. Both gates respond to changes in membrane potential but do so with different voltage sensitivities and time courses.

  These concepts are illustrated in Figure 2–3. (For simplicity, a single Na⁺ channel and Ca²⁺ channel is shown and K⁺ channels are ignored.) In the resting state, with the membrane polarized to approximately −80 mV, the activation gate of the fast Na⁺ channel is closed, but its inactivation gate is open (Figure 2–3A). With a rapid depolarization of the membrane to threshold, the Na⁺ channels will be activated strongly to allow an inrush of positive sodium ions that further depolarizes the membrane and thus accounts for the rising phase of a "fast" response action potential, as illustrated in Figure 2–3B. This occurs because the *activation* gate responds to membrane depolarization by opening more quickly than the *inactivation* gate responds by closing. Thus, a small initial rapid depolarization to threshold is followed by a brief, but strong, period of Na⁺ channel activation wherein the *activation* gate is open, but the *inactivation* gate is yet to close. Within a few milliseconds, however, the inactivation gates of the fast sodium channels close and shut off the inward movement of Na⁺.

After a brief delay, the large membrane depolarization of the rising phase of the fast action potential causes the activation gate of the L-type Ca²⁺ channel to open. This permits the slow inward movement of Ca²⁺ ions, which helps maintain the depolarization through the plateau phase of the action potential (Figure 2–3C). Ultimately, repolarization occurs because of both a delayed inactivation of the Ca²⁺ channel (by closure of the inactivation gates) and a delayed opening of K⁺ channels (which are not shown in Figure 2–3).

The *inactivation* gates of sodium channels remain closed during the plateau phase and the remainder of the action potential, effectively inactivating the Na⁺ channel. This sustained sodium channel inactivation, combined with activation of calcium channels and the delay in opening of potassium channels, accounts for the long plateau phase and the long cardiac refractory period, which lasts until the end of phase 3. With repolarization, both gates of the sodium channel return to their original position and the channel is now ready to be reactivated by a subsequent depolarization.

Multiple factors in addition to membrane voltage can influence the membrane ionic permeability and normal operation of ion channels. For example, high

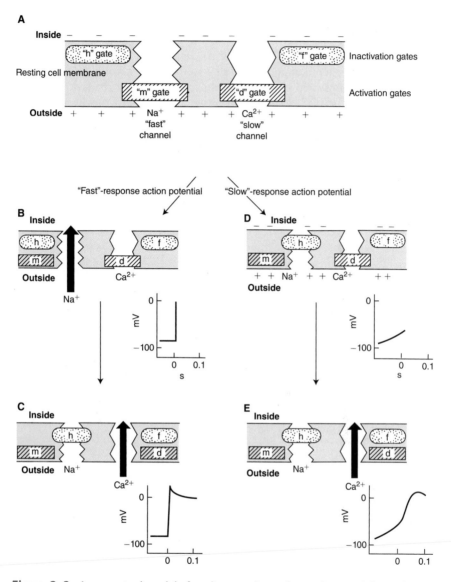

Figure 2–3. A conceptual model of cardiac membrane fast sodium and slow calcium ion channels: at rest (**A**), during the initial phases of the fast-response (**B** and **C**), and the slow-response action potentials (**D** and **E**). "Activation" gates (m and d) are hatched and "inactivation" gates (h and f) are stippled.

intracellular Ca^{2+} concentration during systole contributes to activation of certain K^+ channels and increases the rate of repolarization. Sympathetic and parasympathetic neural input can influence the status of some voltage-gated channels and cause activation or suppression of other ligand-gated channels. In addition, *mechano-gated* and *mechano-modulated channels* may be activated by myocyte stretch or myocyte volume changes and can influence membrane permeability to K^+, Na^+, and Ca^{2+}.

The slow-response action potential shown in the right half of Figure 2–3 differs from the fast-response action potential primarily because of the lack of a strong activation of the fast Na^+ channel at its onset. This accounts for the slow rate of rise of the action potential in these cells. The slow *diastolic* depolarization that occurs in these pacemaker-type cells is primarily a result of an inward current (I_{funny}) flowing through a channel that is an isoform of the family of nonselective cation hyperpolarization-activated, cyclic nucleotide-gated (HCN) channels. This channel is activated at the end of the repolarization phase and promotes a slow sodium, potassium, and calcium influx that gradually depolarizes the cells during diastole. This slow diastolic depolarization gives the inactivating *h* gates of many of the fast sodium channels time to close before threshold is even reached (Figure 2–3D). Thus, in a slow-response action potential, there is no initial period where all the fast sodium channels of a cell are essentially open at once. The depolarization beyond threshold during the rising phase of the action potential in these "pacemaker" cells is slow and caused primarily by the influx of Ca^{2+} through slow L-type channels (Figure 2–3E).

Although cells in certain areas of the heart typically have fast-type action potentials and cells in other areas normally have slow-type action potentials, it is important to recognize that all cardiac cells are potentially capable of having either type of action potential, depending on their maximum resting membrane potential and how fast they depolarize to the threshold potential. As we shall see, rapid depolarization to the threshold potential is usually an event forced on a cell by the occurrence of an action potential in an adjacent cell. Slow depolarization to threshold occurs when a cell itself spontaneously and gradually loses its resting polarization, which normally happens only in the SA or AV node. A *chronic* moderate depolarization of the resting membrane (caused, e.g., by moderately high extracellular K^+ concentrations of 5–7 mM) can inactivate the fast channels (by closing the *h* gates) without inactivating the slow L-type Ca^{2+} channels. Under these conditions, all cardiac cell action potentials will be of the slow type. Large, sustained depolarizations (as might be caused by very high extracellular K^+ concentration such as more than 8 mM), however, can inactivate both the fast and slow channels and thus make the cardiac muscle cells completely inexcitable.

Conduction of Cardiac Action Potentials

Action potentials are initiated at a local site on a cardiac myocyte and then conducted over the surface of individual cells. This occurs because active depolarization in any one area of the membrane produces local currents that pass through the intracellular and extracellular fluids. These currents passively depolarize immediate adjacent areas of the membrane to their voltage thresholds to initiate an action potential at this new site.

In the heart, cardiac muscle cells branch and connect end-to-end with neighboring cells in structures called *intercalated disks*. These disks contain the following:

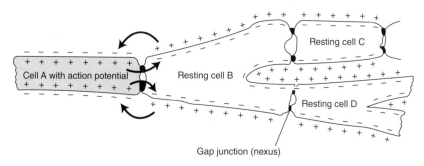

Figure 2–4. Local currents and cell-to-cell conduction of cardiac muscle cell action potentials.

(1) *firm mechanical attachments* between adjacent cell membranes by proteins called *adherins* in structures called *desmosomes* and (2) *low-resistance electrical connections* between adjacent cells through channels formed by proteins called *connexin* in structures called *gap junctions*. Figure 2–4 shows schematically how these gap junctions allow action potential propagation from cell to cell.

Cells B, C, and D are shown in the resting phase with more negative charges inside than outside. Cell A is shown in the plateau phase of an action potential and has more positive charges inside than outside. Because of the gap junctions, electrostatic attraction can cause a local current flow (ion movement) between the depolarized membrane of active cell A and the polarized membrane of resting cell B, as indicated by the arrows in the figure. This ion movement depolarizes the membrane of cell B. Once the local currents from active cell A depolarize the membrane of cell B near the gap junction to the threshold level, an action potential will be triggered at that site and will be conducted over cell B. Because cell B branches (a common morphological characteristic of cardiac muscle fibers), its action potential will evoke action potentials on cells C and D. This process is continued through the entire myocardium. Thus, an action potential initiated at *any* site in the myocardium will be conducted from cell to cell throughout the entire heart.

The speed at which an action potential propagates through a region of cardiac tissue is called the *conduction velocity*. The conduction velocity varies considerably in different areas in the heart and is determined by 3 variables:

1. The diameter of the muscle fiber involved. Thus, conduction over small-diameter cells in the AV node is significantly slower than conduction over large-diameter cells in the ventricular Purkinje system.
2. The intensity of the local depolarizing currents, which are in turn directly determined by the rate of rise of the action potential. Rapid action potential depolarization favors rapid conduction to the neighboring segment or cell.
3. The capacitive and/or resistive properties of the cell membranes, gap junctions, and cytoplasm. Electrical characteristics of gap junctions can be influenced by external conditions that promote phosphorylation or dephosphorylation of the connexin proteins.

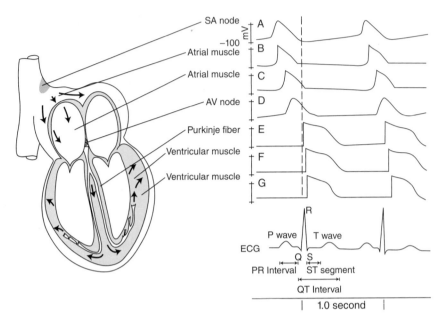

Figure 2–5. Time records of electrical activity at different sites in the heart wall: single-cell voltage recordings (traces A to G) and lead II electrocardiogram.

Details of the overall consequences of the variable cardiac conduction rates are shown in Figure 2–5. As noted earlier, specific electrical adaptations of various cells in the heart are reflected in the characteristic shape of their action potentials that are shown in the right half of Figure 2–5. Note that the action potentials shown in Figure 2–5 have been positioned to indicate the time when the electrical impulse that originates in the SA node reaches other areas of the heart. Cells of the SA node act as the heart's normal pacemaker and determine the heart rate. This is because the slow spontaneous *diastolic* depolarization of the membrane is normally most rapid in SA nodal cells, and therefore, the cells in this region reach their threshold potential and fire before cells elsewhere.

The action potential initiated by an SA nodal cell first spreads progressively throughout the branching and interconnected cardiac muscle cells of the atrial wall. Action potentials from cells in 2 different regions of the atria are shown in Figure 2–5: one close to the SA node and one more distant from the SA node. Both cells have similarly shaped fast response-type action potentials, but their temporal displacement reflects the fact that it takes some time for the impulse to spread over the atria. As shown in Figure 2–5, action potential conduction is greatly slowed as it passes through the AV node. This is because of the small size of the AV nodal cells and the slow rate of rise of their action potentials. Since the AV node delays the transfer of cardiac excitation from the atria to the ventricles, atrial contraction can contribute to ventricular filling before the ventricles begin to contract. Note also that AV nodal cells have a faster spontaneous depolarization during the diastolic period than other cells of the heart except those of the SA node. For this reason, the AV node is sometimes referred to as a *latent* pacemaker, and in many pathological situations, it (rather than the SA node) controls the heart rhythm. This situation is referred to as a "nodal" rhythm as distinguished from the normal "sinus" rhythm.

Because of sharply rising action potentials and other factors, such as large cell diameters, electrical conduction is extremely rapid in Purkinje fibers. This allows the Purkinje system to transfer the cardiac impulse to cells in many areas of the ventricle nearly in unison. Action potentials from muscle cells in 2 areas of the ventricle are shown in Figure 2–5. Because of the high conduction velocity in ventricular tissue, there is only a small discrepancy in their time of onset. Note in Figure 2–5 the ventricular cells that are the last to depolarize have shorter-duration action potentials and thus are the first to repolarize due to increased numbers of repolarizing potassium channels. The physiological importance of this behavior is not clear, but it does have an influence on the ECGs discussed in Chapter 4.

Electrocardiogram (ECG aka EKG)

Fields of electrical potential caused by the electrical activity of the heart extend through the extracellular fluid of the body and can be measured with electrodes placed on the body surface. *Electrocardiography* provides a record of how the voltage between 2 points on the body surface changes with time as a result of the electrical events of the cardiac cycle. At any instant of the cardiac cycle, the ECG indicates the net electrical field, which is the summation of many weak electrical fields being produced by voltage changes occurring on individual cardiac cells at that instant. When a large number of cells are simultaneously depolarizing or repolarizing, large voltages are observed on the ECG. Because the electrical impulse spreads through the heart tissue in a consistent pathway, the temporal pattern of voltage change recorded between 2 points on the body surface is also consistent and repeats itself with each heart cycle.

The lower trace of Figure 2–5 represents a typical recording of the voltage changes normally measured between the right arm and the left leg as the heart goes through 2 cycles of electrical excitation; this record is called a lead II ECG and is discussed in detail in Chapter 4. The major features of an ECG are indicated on this record and include the *P wave*, the PR interval, the *QRS complex*, the QT interval, the ST segment, and the *T wave*. The P wave corresponds to atrial depolarization; the PR interval to the conduction time through the atria and AV node; the QRS complex to ventricular depolarization; the ST segment to the plateau phase of ventricular action potentials; the QT interval to the total duration of ventricular systole; and the T wave to ventricular repolarization. (See Chapters 4 and 5 for further information about ECGs.)

Control of Heart Beating Rate

Normal rhythmic contractions of the heart occur because of spontaneous electrical pacemaker activity (automaticity) of cells in the SA node. The interval between heartbeats (and thus the heart rate) is determined by how long it takes

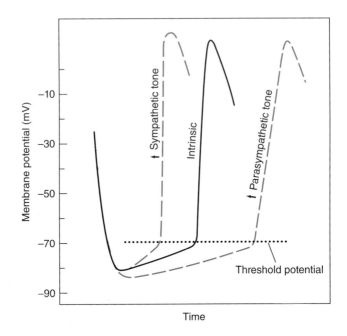

Figure 2-6. The effect of sympathetic and parasympathetic activity on cardiac pacemaker potentials.

the membranes of these pacemaker cells to spontaneously depolarize during the diastolic interval to the threshold level. The SA nodal cells fire at a spontaneous or *intrinsic rate* (≈100 beats/min) in the absence of any outside influences. Outside influences *are* required, however, to increase or decrease automaticity from its intrinsic level.

The 2 most important outside influences on automaticity of SA nodal cells come from the autonomic nervous system. Fibers from both the sympathetic and parasympathetic divisions of the autonomic system terminate on cells in the SA node, and these fibers can modify the intrinsic heart rate. Activating the cardiac sympathetic nerves (increasing cardiac sympathetic *tone*) increases the heart rate. Increasing the cardiac parasympathetic tone slows the heart rate. As shown in Figure 2–6, both the parasympathetic and sympathetic nerves influence the heart rate by altering the course of spontaneous diastolic depolarization of the resting potential in SA pacemaker cells.

Cardiac parasympathetic fibers, which travel to the heart through the *vagus* nerves, release the transmitter substance *acetylcholine* on SA nodal cells. Acetylcholine increases the permeability of the resting membrane to K^+ and decreases the diastolic i_f current flowing through the HCN channels.[8]

---

[8] Acetylcholine interacts with muscarinic receptors (M_2) on the SA nodal cell membrane that in turn are linked to inhibitory G proteins, G_i. The activation of G_i has 2 effects: (1) an increase in K^+ conductance resulting from an increased opening of the K_{Ach} channels; and (2) a suppression of adenylate cyclase leading to a fall in intracellular cyclic adenosine monophosphate, which reduces the inward-going pacemaker current (i_f).

As indicated in Figure 2–6, these changes have 2 effects on the resting potential of cardiac pacemaker cells: (1) they cause an initial hyperpolarization of the resting membrane potential by bringing it closer to the K^+ equilibrium potential and (2) they slow the rate of spontaneous depolarization of the resting membrane. Both of these effects increase the time between beats by prolonging the time required for the resting membrane to depolarize to the threshold level. Because there is normally some continuous *tonic* activity of cardiac parasympathetic nerves, the normal resting heart rate is approximately 70 beats/min, which is significantly slower than the intrinsic rate of ~100 beats/min.

Sympathetic nerves release the transmitter substance *norepinephrine* on cardiac cells. In addition to other effects discussed later, norepinephrine acts on SA nodal cells to increase the inward currents (i_f) carried by Na^+ and by Ca^{2+} through the HCN channels during the diastolic interval.[9] These changes will increase the heart rate by increasing the rate of diastolic depolarization as shown in Figure 2–6.

In addition to sympathetic and parasympathetic nerves, there are many (albeit usually less important) factors that can alter the heart rate. These include a number of ions, circulating hormones, various drugs, and physical influences such as body temperature and atrial wall stretch. All act by altering the time required for the resting membrane to depolarize to the threshold potential. An abnormally high concentration of Ca^{2+} in the extracellular fluid, for example, tends to decrease the heart rate by shifting the threshold potential. Factors that increase the heart rate are said to have a *positive chronotropic effect.* Those that decrease the heart rate have a *negative chronotropic effect.*

Besides their effect on the heart rate, autonomic fibers also influence the conduction velocity of action potentials through the heart. Increases in sympathetic activity increase conduction velocity (have a *positive dromotropic effect*), whereas increases in parasympathetic activity decrease conduction velocity (have a *negative dromotropic effect*). These dromotropic effects are primarily a result of autonomic influences on the initial rate of depolarization of the action potential and/or influences on the conduction characteristics of gap junctions between cardiac cells. These effects are most notable at the AV node and influence the duration of the PR interval of the ECG.

MECHANICAL ACTIVITY OF THE HEART

Contraction of cardiac muscle cells is initiated by a membrane action potential acting on intracellular organelles to evoke tension generation and/or shortening of the cells. In this section, we describe (1) the subcellular processes involved in coupling the excitation to the contraction of the cell (EC coupling) and (2) the mechanical properties of cardiac cells.

---

[9] Norepinephrine interacts with β_1-adrenergic receptors on the SA nodal cell membrane that in turn are linked to stimulatory G proteins, G_s. The activation of G_s increases adenylate cyclase, leading to an increase in intracellular cyclic AMP that increases the open-state probability of the HCN channel and increases the i_f current.

Cardiac Muscle Cell Contractile Apparatus

 Basic histological features of cardiac muscle cells are quite similar to those of skeletal muscle cells. These shared features include:

1. An extensive myofibrillar structure made up of parallel interdigitating thick and thin filaments arranged in serial units called *sarcomeres*, which are responsible for the mechanical processes of shortening and tension development. Proteins making up the thick and thin filaments are collectively referred to as "contractile proteins."

    The *thick filament* consists of a protein called *myosin*, which has a long straight tail with 2 globular heads, each of which contains an ATP-binding site and an actin-binding site; light chains are loosely associated with the myosin heads and their phosphorylation may regulate (or modulate) actin binding.

    The *thin filament* consists of several proteins including *actin*—2 α-helical strands of polymerized subunits (g-actin) extending from the Z lines. Sites along the actin filament interact with the heads of myosin molecules to make deformable cross-bridges with the thick filaments. Thin filaments also contain *tropomyosin*—a regulatory fibrous-type protein lying in the groove of the actin α-helix, which prevents actin from interacting with myosin when the muscle is at rest; and *troponin*—a regulatory protein consisting of 3 subunits (*troponin C*, which binds calcium ions during activation and initiates the configurational changes in the regulatory proteins that expose the actin site for cross-bridge formation; *troponin T*, which anchors the troponin complex to tropomyosin; and *troponin I*, which participates in the inhibition of actin–myosin interaction at rest).

    The giant macromolecule, *titin*, extends from the Z disk to the M line in the middle of each sarcomere and provides a continuous filament network in the sarcomeres extending the length of the cell. It contributes significantly to the passive stiffness of cardiac muscle over its normal working range. Phosphorylation of titin can alter the passive elastic properties of cardiac muscles.

2. A complex internal compartmentation of the myocyte cytoplasm by an intracellular membrane system called the *sarcoplasmic reticulum* (SR). This compartment actively sequesters calcium during the resting phase with the help of the sarco/endoplasmic reticulum Ca^{2+}-ATPase (SERCA) and calcium-binding storage proteins within the SR, the most abundant of which is *calsequestrin*.

3. Regularly spaced, extensive invaginations of the cell membrane (sarcolemma), called *T tubules*. These structures carry the action potential signal to the inner parts of the cell and appear to be connected to parts of the SR ("junctional" SR) by dense strands ("feet").

There are some morphological features that are unique to cardiac muscle cells. The most obvious of these is the large number of mitochondria in the cytoplasm that provide the oxidative phosphorylation pathways needed to ensure a ready supply of adenosine triphosphate (ATP) to meet the very high metabolic needs of the cardiac muscle. Students are encouraged to consult current histological references for specific cellular morphological details.

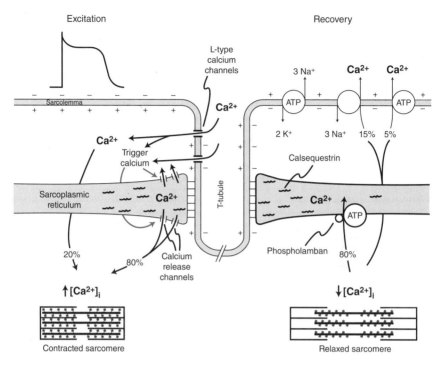

Figure 2–7. Excitation–contraction coupling, sarcomere shortening, and relaxation.

Excitation–Contraction Coupling

Muscle action potentials trigger mechanical contraction through a process called *excitation–contraction coupling*, which is illustrated in Figure 2–7. The major event of excitation–contraction coupling is a dramatic rise in the intracellular free Ca^{2+} concentration. The "resting" intracellular free Ca^{2+} concentration is less than 0.1 μM. In contrast, during maximum activation of the contractile apparatus, the intracellular free Ca^{2+} concentration may reach nearly 1.0 μM. When the wave of depolarization passes over the muscle cell membrane and down the T tubules, Ca^{2+} is released from the SR into the intracellular fluid.

As indicated on the left side of Figure 2–7, the specific trigger for this release appears to be the entry of calcium into the cell via the L-type calcium channels in the t-tubules and an increase in Ca^{2+} concentration just under the sarcolemma of the t-tubular system. Unlike the skeletal muscle, this highly localized increase in calcium is essential for triggering the major release of calcium from the SR. This *calcium-induced calcium release* is a result of opening calcium-sensitive release channels (RyR2) on the junctional SR.[10] Although the amount of Ca^{2+} that enters the cell during a single action potential is quite small compared with that released

---

[10] These channels may be blocked by the plant alkaloid, ryanodine, acting on the RyR2 receptor (often re-ferred to as ryanodine-sensitive calcium release channels), and are activated by the methylxanthine, caffeine. These agents are chemical tools used to assess the properties of these SR channels.

from the SR, it is essential not only for triggering the SR calcium release but also for maintaining adequate levels of Ca^{2+} in the intracellular stores over the long run.

When the intracellular free Ca^{2+} concentration is high (>1.0 μM), links called *cross-bridges* form between the thick and thin filaments found within the muscle. Sarcomere units, as depicted in the lower part of Figure 2–7, are joined end-to-end at Z lines to form *myofibrils*, which run the length of the muscle cell. During contraction, thick and thin filaments slide past one another to shorten each sarcomere and thus the muscle as a whole. The cross-bridges form when the regularly spaced myosin heads from thick filaments attach to regularly spaced sites on the actin molecules in the thin filaments. Subsequent deformation of the bridges pulls actin molecules toward the center of the sarcomere resulting in sarcomere (and muscle) shortening. This actin–myosin interaction requires energy from ATP. In resting muscles, the attachment of myosin to the actin sites is inhibited by troponin and tropomyosin. Calcium causes muscle contraction by interacting with troponin C to cause a configurational change that removes the inhibition of the actin sites on the thin filament. Because a single cross-bridge is a very short structure, gross muscle shortening and tension development requires that cross-bridges repetitively form, produce incremental movement between the myofilaments, detach, and form again at a new actin site, and so on in a cyclic manner.

There are several processes that participate in the reduction of intracellular Ca^{2+} that terminates the contraction. These processes are illustrated on the right side of Figure 2–7. Approximately 80% of this transient calcium increase is actively taken back up into the SR by the action of sarco/endoplasmic reticular calcium ATPase (SERCA) pumps located in the longitudinal part of the SR.[11] About 20% of the calcium is extruded from the cell into the extracellular fluid either via the Na^+–Ca^{2+} exchanger located in the sarcolemma[12] or via sarcolemmal Ca^{2+}-ATPase pumps.

Excitation–contraction coupling in the cardiac muscle differs from that in the skeletal muscle in that it may be modulated, that is, different intensities of actin–myosin interaction (contraction) can result from a single action potential trigger in the cardiac muscle. The mechanism for this is largely dependent on variations in the amount of Ca^{2+} reaching the myofilaments and therefore the number of cross-bridges activated during the contraction. This ability of the cardiac muscle to vary its contractile strength—that is, to change its *contractility*—is extremely important to cardiac function, as discussed in a later section of this chapter.

---

[11] The action of these pumps is regulated by the protein phospholamban. When this protein is phosphorylated (e.g., by the action of norepinephrine), the rate of Ca^{2+} resequestration by the SR is increased and the rate of relaxation is enhanced.

[12] The Na^+–Ca^{2+} exchanger is powered by the sodium gradient across the sarcolemma, which, in turn, is maintained by the Na^+/K^+-ATPase. This exchanger is electrogenic, in that 3 Na^+ ions move into the cell in exchange for each Ca^{2+} ion that moves out. This net inward movement of positive charge may contribute to the maintenance of the plateau phase of the action potential. The cardiac glycoside, digitalis, slows down the Na^+/K^+ pump and thus reduces the sodium gradient across the cell membrane, which, in turn, results in an increase in intracellular Ca^{2+}. This mechanism contributes to the positive therapeutic effect of cardiac glycosides on the contractile force of the failing heart.

The duration of the cardiac muscle cell contraction is approximately the same as that of its action potential. Therefore, the electrical refractory period of a cardiac muscle cell is not over until the mechanical response is completed. Consequently, heart muscle cells cannot be activated rapidly enough to cause a fused (tetanic) state of prolonged contraction. This is fortunate because intermittent contraction and full relaxation of the cardiac muscle cells is essential for the heart's pumping action.

Cardiac Muscle Mechanics

The cross-bridge interaction that occurs after a muscle is activated gives the muscle the potential to develop force and/or shorten. Whether it does one, the other, or some combination of the two depends primarily on what is allowed to happen by the external constraints placed on the muscle during the contraction. For example, activating a muscle whose ends are held rigidly causes it to develop tension, but it cannot shorten. This is called an *isometric* ("fixed length") contraction. The force that a muscle produces during an isometric contraction indicates its maximum ability to develop tension. At the other extreme, activating an unrestrained muscle causes it to shorten without force development because it has nothing to develop force against. This type of contraction is called an *isotonic* ("fixed tension") contraction. Under such conditions, a muscle shortens with its maximum possible velocity (called V_{max}), which is determined by the maximum possible rate of cross-bridge cycling. Adding load to the muscle decreases the velocity and extent of its shortening. Thus, the course of a muscle contraction depends on both the inherent capabilities of the muscle and the external constraints placed on the muscle during contraction. Muscle cells in the ventricular wall operate under different constraints during different phases of each cardiac cycle. To understand ventricular function, the manner in which the cardiac muscle behaves when constrained in several different ways must first be examined.

Isometric Contractions: Length–Tension Relationships

The influence of muscle length on the behavior of the cardiac muscle during isometric contraction is illustrated in Figure 2–8. The top panel shows the experimental arrangement for measuring muscle force at rest and during contraction initiated at 3 different fixed lengths. The middle panel shows time records of active tension developed at each of the 3 fixed lengths in response to a single external stimulus, and the bottom panel shows a graph of how the resting and peak isometric tensions change in response to increases in the resting muscle length.

The first important fact illustrated in Figure 2–8 is that force is required to stretch a resting muscle to different lengths. This force is called the *resting tension*. The lower curve in the graph in Figure 2–8 shows the resting tension measured at different muscle lengths and is referred to as the *resting length–tension curve*. When a muscle is stimulated to contract while its length is held constant, it develops an additional component of tension called *active* or *developed tension*. The *total tension* exerted by a muscle during contraction is the sum of the active and resting tensions.

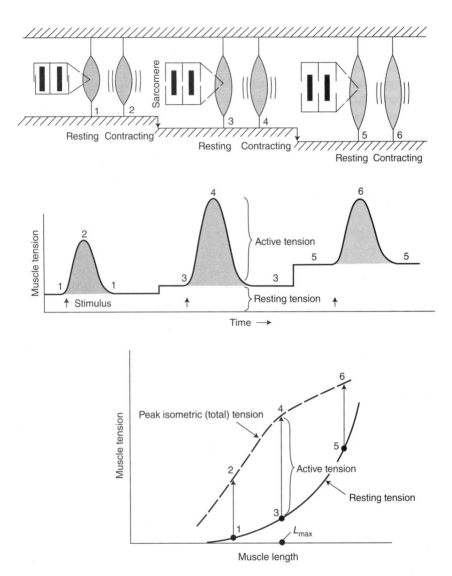

Figure 2–8. Isometric contractions and the effect of muscle length on resting tension and active tension development.

The second important fact illustrated in Figure 2–8 is that the active tension developed by the cardiac muscle during the course of an isometric contraction depends very much on the muscle length at which the contraction occurs. Active tension development is maximal at some intermediate length referred to as L_{max}. Little active tension is developed at very short or very long muscle lengths. Normally, the cardiac muscle operates at lengths well below L_{max} so that increasing muscle length increases the tension developed during an isometric contraction.

There are 3 separate mechanisms that have been proposed to explain the relationship between muscle length and developed tension. The first mechanism to be identified suggests that this relationship depends on the *extent of overlap* of the thick and thin filaments in the sarcomere at rest. Histological studies indicate that the changes in the resting length of the whole muscle are associated with proportional changes in the individual sarcomeres. Peak tension development occurs at sarcomere lengths of 2.2 to 2.3 μm. At sarcomere lengths shorter than approximately 2.0 μm, the opposing thin filaments may overlap or buckle and thus interfere with active tension development, as shown at the top of Figure 2–8. At long sarcomere lengths, the reduced myofilament overlap in the resting muscle cells may be insufficient for optimal cross-bridge formation during contraction.

The second (and perhaps more important) mechanism is based on a length-dependent change in *sensitivity* of the myofilaments to calcium. At short lengths, only a fraction of the potential cross-bridges are apparently activated by a given increase in intracellular calcium. At longer lengths, more of the cross-bridges become activated, leading to an increase in active tension development. This change in calcium sensitivity occurs immediately after a change in length with no time delay. The "sensor" responsible for the length-dependent activation of the cardiac muscle seems to reside within the troponin C molecule, but how it happens is not fully understood.

The third mechanism rests on the observation that within several minutes after increasing the resting length of the cardiac muscle, there is an increase in the *amount* of calcium that is released with excitation, which is coupled to a further increase in force development. It is thought that stretch-sensitive ion channels in the cell membranes may be responsible for this delayed response.

To what extent each of these mechanisms is contributing to the length dependency of cardiac contractile force at any instant is neither clear nor important in this discussion. The important point is that the dependence of active tension development on muscle length is a fundamental property of the cardiac muscle that has extremely powerful effects on heart function.

Isotonic and Afterloaded Contractions

During what is termed *isotonic* ("fixed load") contraction, a muscle shortens against a constant load. A muscle contracts isotonically when it develops sufficient tension to lift a fixed weight such as the 1-g load shown in Figure 2–9. Such a 1-g weight placed on a resting muscle will result in some specific resting (initial) muscle length, which is determined by the muscle's resting length–tension curve. If the ends of the muscle were to be fixed between 2 immoveable objects and the muscle were to be activated at this fixed length, it would contract isometrically and be capable of generating a certain amount of tension, for example, 4.5 g as indicated by the dashed line in the graph in Figure 2–9. A contractile tension of 4.5 g cannot be generated if the muscle is allowed to shorten and actually lift the 1-g weight. When a muscle has contractile potential more than the tension required to move the load, it will shorten. Thus, in an isotonic contraction, muscle length decreases at constant tension, as illustrated by the horizontal arrow from

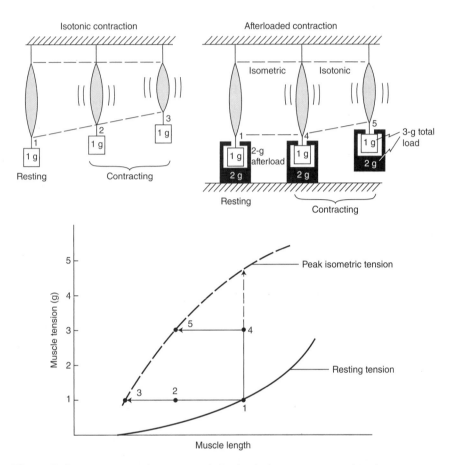

Figure 2-9. Description of isotonic and afterloaded contractions within the constraints of the cardiac muscle length–tension diagram.

point 1 through point 2 to point 3 in Figure 2–9. As the muscle shortens, however, its contractile potential inherently decreases, as indicated by the downward slope of the peak isometric tension curve in Figure 2–9. There exists some short length at which the muscle is capable of generating only 1 g of tension, and when this length is reached, shortening must cease.[13] Therefore, the peak isometric curve on a cardiac muscle length–tension diagram (that indicates how much isometric tension a muscle can develop at various lengths) also establishes the limit on how far muscle shortening can proceed with different loads.

---

[13] In reality, muscle shortening requires some time and the duration of a muscle twitch contraction is limited because intracellular Ca^{2+} levels are elevated only briefly following the initiation of a membrane action potential. For this and possibly other reasons, isotonic shortening may not actually proceed quite as far as the isometric tension development curve on the length–tension diagram suggests is possible. Because this complication does not alter the general correspondence between a muscle's isometric and isotonic performances, we choose to ignore it.

Figure 2–9 also shows a complex type of muscle contraction that is typical of the way cardiac muscle cells actually contract in the heart. This is called an *after-loaded isotonic contraction*, in which the load on the muscle at rest (the *preload*) and the load on the muscle during contraction (the *total load*) are different. In the example of Figure 2–9, the preload is equal to 1 g, and because an additional 2-g weight (the *afterload*) is engaged during contraction, the total load equals 3 g.

Because preload determines the resting muscle length, both contractions shown on the right side at the top of Figure 2–9 begin from the same length. Because of the different loading arrangements, however, the afterloaded muscle must increase its total active tension to 3 g before it can shorten. This initial tension will be developed isometrically and can be represented as going from point 1 to point 4 on the length–tension diagram. Once the muscle generates enough tension to equal the total load, its tension output is fixed at 3 g and it will now shorten isotonically because its contractile potential still exceeds its tension output. This isotonic shortening is represented as a horizontal movement on the length–tension diagram along the line from point 4 to point 5. As in any isotonic contraction, shortening must cease when the muscle's tension-producing potential is decreased sufficiently by the length change to be equal to the load on the muscle. Note that the afterloaded muscle shortens less than the non-afterloaded muscle, even though both muscles began contracting at the same initial length. The factors that affect the extent of cardiac muscle shortening during an afterloaded contraction are of special interest to us, because, as we shall see, stroke volume is determined by how far the cardiac muscle shortens under these conditions.

Cardiac Muscle Contractility

A number of factors in addition to initial muscle length can affect the tension-generating potential of the cardiac muscle. Any intervention that increases the peak isometric tension that a muscle can develop *at a fixed length* is said to increase cardiac muscle contractility. Such an agent is said to have a *positive inotropic effect* on the heart.

The most important physiological regulator of cardiac muscle contractility is norepinephrine. When norepinephrine is released on cardiac muscle cells from sympathetic nerves, it has not only the chronotropic effect on the heart rate discussed earlier but also a pronounced, positive inotropic effect that causes cardiac muscle cells to contract more forcefully and more rapidly.

The positive effect of norepinephrine on the isometric tension-generating potential is illustrated in Figure 2–10A. When norepinephrine is present in the solution bathing the cardiac muscle, the muscle will, *at every length*, develop more isometric tension when stimulated than it would in the absence of norepinephrine. In short, norepinephrine raises the peak isometric tension curve on the cardiac muscle length–tension graph. Norepinephrine is said to increase cardiac muscle *contractility* because it enhances the forcefulness of muscle contraction *even when initial length is constant*. Changes in contractility and initial length can occur simultaneously, but by definition, a change in contractility must involve a shift from one peak isometric length–tension curve to another.

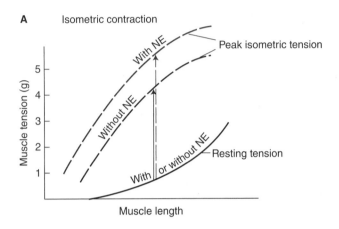

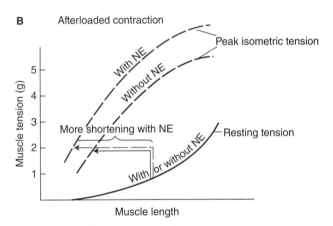

Figure 2–10. The effect of norepinephrine (NE) on isometric (**A**) and afterloaded (**B**) contractions of the cardiac muscle.

Figure 2–10B shows how raising the peak isometric length–tension curve with norepinephrine increases the amount of shortening in afterloaded contractions of the cardiac muscle. With preload and total load constant, *more shortening* occurs in the presence of norepinephrine than in its absence. This is because when contractility is increased, the tension-generating potential is equal to the total load at a *shorter* muscle length. Note that norepinephrine has no effect on the resting length–tension relationship of the cardiac muscle. Thus, norepinephrine causes increased shortening by changing the final but not the initial muscle length associated with afterloaded contractions. The added presence of norepinephrine will increase the *fractional shortening* (i.e., *percent shortening*) of cardiac muscle at any given resting length.

The cellular mechanism of the effect of norepinephrine on contractility is mediated by its interaction with a β_1-adrenergic receptor. The primary signaling pathway involves an activation of the G_s protein–cAMP–protein kinase A, which then phosphorylates the Ca^{2+} channel, increasing the inward calcium current during the plateau of the action potential. This increase in calcium influx not only contributes to the magnitude of the rise in intracellular Ca^{2+} for a given beat but also loads the internal calcium stores, which allows more to be released during subsequent depolarizations. This increase in free Ca^{2+} during activation allows more cross-bridges to be formed and greater tension to be developed (isometrically with any given preload) and more shortening to occur (isotonically with any given preload and afterload).

In addition to its effect on force development and/or shortening, norepineph-rine also has 2 other important effects on the cardiac muscle cell behavior:

1. There is a norepinephrine-induced increase in the rate of muscle relaxation. This is because norepinephrine causes phosphorylation of the regulatory pro-tein, *phospholamban*, on the sarcoplasmic reticular Ca^{2+}-ATPase pump and the rate of calcium retrapping into the SR is enhanced. This is called a *positive lusitropic effect.*
2. There is a norepinephrine-induced decrease in action potential duration. This effect is achieved by a potassium channel alteration, occurring in response to elevated intracellular $[Ca^{2+}]$ that increases potassium permeability, terminates the plateau phase of the action potential, and contributes to early repolariza-tion. Such shortening of the systolic interval by these 2 effects of norepineph-rine is very helpful in the presence of elevated heart rates that might otherwise significantly compromise diastolic filling time.

Enhanced parasympathetic activity has been shown to have a small negative inotropic effect on the heart. In the atria, where this effect is most pronounced, the negative inotropic effect is thought to be due to a shortening of the action potential and a decrease in the amount of Ca^{2+} that enters the cell during the action potential.

Changes in the heart rate that are not associated with autonomic neural input can also influence cardiac contractility. Recall that a small amount of extracel-lular Ca^{2+} enters the cell during the plateau phase of each action potential. As the heart rate increases, more Ca^{2+} enters the cells per minute. There is a buildup of intracellular Ca^{2+} and a greater amount of Ca^{2+} is released into the sarcoplasm with each action potential. Thus, a sudden increase in beating rate is followed by a progressive increase in contractile force to a higher plateau. This behavior is called the *staircase phenomenon* (or treppe). The importance of such rate-dependent modulation of contractility in normal ventricular function is not clear at present.

RELATING CARDIAC MUSCLE CELL MECHANICS TO VENTRICULAR FUNCTION

Certain geometric factors dictate how the length–tension relationships of cardiac muscle fibers in the ventricular wall determine the volume and pressure relationships of the ventricular chamber. The actual relationships are complex because the shape of the ventricle is complex. The ventricle is often modeled as either a cylinder or a sphere, although its actual shape lies somewhere between the two. Because cardiac muscle cells are oriented circumferentially in the ventricular wall, either model can be used to illustrate 3 important functional points:

1. An increase in ventricular volume causes an increase in ventricular circumference and therefore an increase in the length of the individual cardiac muscle cells. Thus, the extent of diastolic filling of the ventricle is the major determinant of cardiac "preload."
2. At any given ventricular volume, an increase in active tension of individual cardiac muscle cells in the wall causes an increase in intraventricular pressure. The intraventricular pressure that must be developed in order to eject blood from the ventricle is largely dependent on the arterial blood pressure, which is, therefore, a major determinant of cardiac "afterload."
3. As the ventricular volume decreases (i.e., as the ventricular radius decreases), a lesser total (collective) active force is required by the muscle cells in the ventricular walls to produce any given intraventricular pressure (and vice versa).

The last point is a reflection of the *law of Laplace* that states the physical relationship that must exist between total wall tension and internal pressure in any hollow vessel with circular containing walls. Regardless of whether the ventricle is envisioned as a hollow cylinder or a hollow sphere or whether it is thick- or thin-walled, the law of Laplace says that the *total* wall tension (T) depends on both intraventricular pressure (P) and its internal radius (r) as $T = P \times r$.

One implication of the law of Laplace is that the muscle cells in the ventricular wall have a somewhat easier job of producing internal pressure at the end of ejection (when the radius is small) than at the beginning of ejection (when the radius is large). More importantly, the law of Laplace has important clinical relevance in pathological situations such as "cardiac dilation" and "cardiac hypertrophy." These are discussed in detail in Chapter 11.

The importance of all these relationships will become more apparent in the subsequent chapter as we consider how cardiac muscle cell behavior determines how the heart functions as a pump.

PERSPECTIVES

It is easy to get overwhelmed by the impressive amount of information that is available concerning the excitation, contraction, and underlying biochemical processes responsible for cardiac muscle cell behavior. Our intent has been to present the basic vocabulary and essential information about excitation and contraction at the cellular level, to introduce areas of promising new information (i.e., channel function, calcium cycling, contractile processes), and perhaps to raise questions about what we *don't* know (e.g., What other cellular processes besides contraction does the calcium oscillation influence? How do these cells sense and adapt to altered pre- and afterloads? How does repair of cell structures and protein synthesis occur in these constantly contracting cells?). However, at this point, we put these questions aside and hope that the student will appreciate the amazing ability of these contracting cells when assembled into a functional pump to effectively move as much as 200 million liters of blood against a substantial pressure during the course of a normal human lifetime.

KEY CONCEPTS

Cardiac myocyte membrane potentials are a result of the relative permeability of the membrane to various ions and their concentration differences across the membrane.

Action potentials of cardiac myocytes have long plateau phases that generate long refractory periods and preclude summated or tetanic contractions.

Action potentials of cardiac myocytes are a result of changes in the membrane's permeability to various ions.

Action potentials are spontaneously generated by pacemaker cells in the SA node and are conducted from cell to cell via gap junctions throughout the entire heart.

The rate of spontaneous diastolic depolarization of the SA nodal cells (and thus the heart rate) is modulated by the autonomic nervous system.

Excitation of the cardiac myocyte initiates a contraction and relaxation cycle by causing a transient increase in cytosolic calcium level that transiently activates the contractile apparatus.

Mechanical response of the myocyte depends on preload (determined by the initial resting length), afterload (determined by the tension that needs to be developed), and contractility (the degree of activation of the contractile apparatus dependent on the amount of calcium released on activation).

The cardiac myocyte length–tension relationships are correlated with changes in volume and pressure in the intact ventricle.

STUDY QUESTIONS

2–1. *Small changes in extracellular potassium ion concentrations have major effects on cell membrane potentials.*

  a. *What will happen to the potassium equilibrium potential of cardiac muscle cells when interstitial [K$^+$] (i.e., [K$^+$]$_o$) is elevated?*

  b. *What effect will this have on the cells' resting membrane potentials?*

  c. *What effect will this have on the cells' excitability?*

2–2. *Cardiac survival during cardiac transplantation is improved by perfusing donor hearts with cardioplegic solutions containing approximately 20 mM KCl. Why is this high potassium concentration helpful?*

2–3. *There are several classes of drugs that are useful for treating various cardiac arrhythmias. Identify the primary effects of each of the following classes of drugs on cardiac myocyte characteristics:*

  a. *What are the effects of sodium channel blockers on the PR interval of the ECG? On the duration of the QRS complex?*

  b. *What are the effects of calcium channel blockers on the rate of firing of SA nodal cells, on the rate of conduction of the action potential through the AV node, and on myocardial contractility?*

  c. *What are the effects of potassium channel blockers on action potential duration? On refractory periods?*

2–4. *Very high sympathetic neural activity to the heart can lead to tetanic contraction of the cardiac muscle. True or false?*

2–5. *An increase in which of the following (with the others held constant) will result in an increase in the amount of active shortening of a cardiac muscle cell?*

  a. *Preload*

  b. *Afterload*

  c. *Contractility*

2–6. *What happens when an intervention promotes early activation of the "delayed rectifier" K$^+$ channel (I_K) in a cardiac muscle?*

  a. *The resting potential is increased (hyperpolarized).*

  b. *The action potential duration is decreased.*

  c. *The action potential amplitude is decreased.*

  d. *The action potential conduction velocity is increased.*

  e. *The absolute refractory period is prolonged.*

2–7. *Action potential conduction velocity in cardiac muscle tissue is influenced by all of the following except*

  a. *cell diameter.*

  b. *resting membrane potential.*

  c. *extracellular potassium concentration.*

  d. *rate of rise (phase 0) of the action potential.*

  e. *duration of the plateau phase (phase 2) of the action potential.*

2–8. The primary route of removal of $[Ca^{2+}]$ from the sarcoplasm during the relaxation of a cardiac muscle cell is by

a. active transport out of the cell.

b. passive exchange with extracellular sodium.

c. active transport into the sarcoplasmic reticulum.

d. trapping of calcium by troponin in the myofilaments.

e. passive movement out of the cell via L-type calcium channels.

The Heart Pump

3

The repetitive, synchronized contraction and relaxation of the cardiac muscle cells provide the forces necessary to pump blood through the systemic and pulmonary circulations. In this chapter, we describe (1) basic mechanical features of this cardiac pump, (2) factors that influence and/or regulate the cardiac output, and (3) sources of energy and energy costs required for myocardial activity.

CARDIAC CYCLE

Left Pump

A cardiac cycle is defined as one complete sequence of cardiac filling, cardiac muscle excitation and contraction, with ejection of blood and then muscle relaxation (diastole and systole). Graphs of several normal events of a single cycle of the left heart pump are plotted on the same timeline in Figure 3–1. Changes in electrical activity, muscle contractions, pressures, volume, valve position, heart sounds, and aortic flow are shown so that events that are occurring simultaneously in different parts of the cycle can be assessed. This important figure summarizes a great deal of information and should be studied carefully.

VENTRICULAR DIASTOLE

The *diastolic phase*[1] of the cardiac cycle begins with the opening of the atrioventricular (AV) valves. As shown in Figure 3–1, the mitral valve passively opens when left ventricular pressure falls below left atrial pressure and the period of ventricle filling begins. Blood that had previously accumulated in the atrium behind the closed mitral valve empties rapidly into the ventricle, and this causes an initial drop in atrial pressure. Later, the pressures in both chambers slowly rise together as the atrium and ventricle continue passively filling in unison with blood returning to the heart through the veins.

Proper filling of the ventricles depends on 3 conditions: (1) the filling pressure of blood returning to the heart and atria; (2) the ability of the AV valves to open fully (not be stenotic); and (3) the ability of the ventricular wall to expand passively with little resistance (i.e., to have high *compliance*). The healthy heart is very compliant during diastole so that filling normally occurs with only small increases in ventricular pressure.

Atrial contraction is initiated near the end of ventricular diastole by the depolarization of the atrial muscle cells, which coincides with the P wave of the ECG. As the atrial muscle cells develop tension and shorten, atrial pressure rises, and an additional amount of blood is forced into the ventricle. At normal resting heart rates (HRs) in healthy young individuals, atrial contraction is not essential for adequate ventricular filling. This is evident in Figure 3–1 from the fact that the ventricle has nearly reached its maximum or *end-diastolic volume* before atrial

---

[1] The atria and ventricles do not beat simultaneously. Usually, and unless otherwise noted, in this discussion, systole and diastole denote phases of ventricular operation.

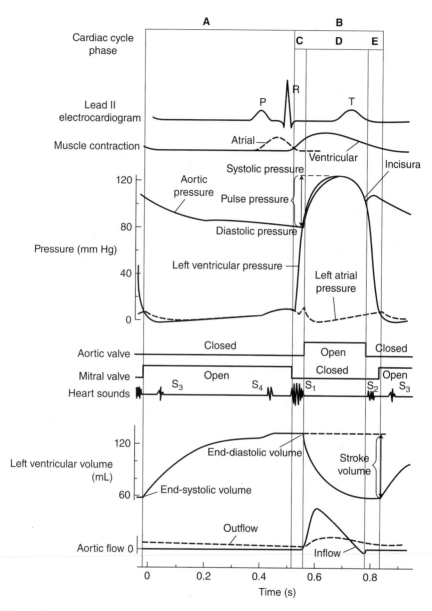

Figure 3–1. Cardiac cycle—left heart pump. Cardiac cycle phases: **A**, diastole; **B**, systole that is divided into 3 periods; **C**, isovolumetric contraction; **D**, ejection; and **E**, isovolumetric relaxation.

contraction begins. Atrial contraction plays an increasingly significant role in ventricular filling as HR increases because the time interval between beats for passive filling becomes progressively shorter with increased HR. Atrial contraction also plays a more important role as ventricular stiffness increases with age or disease.

Note that throughout diastole, atrial and ventricular pressures are nearly identical. This is because a normal open mitral valve has very little resistance to flow and thus only a very small atrial–ventricular pressure difference is necessary to produce ventricular filling.

VENTRICULAR SYSTOLE

Ventricular systole begins when the action potential passes through the AV node and sweeps over the ventricular muscle—an event heralded by the QRS complex of the electrocardiogram (ECG). Contraction of ventricular muscle cells causes intraventricular pressure to rise above that in the atrium. Because of the valve structure, the increased pressure behind the leaflets in the ventricle causes abrupt closure of the AV valve.

Pressure in the left ventricle continues to rise sharply as ventricular contraction intensifies. When left ventricular pressure exceeds that in the aorta, the aortic valve passively opens. The period between mitral valve closure and aortic valve opening is referred to as the *isovolumic* (or isovolumetric) *contraction phase* because during this interval, the ventricle is a closed chamber with a fixed volume. Ventricular ejection begins with the opening of the aortic valve. In early ejection, blood enters the aorta rapidly and causes the pressure there to rise. Pressure builds up simultaneously in both the ventricle and the aorta as the ventricular muscle cells continue to contract in early systole. This interval is often called the *rapid ejection period.*

Left ventricular and aortic pressures ultimately reach a maximum called *peak systolic pressure.* At this point, the strength of ventricular muscle contraction begins to wane. Muscle shortening and ejection continue, but at a reduced rate. Aortic pressure begins to fall because blood is leaving the aorta and large arteries faster than blood is entering from the left ventricle. Throughout ejection, very small pressure differences exist between the left ventricle and the aorta because the aortic valve orifice is so large that it presents very little resistance to flow.

Eventually, the strength of the ventricular contraction diminishes to the point where intraventricular pressure falls below aortic pressure. Because of the aortic valve structure, the increased pressure behind the leaflets in the aorta causes abrupt closure of the aortic valve. A dip, called the *incisura* or *dicrotic notch,* appears in the aortic pressure trace because a small volume of aortic blood must flow backward to fill the space behind the aortic valve leaflets as they close.[2] After aortic valve closure, intraventricular pressure falls rapidly as the ventricular muscle relaxes. For a brief interval, called the *isovolumetric relaxation phase*, the mitral valve is also closed. Ultimately, intraventricular pressure falls below atrial pressure, the AV valve opens, and a new cardiac cycle begins.

---

[2] Some choose to identify this event as the beginning of diastole, as it is easily demarked on the arterial pressure record of the mitral valve as part of ventricular systole or diastole. For clinical purposes, the incisura is a convenient and easily attainable marker of the end of ventricular ejection (but not of ventricular relaxation). The debate involves whether to include the short isovolumic relaxation period that occurs between the closure of the aortic valve and the opening of the mitral valve. We don't care.

Note that atrial pressure progressively rises during ventricular systole because blood continues to return to the heart and fill the atrium behind the closed AV valve. The elevated atrial pressure at the end of systole promotes rapid ventricular filling once the AV valve opens to begin the next heart cycle.

The ventricle reaches its minimum, or *end-systolic volume*, at the time of aortic valve closure. The amount of blood ejected from the ventricle during a single beat, the *stroke volume*, is equal to ventricular end-diastolic volume (EDV) minus ventricular end-systolic volume. Note that under normal conditions, the heart ejects only about 60% of its EDV.

The aorta distends or balloons out during systole because more blood enters the aorta than leaves it. During diastole, the arterial pressure is maintained by the elastic recoil of walls of the aorta and other large arteries. Aortic pressure gradually falls during diastole as the aorta supplies blood to the systemic vascular beds. The lowest aortic pressure, reached at the end of diastole, is called *arterial diastolic pressure*. The difference between diastolic and peak systolic pressures in the aorta is called the arterial *pulse pressure*. Typical values for systolic and diastolic pressures in the aorta are 120 and 80 mm Hg, respectively.

At a normal resting HR of approximately 70 beats/min, the heart spends approximately two-thirds of the cardiac cycle in diastole and one-third in systole. When increases in the HR occur, both diastolic and systolic intervals become shorter. Action potential durations are shortened, and conduction velocity is increased. Contraction and relaxation rates are also enhanced. This shortening of the systolic interval tends to blunt the potential adverse effects of increases in the HR on diastolic filling time.

Right Pump

Because the entire heart is served by a single electrical excitation system, similar mechanical events occur essentially simultaneously in both the left and right sides of the heart. Both ventricles have synchronous systolic and diastolic periods, and the valves of the right and left sides of the heart normally open and close nearly in unison. Because the 2 sides of the heart are arranged in series in the circulation, they must pump the same amount of blood and therefore must have identical SVs.

The major difference between the right and left pumps is in the magnitude of the peak systolic pressure. The pressures developed by the right side of the heart, as shown in Figure 3–2, are considerably lower than those for the left side of the heart (Figure 3–1). This is because the lungs provide considerably less resistance to blood flow than that offered collectively by the systemic organs. Therefore, less arterial pressure is required to drive the cardiac output through the lungs than through the systemic organs. Typical pulmonary artery systolic and diastolic pressures are 24 and 8 mm Hg, respectively.

The pressure pulsations that occur in the right atrium are transmitted in a retrograde fashion to the large veins near the heart. These pulsations, shown on the atrial pressure trace in Figure 3–2, can be visualized in the neck over the jugular veins in a recumbent individual. They are collectively referred to as the *jugular*

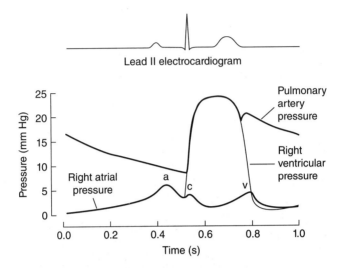

Lead II electrocardiogram

Figure 3–2. Cardiac cycle—right heart pump.

venous pulse and can provide clinically useful information about the heart. Atrial contraction produces the first pressure peak called the *a* wave. The *c* wave, which follows shortly thereafter, coincides with the onset of ventricular systole, and is caused by an initial bulging of the tricuspid valve into the right atrium. Right atrial pressure falls after the *c* wave because of atrial relaxation and a downward displacement of the tricuspid valve during ventricular emptying. Right atrial pressure then begins to increase toward a third peak, the *v* wave, as the central veins and right atrium fill behind a closed tricuspid valve with blood returning to the heart from the peripheral organs. With the opening of the tricuspid valve at the conclusion of ventricular systole, right atrial pressure again falls as blood moves into the relaxed right ventricle. Shortly afterward, right atrial pressure begins to rise once more toward the next *a* wave, as returning blood fills the central veins, the right atrium, and the right ventricle together during diastole.

Heart Sounds

Phonocardiography of the heart sounds, which occurs in the cardiac cycle, is included in Figure 3–1. These sounds are normally heard by *auscultation* with a stethoscope placed on the chest. The first heart sound, S_1, occurs at the beginning of systole because of the abrupt closure of the AV valves, which produces vibrations of the cardiac structures and the blood in the ventricular chambers. S_1 can be heard most clearly by placing the stethoscope over the apex of the heart. Note that this sound occurs immediately after the QRS complex of the ECG.

The second heart sound, S_2, arises from the closure of the aortic and pulmonic valves at the beginning of the period of isovolumetric relaxation. This sound is heard near the end of the T wave in the ECG. The pulmonic valve usually closes slightly after the aortic valve. Because this discrepancy is enhanced during the inspiratory phase of the respiratory cycle, inspiration causes what is referred to as the *physiological splitting of the second heart sound*. The discrepancy in valve closure during inspiration may range from 30 to 60 ms. There are at least 2 factors that lead to this prolonged ejection time from the right ventricle during inspiration. The first is related to an inspiration-induced decrease in intrathoracic pressure and increased filling of the right side of the heart. This extra volume will be ejected, but a little extra time is required to do so. The second factor is related to the inspiration-induced decrease in pulmonary vascular resistance, which transiently reduces pulmonary artery pressure and right ventricular afterload. With reduced afterload, ventricular ejection can go on for a slightly longer period.

The third and fourth heart sounds, shown in Figure 3–1, are not normally present in adults. When they are present, however, they, along with S_1 and S_2, produce what are called *gallop rhythms* (resembling the sound of a galloping horse). When present, the third heart sound occurs shortly after S_2 during the period of rapid passive ventricular filling and, in combination with heart sounds S_1 and S_2, produces what is called *ventricular gallop rhythm*. Although S_3 may sometimes be detected in normal children, it is heard more commonly in patients with left ventricular failure. The fourth heart sound, which occasionally is heard shortly before S_1, is associated with atrial contraction and rapid active filling of the ventricle. Thus, the combination of S_1, S_2, and S_4 sounds produces what is called an *atrial gallop rhythm*. The presence of S_4 often indicates an increased ventricular diastolic stiffness, which can occur with several cardiac disease states.

There may be other sounds associated with the cardiac cycle that usually indicate abnormal conditions. Murmurs can occur during systole or diastole and usually indicate turbulent flow through cardiac valves that either do not fully open or completely close. (These are described in more detail in Chapter 5.) Information about other abnormal sounds, including rubs, snaps, and clicks, can be obtained in more specific clinical references.

Cardiac Cycle Pressure–Volume and Length–Tension Relationships

Intraventricular pressure and volume are intimately linked to the tension and length of the cardiac muscle cells in the ventricular wall through purely geometric and physical laws. Figure 3–3A and 3–3B shows the correspondence between a ventricular pressure–volume loop and a cardiac muscle length–tension loop during a single cardiac cycle. These 2 loops indicate that cardiac muscle length–tension behavior is the underlying basis for ventricular function. Note that in Figure 3–3, each major phase of the ventricular cardiac cycle (panel A) has a corresponding phase of cardiac muscle length and tension change (panel B). During diastolic ventricular filling, for example, the progressive increase in ventricular pressure causes a corresponding increase in muscle tension, which passively stretches the resting cardiac muscle to greater lengths along its resting length–tension curve. End-diastolic ventricular pressure is referred to as *ventricular preload* because it sets the end-diastolic ventricular volume and, therefore, the resting length of the cardiac muscle fibers at the end of diastole.

A

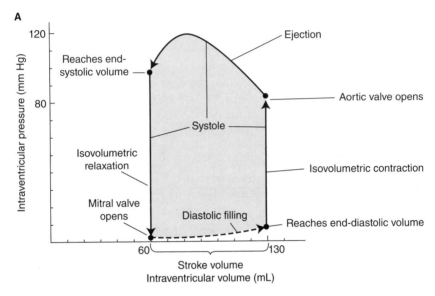

B

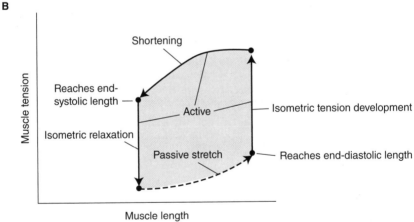

Figure 3–3. (**A**) Left ventricular pressure–volume cycle and (**B**) corresponding cardiac muscle length–tension cycle.

At the onset of systole, the ventricular muscle cells develop tension isometrically and intraventricular pressure rises accordingly. After the intraventricular pressure rises sufficiently to open the outlet valve, ventricular ejection begins because of ventricular muscle shortening. Systemic arterial pressure is often referred to as the *ventricular afterload* because it determines the tension that must be developed by cardiac muscle fibers before they can shorten.[3]

---

[3] This designation is somewhat misleading for at least 3 reasons. First, arterial pressure is more analogous to ventricular total load than to ventricular afterload. Second, because of the law of Laplace, the actual wall

During cardiac ejection, the cardiac muscle is simultaneously generating active tension *and* shortening (i.e., an afterloaded isotonic contraction). The magnitude of ventricular volume change during ejection (i.e., stroke volume) is determined by how far ventricular muscle cells shorten during contraction. This, as already discussed, depends on the length–tension relationship of the cardiac muscle cells and the load against which they are shortening. Once shortening ceases and the output valve closes, the cardiac muscle cells relax isometrically. Ventricular wall tension and intraventricular pressure fall in unison during isovolumetric relaxation.

DETERMINANTS OF CARDIAC OUTPUT

Cardiac output (liters of blood pumped by *each* of the ventricles per minute) is an extremely important cardiovascular variable that is continuously adjusted so that the cardiovascular system operates to meet the body's moment-to-moment transport needs. In going from rest to strenuous exercise, for example, the cardiac output of an average person may increase from approximately 5.5 to as much as 15 L/min. The extra cardiac output provides the exercising skeletal muscles with the additional nutritional supply needed to sustain an increased metabolic rate. To understand the cardiovascular system's response not only to exercise but also to all other physiological or pathological demands placed on it, one must understand what determines and controls cardiac output.

As stated in Chapter 1, cardiac output is the product of the heart rate and stroke volume (CO = HR × SV). Therefore, all changes in cardiac output must be produced by changes in the HR and/or SV.

Factors influencing the HR do so by altering the characteristics of the diastolic depolarization of the pacemaker cells, as discussed in Chapter 2 (Figure 2–6). Recall that variations in activity of the sympathetic and parasympathetic nerves leading to cells of the sinoatrial (SA) node constitute the most important regulators of the HR. An increase in sympathetic activity increases the HR, whereas an increase in parasympathetic activity decreases the HR. These neural inputs have immediate effects (within 1 beat) and, therefore, can cause very rapid adjustments in cardiac output.

INFLUENCES ON STROKE VOLUME

Effect of Changes in Ventricular Preload: The Frank–Starling Law of the Heart

The volume of blood that the heart ejects with each beat can vary significantly. One of the most important factors responsible for these variations in stroke volume is the extent of cardiac filling during diastole.

---

tension that needs to be generated to attain a given intraventricular pressure also depends on the ventricular radius (tension = pressure × radius). Thus, the larger the EDV, the greater the tension required to develop sufficient intraventricular pressure to open the outflow valve. Third, inertial factors associated with acceleration of blood flow during ejection also contribute to ventricular afterload. We choose, however, to ignore these complications.

This concept was introduced in Chapter 1 (Figure 1–7) and is known as the Starling law of the heart. To review (and to reemphasize its importance), this law states that, with other factors equal, *stroke volume increases as cardiac filling increases*. As discussed in the following section, this phenomenon is based on the intrinsic mechanical properties of myocardial muscle.

Figure 3–4A illustrates how increasing muscle preload will increase the extent of shortening during a subsequent contraction with a fixed total load. Recall from the nature of the resting length–tension relationship that an increased preload is necessarily accompanied by increased initial muscle fiber length. As described in Chapter 2, when a muscle starts from a greater length, it has more distance to shorten before it reaches the length at which its tension-generating capability is no longer greater than the load on it. The same behavior is exhibited by cardiac muscle cells when they are operating in the ventricular wall. Increased ventricular preload (i.e., diastolic filling) increases both EDV and stroke volume almost equally, as illustrated in Figure 3–4B.

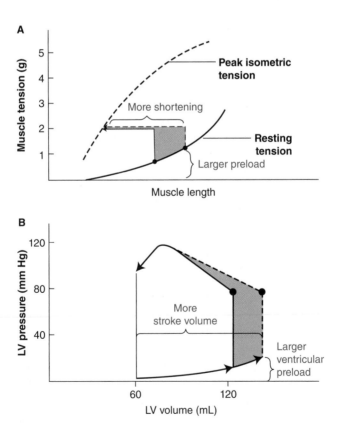

Figure 3–4. The effect of an increase in preload on (**A**) cardiac muscle shortening during afterloaded contractions and (**B**) ventricular stroke volume.

The precise relationship between cardiac diastolic filling pressure and EDV has especially important physiological and clinical consequences. Although the actual relationship is somewhat curvilinear, especially at very high filling pressures, it is nearly linear over the normal operating range of the normal heart. The low slope of this relationship indicates the substantial compliance of the normal ventricle during diastole (e.g., a change in filling pressure of only 1 mm Hg normally will change EDV by approximately 25 mL). As will be discussed in Chapter 11, one major form of cardiac failure is called "diastolic failure" and is characterized by a low ventricular compliance and a decidedly abnormal relationship between cardiac filling pressure and EDV.[4]

It should be noted in Figure 3–4A that increasing preload increases initial muscle length without significantly changing the final length to which the muscle shortens against a constant total load. Thus, increasing ventricular filling pressure increases stroke volume, primarily by increasing EDV. As shown in Figure 3–4B, this is not accompanied by a significant alteration in end-systolic volume.

Effect of Changes in Ventricular Afterload

As stated previously, systemic arterial pressure is usually taken to be the left ventricular "afterload." A slight complication is that arterial pressure varies between a diastolic value and a systolic value during each cardiac ejection. Usually, however, we are interested in *mean* ventricular afterload and take this to be *mean* arterial pressure (MAP).

Figure 3–5A shows how increased afterload, at constant preload, has a negative effect on cardiac muscle cell shortening. Again, this is simply a consequence of the fact that muscle cannot shorten beyond the length at which its peak isometric tension-generating potential equals the total load on it. Thus, shortening must stop at a greater muscle length when afterload is increased.

Normally, mean ventricular afterload is quite constant because MAP is held within tight limits by the cardiovascular control mechanisms described later. In many pathological situations such as hypertension and aortic valve obstruction, however, ventricular function is adversely influenced by abnormally high ventricular afterload. When this occurs, stroke volume may be decreased, as shown by the changes in the pressure–volume loop in Figure 3–5B. Under these conditions, note that stroke volume is decreased because end-systolic volume is increased.

The relationship between end-systolic pressure and end-systolic volume obtained at a constant preload but different afterloads is indicated by the dotted line in Figure 3–5B. In a normally functioning heart, the effect of changes in afterload on end-systolic volume (and therefore stroke volume) is quite small (approximately 0.5 mL/mm Hg). However, in what is termed "systolic cardiac failure," the effect of changes in afterload on end-systolic volume is greatly exaggerated such

---

[4] This is also more commonly called "heart failure with preserved ejection fraction."

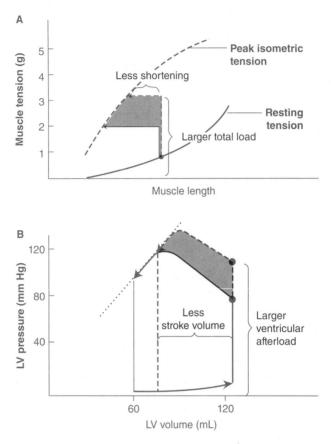

Figure 3-5. The effect of an increase in afterload on (**A**) cardiac muscle shortening during afterloaded contractions and (**B**) ventricular stroke volume.

that a small increase in arterial pressure can significantly reduce stroke volume. Thus, the slope of this line can be used clinically to assess the systolic function of the heart, as discussed further in Chapter 11.

Effect of Changes in Cardiac Muscle Contractility

Recall that activation of the sympathetic nervous system results in release of norepinephrine (NE) from cardiac sympathetic nerves, which increases contractility of the individual cardiac muscle cells. This results in an upward shift of the peak isometric length–tension curve. As shown in Figure 3–6A, such a shift will result in an increase in the shortening of a muscle contracting with constant preload and total load. Thus, as shown in Figure 3–6B, the NE released by sympathetic nerve stimulation will increase ventricular stroke volume by decreasing the end-systolic volume, without directly influencing the EDV.

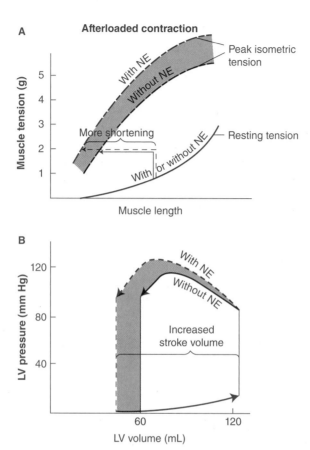

Figure 3-6. The effect of an increase in contractility by norepinephrine (NE) on (**A**) cardiac muscle shortening during afterloaded contractions and (**B**) ventricular stroke volume.

The term *ejection fraction* is a clinically useful variable used to assess cardiac muscle contractility. It is the fraction of the blood in the ventricle at the end of diastole that is ejected during systole. It is defined as the ratio of stroke volume (SV) to end-diastolic volume (EDV):

$$EF = SV/EDV$$

Because increased myocardial contractility causes an increase in ventricular ejection fraction, measurements of ejection fraction are often used clinically to assess the state of myocardial contractility.[5]

---

[5] Ejection fraction is commonly expressed as a percentage and normally ranges from 55% to 80% (mean 67%) under resting conditions. Ejection fractions of less than 50% to 55% indicate depressed myocardial contractility. Changes in preload and afterload can also influence ejection fraction but can be taken into account during the clinical assessment.

In addition to this change in the *extent* of myocyte shortening, an increase in contractility will also cause an increase in the *rates* of myocyte tension development and of shortening. This will result in an increase in the *rate* of isovolumetric pressure development and the *rate* of ejection during systole.

SUMMARY OF DETERMINANTS OF CARDIAC OUTPUT

The major influences on cardiac output are summarized in Figure 3–7. The HR is controlled by chronotropic influences on the spontaneous electrical activity of SA nodal cells. Cardiac parasympathetic nerves have a negative chronotropic effect, and sympathetic nerves have a positive chronotropic effect on the SA node. Stroke volume is controlled by influences on the contractile performance of the ventricular cardiac muscle—in particular, its degree of shortening in the afterloaded situation. The 3 distinct influences on stroke volume are contractility, preload, and afterload. Increased cardiac sympathetic nerve activity tends to increase stroke volume by increasing the contractility of the cardiac muscle. Increased arterial pressure tends to decrease stroke volume by increasing the afterload on cardiac muscle fibers. Increased ventricular filling pressure increases EDV, which tends to increase stroke volume through the Starling law.

It is important to recognize at this point that both the HR and stroke volume are subject to more than one influence. Thus, the fact that increased contractility tends to increase stroke volume should not be taken to mean that, in the intact cardiovascular system, stroke volume is always high when contractility is high. Following blood loss caused by hemorrhage, for example, stroke volume may be low despite a high level of sympathetic nerve activity and increased contractility. The only other possible causes for low stroke volume are high arterial pressure and low cardiac filling pressure. Because arterial pressure is normal or low following

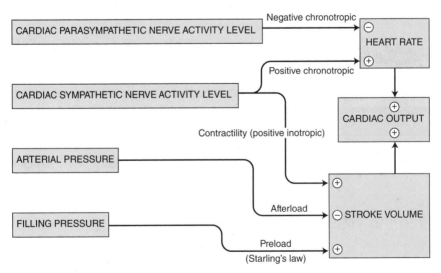

Figure 3–7. Summary of influences on cardiac output.

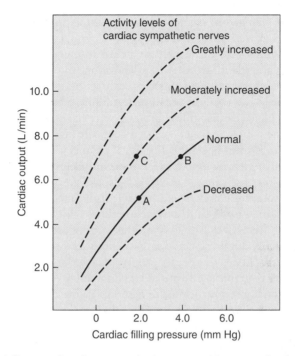

Figure 3–8. Influence of cardiac sympathetic nerve activity on cardiac function curves.

hemorrhage, the low stroke volume associated with severe blood loss must be (and is) the result of low cardiac filling pressure.

Cardiac Function Curves

One very useful way to summarize the influences on cardiac function and the interactions between them is by cardiac function curves such as those shown in Figure 3–8.

 In this case, cardiac output is treated as the dependent variable and is plotted on the vertical axis in Figure 3–8, while cardiac filling pressure is plotted on the horizontal axis.[6]

Different curves are used to show the influence of alterations in cardiac sympathetic nerve activity. Thus, Figure 3–8 shows how the cardiac filling pressure, and the activity level of cardiac sympathetic nerves interact to determine cardiac output. When the cardiac filling pressure is 2 mm Hg and the activity of cardiac sympathetic nerves is normal, the heart will operate at point A and have a cardiac output of 5 L/min. Each single curve in Figure 3–8 shows how cardiac

---

[6] Other variables may appear on the axes of these curves. The vertical axis may be designated as stroke volume or stroke work, whereas the horizontal axis may be designated as central venous pressure, right (or left) atrial pressure, or ventricular EDV (or pressure). In all cases, the curves describe the relationship between preload and cardiac function.

output would be changed by changes in cardiac filling pressure if cardiac sympathetic nerve activity were held at a fixed level. For example, if cardiac sympathetic nerve activity remained normal, increasing cardiac filling pressure from 2 to 4 mm Hg would cause the heart to shift its operation from point A to point B on the cardiac function diagram. In this case, cardiac output would increase from 5 to 7 L/min solely as a result of the increased filling pressure (the Starling law). If, on the other hand, cardiac filling pressure were fixed at 2 mm Hg while the activity of cardiac sympathetic nerves was moderately increased from normal, the heart would change from operating at point A to operating at point C. Cardiac output would again increase from 5 to 7 L/min. In this instance, however, cardiac output does not increase through the length-dependent mechanism because cardiac filling pressure did not change. Cardiac output increases at constant filling pressure with an increase in cardiac sympathetic activity for 2 reasons. First and most importantly, increased cardiac sympathetic nerve activity increases the HR. Second, increased sympathetic nerve activity increases stroke volume by increasing cardiac contractility.[7]

Cardiac function graphs thus consolidate knowledge of many mechanisms of cardiac control and are most helpful in describing how the heart interacts with other elements in the cardiovascular system. Furthermore, these graphs reemphasize the important point that a change in cardiac filling pressure alone will have a very potent effect on cardiac output at any level of sympathetic activity.

SUMMARY OF SYMPATHETIC NEURAL INFLUENCES ON CARDIAC FUNCTION

Because of its importance in overall control of cardiac function, it is appropriate at this point to summarize the major direct effects that the sympathetic nervous system exerts on electrical and mechanical properties of the cardiac muscle and thus on cardiac pumping ability. These effects are initiated by NE interaction with β_1-adrenergic receptors on cardiac muscle cells, resulting in a cascade of events involving the G_s activation of adenylate cyclase, formation of cAMP, and activation of protein kinase A with subsequent phosphorylation of many molecules that play key regulatory roles in intracellular processes. These cellular events resulting from increase in sympathetic neural activity to the heart combine to evoke improvements in pumping capabilities of the heart. These improvements include the following:

1. An increase in the HR (positive chronotropic effect) by activating the inward-going i_f current in SA nodal cells.
2. A decrease in cardiac action potential duration by early activation of the delayed i_K current in cardiac myocytes, which minimizes the detrimental effect of high HRs on diastolic filling time.

---

[7] Decreases in cardiac afterload (i.e., arterial pressure) can also shift the position of the curve upward by allowing more shortening to occur at a given preload. This effect is normally not important because afterload (i.e., arterial pressure) is usually kept constant.

3. An increase in the rate of action potential conduction, particularly evident in the AV node (positive dromotropic effect) by altering conductivity of gap junctions and by increasing the rate of initial depolarization of the action potential.

4. An increase in cardiac contractility (positive inotropic effect) by activating the $^i{}_{Ca^{2+}}$ current and increasing Ca^{2+} release from the sarcoplasmic reticulum, which increases the contractile ability of the cardiac muscle at any given preload.

5. An increase in the rate of cardiac relaxation (positive lusitropic effect) by increasing Ca^{2+} uptake by the sarcoplasmic reticulum, which also helps minimize the detrimental effect of high HRs on diastolic filling time.[8,9]

As will be presented in subsequent chapters, increases in sympathetic activity can have *indirect* influences on cardiac function that are a consequence of sympathetic-induced alterations in arteriolar and venous tone (i.e., alterations in afterload and preload, respectively). It should also be noted that increases in sympathetic drive can have negative effects on the heart primarily as a consequence of the catecholamine-induced increased metabolic demands on the heart.

CARDIAC ENERGETICS
Energy Sources and Chemical Efficiency

 For the heart to operate properly, it must have an adequate supply of chemical energy in the form of adenosine triphosphate (ATP). The relatively low ATP content of cardiac tissue combined with a relatively high rate of ATP hydrolysis at rest suggests that the myocardial ATP pool will completely turn over every 10 seconds.

The substrates from which ATP is formed by the heart depend partly on which substrates are in the greatest supply at a particular instant. For example, after a high carbohydrate meal, the heart will take up and metabolize glucose and pyruvate, whereas between meals, the heart can switch to metabolize free fatty acids, triglycerides, and ketones. Unlike skeletal muscle, cardiac muscle can utilize lactate as an energy source, which is beneficial during strenuous exercise when skeletal muscles are producing lactate. In addition, the choice of substrate depends on the metabolic phenotype of the cardiac muscle. Fetal and newborn hearts derive most of their ATP from metabolism of glucose and lactate, whereas within a few weeks of birth, a switch toward fatty acid oxidation occurs so that by adulthood, 60% to 90% of cardiac ATP is derived from fatty acids. A switch

---

[8] Most catecholamine effects on the heart are a result of increases in sympathetic neural activity. Although circulating catecholamines of adrenal origin can potentially evoke similar effects, their concentrations are normally so low that their contributions are negligible.

[9] Specific drugs called β-adrenergic receptor blockers can block all the effects of catecholamines on cardiac muscle. The drugs may be useful in the treatment of coronary artery disease to thwart increased metabolic demands placed on the heart by activity of sympathetic nerves.

back toward the fetal phenotype accompanies severe heart failure. Glycogen is stored in myocardial cells as a reserve energy supply and can be mobilized via the glycolytic pathway to provide extra substrate under conditions of increased sympathetic stimulation.

The end product of metabolism of glycogen, glucose, fatty acids, triglycerides, pyruvate, and lactate is acetyl CoA, which enters the citric acid (Krebs) cycle in the mitochondria, where, by a process of oxidative phosphorylation, the molecules are degraded to carbon dioxide and water and the energy is converted to ATP. (The student is encouraged to consult a biochemistry textbook for further details of these important metabolic pathways.)

The anaerobic sources of energy in the heart (e.g., glycolysis and creatine phosphate) are not adequate to sustain the metabolic demand for more than a few minutes. The heavy (nearly total) reliance of the heart on the aerobic pathways for ATP production is evident by (1) the high number of mitochondria and (2) the presence of high concentrations of the oxygen-binding protein myoglobin within the cardiac muscle cells. Myoglobin can release its oxygen to the mitochondrial cytochrome oxidase system when intracellular oxygen levels are lowered. In this regard, the cardiac muscle resembles "red" skeletal muscle that is adapted for sustained contractile activity as opposed to "white" skeletal muscle that is adapted for high-intensity, short-duration contractile activity.

The heart uses this chemical energy for basic "housekeeping" functions (e.g., ion pumps, repair processes) and for doing external "work" (e.g., pumping blood through the circulation). The heart's *chemical* efficiency can be described as the proportion of chemical energy supplied that actually does "work," and in normal conditions, the heart operates with an impressive overall efficiency of more than 30%. (For comparison, internal combustion engines are only 20–25% efficient.) The excess expended chemical energy is lost as heat that is ultimately carried away by coronary blood flow.

Determinants of Cardiac Energy Demand: Myocardial Oxygen Consumption

Because the heart derives its energy almost entirely from aerobic metabolism, myocardial oxygen consumption is directly related to myocardial ATP production and use. Therefore, changes in myocardial oxygen consumption closely parallel changes in myocardial external work rate.

In many pathological situations, such as obstructive coronary artery disease, the oxygen requirements of the myocardial tissue may exceed the capacity of coronary blood flow to deliver oxygen to the heart muscle. It is important to understand what factors determine the energy costs and, therefore, the myocardial oxygen consumption rate because, if oxygen delivery is compromised, reduction of the oxygen demand may be of significant clinical benefit to the patient.

The *basal metabolism* of the heart tissue required for basic "housekeeping" functions (e.g., energy-dependent ion pumping) normally accounts for approximately

25% of myocardial ATP use and therefore 25% of myocardial oxygen consumption in a resting individual.[10] Because basal metabolism represents the energy consumed in cellular processes other than contraction, little can be done to reduce it.

The processes associated with *muscle contraction* account for approximately 75% of myocardial energy use. Primarily, this reflects ATP splitting associated with cross-bridge cycling during the isovolumetric contraction and ejection phases of the cardiac cycle. Some ATP is also used for Ca^{2+} sequestration at the termination of each contraction.

The energy expended during the isovolumetric contraction phase of the cardiac cycle accounts for the largest portion ($\sim$50%) of total myocardial oxygen consumption despite the fact that the heart does no *external* work during this period. The energy needed for isovolumetric contraction depends heavily on the intraventricular pressure that must develop during this time, that is, on the cardiac afterload. *Cardiac afterload* is then a major determinant of myocardial oxygen consumption. Reductions in cardiac afterload can produce clinically significant reductions in myocardial energy requirements and, therefore, myocardial oxygen consumption.

Energy utilization during isovolumetric contraction is actually more directly related to isometric *wall tension* development than to intraventricular pressure development. Recall that wall tension is related to intraventricular pressure *and* ventricular radius through the law of Laplace ($T = P \times r$). Consequently, reductions in cardiac preload (i.e., EDV and radius) will also tend to reduce the energy required for isovolumetric contraction per beat.[11]

It is during the ejection phase of the cardiac cycle when the heart actually performs useful *external work*. The energy the heart expends during ejection depends on how much work it is doing during ejection. In a fluid system, work (force $\times$ distance) is equal to pressure (force/distance^2) $\times$ volume (distance^3). The external physical work done by the left ventricle in 1 beat, called *stroke work*, is equal to the area enclosed by the left ventricular pressure–volume loop (see Figure 3–3). Stroke work is increased either by an increase in stroke volume (increased "volume" work) or by an increase in afterload (increased "pressure" work). In terms of ATP utilization and oxygen consumption, increases in the pressure work of the heart are more costly than increases in volume work. Thus, reductions in afterload are especially helpful in reducing the myocardial oxygen requirements for doing external work.

Changes in *myocardial contractility* can have important consequences on the oxygen requirement for basal metabolism, isovolumic wall tension generation, and external work. Heart muscle cells use more energy in rapidly developing a given tension and shortening by a given amount than in doing the same thing more slowly.

---

[10] Indeed, many of these "housekeeping" functions increase their energy demands during exercise.

[11] This fact is especially important in congestive heart failure when the heart is distended and has an abnormally large ventricular radius. In this situation, the heart *muscle* itself will have an elevated "afterload" even when the MAP may be normal. In a sense, reduction of the EDV will reduce both preload and afterload.

Also, with increased contractility, more energy is expended in active Ca^{2+} transport. The net result of these influences is often referred to as the "energy wasting" effect of increased contractility.

The *heart rate* is one of the most important determinants of myocardial oxygen consumption because the energy cost per minute must equal the energy cost per beat times the number of beats per minute. In general, it has been found that it is more efficient (i.e., less oxygen is required) to achieve a given cardiac output with the low HR and high stroke volume than with the high HR and low stroke volume. This again appears to be related to the relatively high energy cost of the pressure development phase of the cardiac cycle.

External Work of the Heart and Mechanical Efficiency

The left heart does the work needed to pump blood through the systemic organs. For any pump, the *rate* of doing external work is equal to the flow it is producing *times* the pressure into which it is delivering flow. The output flow of the left heart is the cardiac output (CO). It delivers that flow into the aorta with an arterial pressure that has an average value over time called the *mean arterial pressure* (MAP). Thus, to a rough approximation, the work rate (WR) of the left heart pump can be calculated as:

$$WR = CO \times MAP$$

This equation shows that the WR of the left heart is increased by any increases in CO or MAP. One may use this equation to estimate how much work the left heart is doing per time in any given situation with a known CO and MAP. For example, a normal adult has a resting CO of about 5 L/min and a MAP of about 100 mm Hg. So, for a normal adult at rest, their left heart pump is doing work at a rate of about 500 (L × mm Hg)/min. This is the amount of energy the heart is delivering/time to the peripheral circulation. By appropriate unit conversion, it can be shown that this is a WR of about 20 calories/day. Note that with a standard recommended daily dietary caloric input of ~2000 calories, only a very small percentage of our ingested energy is needed to do the work of blood circulation in a resting individual. This observation emphasizes the fact that, under normal conditions, the cardiovascular system operates with astounding efficiency.

During heavy exercise, the metabolic rate of the body may increase about 3-fold over that at rest. To sustain that increased metabolic rate, tissue blood flow (i.e., CO) must increase by roughly an equal amount. Recall from the basic flow equation ($Q = \Delta P/R$) that an increase in tissue blood flow can only be caused by either an increase in ΔP (i.e., MAP) or a decrease in TPR (the "*total peripheral resistance*" to flow through the systemic circulation). If the 3-fold increase in flow during heavy exercise were caused solely by a 3-fold increase in MAP, both CO and MAP would each increase by 3-fold. Thus, the WR of the heart would increase 9-fold over rest during heavy exercise. At the opposite extreme, if the 3-fold increase in tissue blood flow were accomplished by a decrease in systemic vascular resistance to one-third of its resting value with no change in MAP, the WR of the heart would increase only 3-fold over rest during heavy exercise. It is little wonder why our cardiovascular systems have evolved to operate very efficiently with nearly constant arterial pressure and to regulate flow by varying the vascular resistance to flow through the blood vessels within the body.

The cardiac WR equation also has important implications for the normal overall operation of the cardiovascular system. Recall that the primary task of the cardiovascular system is to maintain homeostasis in organs throughout the body by supplying each organ with sufficient blood flow to meet its current metabolic needs. To accomplish this with a minimum effort by the heart in any given situation requires 2 things:

1. Supply each organ with just enough blood flow to meet its current needs. Collectively, this minimizes the cardiac output necessary in any situation.
2. Maintain an arterial pressure that is sufficient (but not excessive) to cause that tissue blood flow.

As will be described in detail in subsequent chapters, the first of these goals is accomplished primarily via mechanisms that operate on blood vessels to change their diameter and resistance to flow. The second goal is accomplished primarily by mechanisms that operate on the heart to appropriately adjust HR and SV so as to maintain near-constant arterial pressure regardless of what is happening in the periphery.

PERSPECTIVES

The job of the heart is to establish the pressure that drives blood passively through the pulmonic and systemic circulations. This is a remarkable, highly efficient, adaptable, and long-lasting pump that we, despite our best efforts, are unable to duplicate with any significant degree of success. When it breaks down, we suffer rather immediate adverse consequences.

As might be expected, support of this pump is highly dependent on the maintenance of coronary flow to the ventricular wall. Much of our current medical interventions are aimed at the coronary vasculature. Description of coronary flow is presented in more detail in Chapter 7.

In this book, we have ignored the extracellular structures of the heart, that is, the fibrous valves, the connective tissue frame (cardiac skeleton) that functions to electrically isolate the atria from the ventricles, and the extracellular matrix that forms a dynamic scaffolding surrounding the contractile cells. These structures are made primarily of collagen from the fibroblasts and not only maintain the structural integrity of the heart but also appear to participate importantly in dynamic adaptations to changing conditions.

KEY CONCEPTS

 Effective cardiac pumping of blood requires coordinated filling of the chambers, excitation and contraction of the cardiac muscle cells, pressure generation within the chambers, opening and closing of cardiac valves, and one-way movement of blood through the chambers into the aorta or pulmonary artery.

 Except for lower ejection pressures, events of the right side of the heart are identical to those of the left side.

 Heart sounds associated with valve movements and detected on auscultation can be used to identify the beginnings of diastolic and systolic phases of the cardiac cycle.

 The events of a single ventricular cardiac cycle can be displayed as records of electrical, mechanical, pressure, sound, or flow changes against time or as a record of volume against pressure.

 Cardiac output is defined as the amount of blood pumped by either of the ventricles per minute and is determined by the product of the heart rate and stroke volume.

 Stroke volume can be altered by changes in ventricular preload (filling), ventricular afterload (arterial pressure), and/or cardiac muscle contractility.

 Ventricular "ejection fraction" describes the fraction of end-diastolic volume of blood in the ventricle that is ejected per beat and is an index of cardiac contractility.

 A cardiac function curve describes the relationship between ventricular filling and cardiac output and can be shifted up (left) or down (right) by changes in sympathetic activity to the heart or by changes in cardiac muscle contractility.

 Energy for cardiac muscle contraction is derived primarily from aerobic metabolic pathways such that myocardial oxygen consumption is tightly related to cardiac work.

 The heart is highly efficient (>30%) at turning chemical energy into the energy of external work.

 In any given situation, the heart is doing external work at a rate given by CO × MAP.

 To produce an increase in tissue blood flow while minimizing the external workload of the heart, it is much more efficient to reduce tissue resistance to blood flow than to increase arterial blood pressure.

STUDY QUESTIONS

3–1. If pulmonary artery pressure is 24/8 mm Hg (systolic/diastolic), what are the respective systolic and diastolic pressures of the right ventricle?

3–2. Which of the following interventions will increase cardiac stroke volume?

  a. Increased ventricular filling pressure

  b. Decreased arterial pressure

  c. Increased activity of cardiac sympathetic nerves

  d. Increased circulating catecholamine levels

3–3. In which direction will cardiac output change if central venous pressure is lowered while cardiac sympathetic tone is increased?

3–4. Increases in sympathetic neural activity to the heart will result in an increase in stroke volume by causing a decrease in end-systolic volume for any given end-diastolic volume. True or false?

3–5. Four of these conditions exist during the same phase of the cardiac cycle and one does not. Which one is the odd one?

  a. The mitral valve is open.

  b. The ST segment of the ECG is occurring.

  c. Ventricular volume is increasing.

  d. Aortic pressure is falling.

3–6. With all other factors equal, myocardial oxygen demands will be increased to the greatest extent by which of the following?

  a. Increases in the heart rate

  b. Increases in coronary flow

  c. Increases in end-diastolic volume

  d. Decreases in arterial pressure

  e. Decreases in cardiac contractility

3–7. Sympathetic neural activation of the heart will decrease which of the following?

  a. Heart rate

  b. PR interval on the ECG

  c. Metabolic demands

  d. Coronary flow rate

  e. Cardiac contractility

3–8. An increase in total peripheral resistance (TPR) normally results in an increase in the external work rate required by the heart. True or false?

3–9. The metabolic requirement of the heart muscle in any situation is always equal to how much external work the heart is doing in that situation. True or false?

Measurements of Cardiac Function

4

OBJECTIVES

The student recognizes several techniques of assessing cardiac mechanical activity:

▶ Describes echocardiography and other cardiac visualization techniques for estimating cardiac ejection fraction.

▶ Describes the end-systolic pressure–volume relationship and how it reflects cardiac contractility.

▶ Given data, calculates cardiac output using the Fick principle.

▶ Defines cardiac index.

The student understands the physiological basis of the electrocardiogram:

▶ States the relationship between electrical events of cardiac excitation and the P, QRS, and T waves, the PR and QT intervals, and the ST segment of the electrocardiogram.

▶ States Einthoven's basic electrocardiographic conventions and, given data, determines the mean electrical axis of the heart.

▶ Describes the standard 12-lead electrocardiogram.

There are a variety of methods available to assess cardiac function. Some of these are noninvasive (e.g., auscultation of the chest to evaluate valve function, electrocardiography to evaluate electrical characteristics, and various imaging techniques to assess mechanical pumping action) and others require some invasive instrumentation. This chapter provides a brief overview of some of these commonly used clinical tools.

MEASUREMENT OF MECHANICAL FUNCTION

Imaging Techniques

Advances in several noninvasive imaging techniques have made it possible to obtain 2- and 3-dimensional images of the heart throughout the cardiac cycle. Visual or computer-aided analysis of such images provides information useful in clinically evaluating cardiac function. These techniques are especially suited for detecting abnormal operation of cardiac valves or abnormal wall motion. Estimates of cardiac chamber volumes at different times in the cardiac cycle can be used to assess cardiac ejection fraction (i.e., stroke volume divided by end-diastolic volume, SV/EDV), and displacement or deformation imaging can be used to assess cardiac wall strain or strain rate.

Echocardiography is the most widely used of the cardiac imaging techniques currently available. This noninvasive technique is based on the fact that sound waves reflect back toward the source when encountering abrupt changes in the density of the medium through which they travel. A transducer, placed at specified locations on the chest, generates pulses of ultrasonic waves and detects reflected waves that bounce off the cardiac tissue interfaces. The longer the time between the transmission of the wave and the arrival of the reflection, the deeper the structure is in the thorax. Such information can be reconstructed by a computer in various ways to produce a continuous image of the heart and its chambers throughout the cardiac cycle. Doppler echocardiography can provide additional information about blood flow velocity and direction across the cardiac valves. It is particularly useful in detecting valve stenosis or insufficiency.

Other imaging techniques are available for assessing cardiac function. *Cardiac angiography* involves the placement of catheters into the right or left ventricle and injection of radiopaque contrast medium during high-speed x-ray filming (cine-radiography). This is often done in conjunction with coronary angiography for assessing the integrity of the large coronary arteries. *Radionuclide ventriculography* (also known as multigated acquisition scan or MUGA scan) involves the intravenous injection of a radioactive isotope that stays in the vascular space (usually technetium that binds to red blood cells) with measurement of the changes in intensity of radiation detected over the ventricles during the cardiac cycle. A gamma camera is used to obtain images collected at (i.e., gated to) different times in the cardiac cycle. *Positron emission tomography* (PET) scans, *computed tomography angiography* (CTA) scans, and *magnetic resonance imaging* (MRI) all use other imaging modalities to get estimations of mechanical behavior of the heart.

Left Ventricular Pressure–Volume Loops and End-Systolic Pressure–Volume Relationship

As shown in Figures 3–4, 3–5, and 3–6 (also in Figures 11–4 and 11–5) complete left ventricular pressure–volume loops can reveal significant information about loading conditions and cardiac function. A variety of visualization strategies can be used to obtain the volume information, but detailed pressure information usually requires an invasive intraventricular cannulation.

However, the *end-systolic* pressure–volume relationship can be used to assess cardiac contractility. End-systolic volume for a given cardiac cycle is estimated by one of the imaging techniques described above, whereas end-systolic pressure for that cardiac cycle can be obtained from the arterial pressure recorded at the point of closure of the aortic valve (the incisura). Values for several different cardiac cycles may be obtained during infusion of a vasoconstrictor (which increases afterload), and the data plotted as in Figure 4–1 in the context of overall ventricular pressure–volume loops. As shown, increases in myocardial contractility are associated with a leftward rotation in the end-systolic

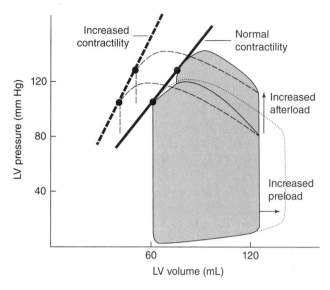

Figure 4-1. The effect of increased contractility on the left ventricular end-systolic pressure–volume relationship.

pressure–volume relationship. Decreases in contractility (as may be caused by heart failure) are associated with a downward shift of the line, discussed further in Chapter 11. This method of assessing cardiac function is particularly important because it provides an estimate of contractility that is independent of the EDV (preload). (Recall from Figure 3–4 and from the pressure–volume loop described by the dotted line in Figure 4–1 that increases in preload cause increases in stroke volume without changing the end-systolic volume. Thus, only alterations in contractility will cause shifts in the end-systolic pressure–volume relationship.)

Note in Figure 4–1 that both the "normal" and "increased contractility" end-systolic pressure–volume lines nearly project to the origin of zero pressure, zero volume. Thus, it is possible to get a reasonable clinical estimate of the slope of the end-systolic pressure–volume relationship (read "myocardial contractility") from a single measurement of end-systolic pressure and volume. This avoids the need to perform multiple tests with vasodilator or vasoconstrictor infusions.

Measurement of Cardiac Output

Fick principle: The most accurate (but unfortunately somewhat invasive) way of measuring how much blood is pumped by the heart per minute is by the use of the Fick principle described in Chapter 1. Recall that the amount of a substance *consumed* by an organ or tissues, $\dot{X}_{tc}$, is equal to what goes *in* minus what goes *out*, which is the arterial–venous concentration difference in the substance $([X]_a - [X]_v)$ times the blood flow rate, $\dot{Q}$.

$$\dot{X}_{tc} = \dot{Q}([X]_a - [X]_v)$$

This relationship can be algebraically rearranged to solve for blood flow through a given organ:

$$\dot{Q} = \frac{(\dot{X}_{tc})}{[X]_a - [X]_v}$$

A common method of determining cardiac output is to use the Fick principle to calculate the collective flow through *all* systemic organs from (1) the whole-body oxygen consumption rate $\dot{X}_{tc}$ (by monitoring the oxygen uptake from inspired air), (2) the oxygen concentration in arterial blood ($[X]_a$) obtained from any convenient arterial puncture, and (3) the concentration of oxygen in *mixed* venous blood ($[X]_v$) (which is the most difficult to obtain). Generally, the sample for *mixed* venous blood oxygen measurement must be taken from venous catheters positioned in the right ventricle or the pulmonary artery to ensure that it is a well-mixed sample of venous blood from *all* systemic organs.

The calculation of cardiac output from the Fick principle is best illustrated by an example. Suppose that a patient is consuming 250 mL of O_2 per minute when his or her systemic arterial blood contains 200 mL of O_2 per liter and the right ventricular blood contains 150 mL of O_2 per liter. This means that, on an average, each liter of blood loses 50 mL of O_2 as it passes through the systemic organs. For 250 mL of O_2 to be consumed per minute, 5 L of blood must pass through the systemic circulation each minute:

$$\dot{Q} = \frac{250\,\text{mL}\,O_2/\min}{200 - 150\,\text{mL}\,O_2/\text{L blood}}$$

$$\dot{Q} = 5\,\text{L blood/min}$$

③ *Indicator dilution techniques*: Another method of estimating cardiac output is to determine how much a given substance is diluted by the blood that passes through the heart in a given period of time. In these methods, a known quantity of indicator (a dye or a thermal change induced by a bolus of heated or cooled fluid) is rapidly injected into the blood as it enters the right side of the heart and appropriate detectors are arranged to continuously record the concentration of the indicator in blood as it leaves the left side of the heart. It is possible to estimate the cardiac output from the quantity of indicator injected and the time record of indicator concentration in the blood that leaves the left side of the heart.

Echocardiography: Cardiac output can be estimated noninvasively by this very useful visualization technique. Ultrasound imaging of the changing chamber sizes in diastole and systole can be used to estimate stroke volume. *Doppler shifts* of the echo from blood flow through the aortic (or mitral) valve allow assessment of blood flow velocity and can be used to estimate stroke volume. Information about cardiac output can be obtained from the product of these estimates of stroke volume and heart rate (HR).

A variety of other methods for estimating cardiac output have been used and may provide useful assessments under various conditions. These include *impedance cardiography, MRI*, and *pulse pressure evaluations*.

Cardiac Index

Normal cardiac outputs are directly dependent on an individual's size. For example, the cardiac output of a 50 kg woman will be significantly lower than that of a 90 kg man. *Cardiac index* is equal to cardiac output corrected for the individual's size and is commonly used for clinical comparisons with normal values. It has been found, however, that cardiac output correlates better with body surface area than with body weight. Therefore, it is common to express the cardiac output per square meter of surface area. Under resting conditions, the cardiac index is normally approximately 3 L/min/m². (Nomograms are available for determining body surface area from height and weight measurements.)

MEASUREMENT OF CARDIAC EXCITATION— THE ELECTROCARDIOGRAM

The electrocardiogram (ECG) is a powerful clinical tool that is used to evaluate cardiac electrical properties such as excitation rate, rhythm, and conduction characteristics. It does not provide specific information about mechanical activity. As briefly described in Chapter 2, the ECG is the result of currents propagated through the extracellular fluid that are generated by the spread of the wave of excitation throughout the heart. Electrodes placed on the surface of the body record the small potential differences between various recording sites that vary over the time course of the cardiac cycle.

A typical electrocardiographic record is indicated in Figure 4–2. The major features of the ECG are the P, QRS, and T waves that are caused by atrial depolarization, ventricular depolarization, and ventricular repolarization, respectively. The period from the initiation of the P wave to the beginning of QRS complex is designated as the PR interval and indicates the time it takes for an action potential to spread through the atria and the atrioventricular (AV) node. During the latter portion of the PR interval (PR segment), no voltages are detected on the body surface. This is because atrial muscle cells are depolarized (in the plateau phase of their action potentials), ventricular cells are still resting, and the electrical field set up by the action potential progressing through the small AV node is not intense enough to be detected. The duration of the normal PR interval ranges from 120 to 200 ms. Shortly after the cardiac impulse breaks out of the AV node and into the rapidly conducting Purkinje system, all the ventricular muscle cells depolarize within a very short period and cause the QRS complex. The R wave is the largest event in the ECG because ventricular muscle cells are numerous, and they depolarize nearly in unison. The normal QRS complex lasts between 60 and 100 ms. (The repolarization of atrial cells also occurs during the period in which ventricular depolarization generates the QRS complex on the ECG [see Figure 2–5].) Atrial repolarization is not evident on the ECG because it is a poorly synchronized

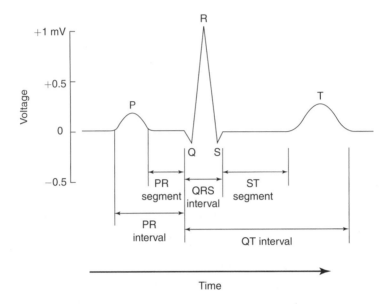

Figure 4–2. Typical electrocardiogram of a single cardiac cycle.

event in a relatively small mass of heart tissue and is completely overshadowed by the major electrical events occurring in the ventricles at this time.

The QRS complex is followed by the *ST segment*. Normally, no electrical potentials are measured on the body surface during the ST segment because no rapid changes in membrane potential are occurring in any of the cells of the heart; atrial cells have already returned to the resting phase, whereas ventricular muscle cells are in the plateau phase of their action potentials. (Myocardial injury or inadequate blood flow, however, can produce elevations or depressions in the ST segment.) When ventricular cells begin to repolarize, a voltage difference once again appears on the body surface and is measured as the T wave of the ECG. The T wave is broader and not as large as the R wave because ventricular repolarization is less synchronous than depolarization. At the conclusion of the T wave, all the cells in the heart are in the resting state. The *QT interval* roughly approximates the duration of ventricular myocyte action potential and thus the period of ventricular systole. At a normal HR of 60 beats/min, the QT interval is normally less than 380 ms. No body surface potential is measured until the next impulse is generated by the sinoatrial (SA) node.

It should be recognized that the operation of the specialized conduction system is a primary factor in determining the normal electrocardiographic pattern. For example, the AV nodal transmission time determines the PR interval. Also, the effectiveness of the Purkinje system in synchronizing ventricular depolarization is reflected in the large magnitude and short duration of the QRS complex. It should also be noted that nearly every heart muscle cell is inherently capable of rhythmicity and that all cardiac cells are electrically interconnected through gap junctions.

Thus, a functional heart rhythm can, and often does, occur without the involvement of part or all of the specialized conduction system. Such a situation is, however, abnormal, and the existence of abnormal conduction pathways would produce an abnormal ECG.

Basic Electrocardiographic Conventions

Recording ECGs is a routine diagnostic procedure, which is standardized by universal application of certain conventions. The conventions for recording and analysis of ECGs from the 3 standard bipolar limb leads are briefly described here.

Recording electrodes are placed on both arms and the left leg—usually at the wrists and the ankle. The appendages are assumed to act merely as extensions of the recording system, and voltage measurements are assumed to be made between points that form an equilateral triangle over the thorax, as shown in Figure 4–3. This conceptualization is called the *Einthoven triangle* in honor of the Dutch physiologist who devised it in the early 20th century. Any single electrocardiographic trace is a recording of the voltage difference measured between any 2 vertices of the Einthoven triangle. An example of the lead II ECG measured between the right arm and the left leg has already been shown in Figure 4–2. Similarly, lead I and lead III ECGs represent voltage measurements taken along the other 2 sides of the Einthoven triangle, as indicated in Figure 4–3. The "+" and "−" symbols in Figure 4–3 indicate polarity conventions that have been universally adopted.

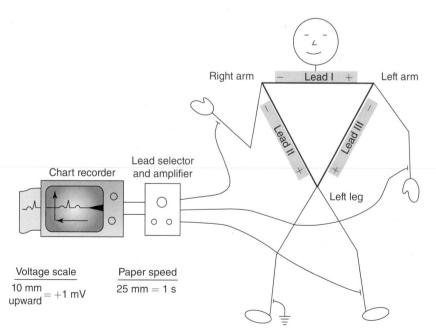

Figure 4–3. Einthoven's electrocardiographic conventions.

For example, an upward deflection in a lead II ECG (as normally occurs during the P, R, and T waves) indicates that an electrical potential exists at that instant between the left leg and the right shoulder electrodes, with the left leg electrode being positive. Conversely, a downward deflection in a lead II record indicates that a polarity exists between the electrodes at that instant, with the left leg electrode being negative. Similar polarity conventions have been established for lead I and lead III recordings and are indicated by the "+" and "−" symbols in Figure 4–3. In addition, electrocardiographic recording equipment is often standardized so that a 1-cm deflection on the vertical axis always represents a potential difference of 1 mV, and that 25 mm on the horizontal axis of any electrocardiographic record represents 1 second. Most electrocardiographic records contain calibration signals so that abnormal rates and wave amplitudes can be easily detected.

As shown in the next chapter, many cardiac electrical abnormalities can be detected in recordings from a single electrocardiographic lead. However, certain clinically useful information can be derived only by combining the information obtained from 2 electrocardiographic leads. To understand these more complex electrocardiographic analyses, a close examination of how voltages appear on the body surface as a result of the cardiac electrical activity must be done.

Cardiac Dipoles and Electrocardiographic Records

Einthoven's conceptualization of how cardiac electrical activity causes potential differences on the surface of the body is illustrated in Figure 4–4. In this example, the heart is shown at one instant in the atrial depolarization phase. The cardiac impulse, after having arisen in the SA node, is spreading as a wavefront of depolarization through the atrial tissue. At each point along this wavefront of electrical activity, a small charge separation exists in the extracellular fluid between polarized membranes (positive outside) and depolarized membranes (negative outside). Thus, the wavefront may be thought of as a series of individual *electrical dipoles* (regions of charge separation). Each individual dipole is oriented in the direction of local wavefront movement. The large, black arrow in Figure 4–4

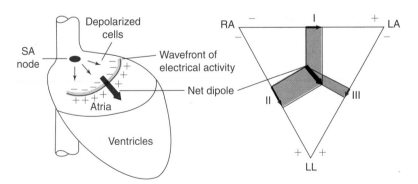

Figure 4–4. Net cardiac dipole during atrial depolarization and its components on the limb leads.

represents the total *net* dipole created by the summed contributions of all the individual dipoles distributed along the wavefront of atrial depolarization. The salty extracellular fluid acts as an excellent conductor, allowing these instantaneous net dipoles, generated on the surface of the heart muscle, to be recorded by electrodes on the surface of the body.

The net dipole that exists at any instant during depolarization is oriented (i.e., points) in the general direction of wavefront movement at that instant. The magnitude or strength of the dipole (represented here by the arrow length) is determined by (1) how extensive the wavefront is (i.e., how many cells are simultaneously depolarizing at the instant in question) and (2) the consistency of orientation between individual dipoles at different points in the wavefront (dipoles with the same orientation reinforce each other; dipoles with the opposite orientation cancel each other).

The net dipole in the example in Figure 4–4 causes the lower-left portion of the body to be generally positive with respect to the upper-right portion. This particular dipole will cause positive voltages to exist on all 3 of the ECG limb leads. As shown in the right half of Figure 4–4, this can be deduced from the Einthoven triangle by observing that the net dipole has some component that points in the positive direction of leads I, II, and III. As illustrated in Figure 4–4, the component that a cardiac dipole has on a given ECG lead is found by drawing perpendicular lines from the appropriate side of the Einthoven triangle to the tip and tail of the dipole. (It may be helpful to think of the component on each lead as the "shadow" cast by the dipole on that lead as a result of a "sun" located far beyond the corner of the Einthoven triangle that is opposite the lead.) Note that the dipole in this example is most parallel to lead II and, therefore, has a large component in the lead II direction. Thus, it will create a larger voltage on lead II than on lead I or lead III. This dipole has a rather small component on lead III because it is oriented nearly perpendicular to lead III.

The limb lead configuration may be thought of as a way to view the heart's electrical activity from 3 different perspectives (or axes). The vector representing the heart's instantaneous dipole strength and orientation is the object under observation, and its appearance depends on the position from which it is viewed. The instantaneous voltage measured on the axis of lead I, for example, indicates how the dipole being generated by the heart's electrical activity at that instant appears when viewed directly from above. A cardiac dipole that is oriented horizontally appears large on lead I, whereas a vertically oriented cardiac dipole, however large, produces no voltage on lead I. Thus, it is necessary to have views from 2 directions to establish the magnitude and orientation of the heart's dipole. A vertically oriented dipole would be invisible on lead I but would be readily apparent if viewed from the perspective of lead II or lead III.

It is important to emphasize that the example in Figure 4–4 pertains only to one instant during atrial depolarization. The net cardiac dipole continually changes in magnitude and orientation during the course of atrial depolarization. The nature of these changes will determine the shape of the P wave on each of the ECG leads.

The P wave terminates when the wave of depolarization, as illustrated in Figure 4–4, reaches the nonmuscular border between the atria and the ventricles and the number of individual dipoles becomes very small. At this time, the cardiac impulse is still being slowly transmitted toward the ventricles through the AV node. However, the electrical activity in the AV node involves so few cells that it generates no detectable net cardiac dipole. Thus, no voltages are measured on the surface of the body for a brief period following the P wave. A net cardiac dipole reappears only when the depolarization completes its passage through the AV node, enters the Purkinje system, and begins its rapid passage over the ventricular muscle cells. Because the Purkinje fibers initially pass through the intraventricular septum and to the endocardial layers at the apex of the ventricles, ventricular depolarization occurs first in these areas and then proceeds outward and upward through the ventricular myocardium.

Ventricular Depolarization and the QRS Complex

It is the rapid and large changes in the magnitude and direction of the net cardiac dipole that occur during ventricular depolarization that cause the QRS complex of the ECG. The normal process is illustrated in Figure 4–5. The initial ventricular depolarization usually occurs on the left side of the intraventricular septum, as illustrated in the upper panel of the figure. Analysis of the cardiac dipole formed by this initial ventricular depolarization with the aid of the Einthoven triangle shows that this dipole has a negative component on lead I, a small negative component on lead II, and a positive component on lead III. The upper-right panel shows the actual deflections on each of the electrocardiographic limb leads that will be produced by this dipole. Note that it is possible for a given cardiac dipole to produce opposite deflections on different leads. For example, in Figure 4–5, Q waves appear on leads I and II but not on lead III.

The second row of panels in Figure 4–5 shows the ventricles during the instant in ventricular depolarization when the number of individual dipoles is greatest and/or their orientation is most similar. This phase generates the large net cardiac dipole, which is responsible for the R wave of the ECG. In Figure 4–5, this net cardiac dipole is nearly parallel to lead II. As indicated, such a dipole produces large positive R waves on all 3 limb leads.

The third row in Figure 4–5 shows the situation near the end of the spread of depolarization through the ventricles and indicates how the small net cardiac dipole present at this time produces the S wave. Note that an S wave does not necessarily appear on all ECG leads (as in lead I of this example).

The bottom row in Figure 4–5 shows that during the ST segment, all ventricular muscle cells are in a depolarized state. There are no waves of electrical activity moving through the heart tissue. Consequently, no net cardiac dipole exists at this time and no voltage differences exist between points on the body surface. All electrocardiographic traces will be flat at the *isoelectric* (zero voltage) level.

Ventricular Repolarization and the T Wave

As illustrated in Figure 4–2, the T wave is normally positive on lead II as is the R wave. This indicates that the net cardiac dipole generated during ventricular

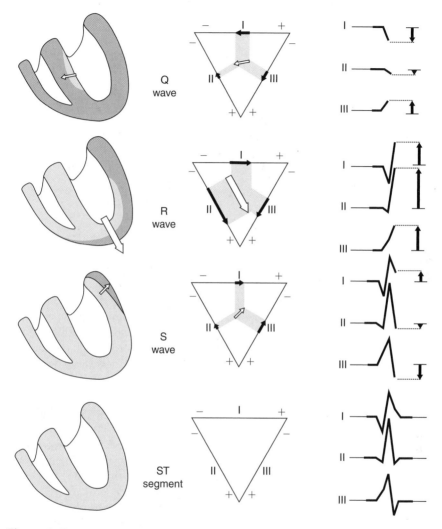

Figure 4–5. Ventricular depolarization and the generation of the QRS complex.

repolarization is oriented in the same general direction as that existing during ventricular depolarization. This may be somewhat surprising. However, recall from Figure 2–5 that the *last ventricular cells to depolarize are the first to repolarize.* The reasons for this are not well understood, but the result is that the wavefront of electrical activity during ventricular repolarization tends to retrace, in *reverse direction*, the course followed during ventricular depolarization. Therefore, the dipole formed during repolarization has the *same* polarity as that during depolarization. This reversed wavefront propagation pathway during ventricular repolarization results in a positive T wave recorded, for example, on lead II. The T wave is broader and smaller than the R wave because the repolarization of ventricular muscle cells is less well synchronized than is their depolarization.

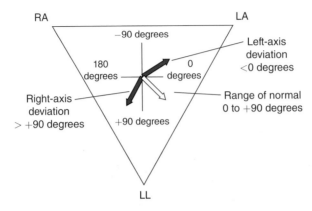

Figure 4-6. Mean electrical axis and axis deviations.

Mean Electrical Axis and Axis Deviations

The orientation of the cardiac dipole during the most intense phase of ventricular depolarization (i.e., at the instant the R wave reaches its peak) is called the *mean electrical axis* of the heart. It is used clinically as an indicator of whether ventricular depolarization is proceeding over normal pathways. The mean electrical axis is reported in degrees according to the convention indicated in Figure 4–6. (Note that the downward direction corresponds to *plus* 90 degrees in this polar coordinate system.) As indicated, a mean electrical axis that lies anywhere in the patient's lower left-hand quadrant is considered normal. A *left-axis deviation* exists when the mean electrical axis falls in the patient's upper left-hand quadrant and may indicate a physical displacement of the heart to the left, left ventricular hypertrophy, or loss of electrical activity in the right ventricle. A *right-axis deviation* exists when the mean electrical axis falls in the patient's lower right-hand quadrant and may indicate a physical displacement of the heart to the right, right ventricular hypertrophy, or loss of electrical activity in the left ventricle.

The mean electrical axis of the heart can be determined from the ECG. The process involves determining what single net dipole orientation will produce the R-wave amplitudes recorded on any 2 leads. For example, if the R waves on leads II and III are both positive (upright) and of equal magnitude, the mean electrical axis must be +90 degrees. As should be obvious, in this case, the amplitude of the R wave on lead I will be zero.[1] Alternatively, one can scan the electrocardiographic records for the lead tracing with the largest R waves and then deduce that the mean electrical axis must be nearly parallel to that lead. In Figure 4–5, for

---

[1] An accurate, albeit tedious, way to determine the mean electrical axis is to follow these steps: (1) determine the algebraic sum of the R- and S-wave amplitudes on each of the 2 leads; (2) plot these magnitudes as components on the appropriate sides of Einthoven's equilateral triangle according to the standardized polarity conventions; (3) project perpendicular lines from the heads and tails of these components into the interior of the triangle to find the position of the head and tail of the cardiac dipole, which produced the R waves; and (4) measure the angular orientation of this dipole.

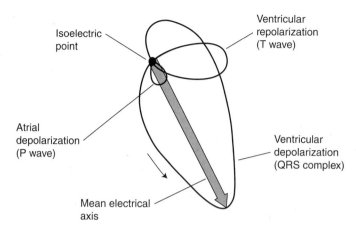

Figure 4-7. Typical vectorcardiogram.

example, the largest R wave occurs on lead II. Lead II has an orientation of +60 degrees, which is very close to the actual mean electrical axis in this example.

Another analysis technique called *vectorcardiography* is based on continuously following the magnitude and orientation of the heart's dipole throughout the cardiac cycle. A typical vectorcardiogram is illustrated in Figure 4–7 and is a graphical record of the dipole amplitude in the x and y directions throughout a single cardiac cycle. If one imagines the heart's electrical dipole as a vector with its tail always positioned at the center of the Einthoven triangle, then the vectorcardiogram can be thought of as a complete record of all the various positions that the head of the dipole assumes during the course of 1 cardiac cycle. A vectorcardiogram starts from an isoelectric diastolic point and traces 3 loops during each cardiac cycle. The first small loop is caused by atrial depolarization, the second large loop is caused by ventricular depolarization, and the final intermediate-sized loop is caused by ventricular repolarization. The mean electrical axis of the ventricle is immediately apparent in a vectorcardiographic record as the orientation of the largest deviation from the isoelectric point during ventricular depolarization. Analogous "mean axes" can similarly be defined for the P wave and T wave but are not commonly used.

The Standard 12-Lead Electrocardiogram

The standard clinical ECG involves voltage measurements recorded from 12 different leads. Three of these are the bipolar limb leads I, II, and III, which have already been discussed. The other 9 leads are unipolar leads. Three of these leads are generated by using the limb electrodes. Two of the electrodes are electrically connected to form an *indifferent electrode*, whereas the third limb electrode is made the positive pole of the pair. Recordings made from these electrodes are called *augmented unipolar limb leads.* The voltage record obtained between the electrode on the right arm and the indifferent electrode is called a lead aVR ECG. Similarly, lead aVL is recorded from the electrode on the left arm, and lead aVF is recorded from the electrode on the left leg.

The standard limb leads (I, II, and III) and the augmented unipolar limb leads (aVR, aVL, and aVF) record the electrical activity of the heart as it appears from 6 different "perspectives," all in the frontal plane. As shown in Figure 4–8A, the axes for leads I, II, and III are those of the sides of the Einthoven triangle, whereas those for aVR, aVL, and aVF are specified by lines drawn from the center of the Einthoven triangle to each of its vertices. As indicated in Figure 4–8B, these 6 limb leads can be thought of as a hexaxial reference system for observing the cardiac vectors in the frontal plane.

The other 6 leads of the standard 12-lead ECG are also unipolar leads that "look" at the electrical vector projections in the transverse plane. These potentials are obtained by placing an additional (*exploring*) electrode in 6 specified positions on the chest wall, as shown in Figure 4–8C. The indifferent electrode in this case is formed by electrically connecting the limb electrodes. These leads are identified

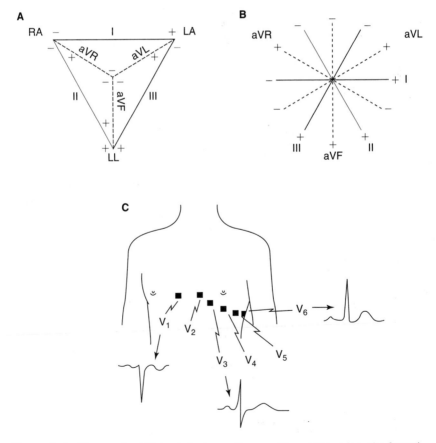

Figure 4–8. The standard 12-lead electrocardiogram. (**A** and **B**) Leads in the frontal plane. (**C**) Electrode positions for precordial leads in the transverse plane.

as *precordial* or *chest* leads and are designated as V1 through V6. As shown in this figure, when the positive electrode is placed in position 1 and the wave of ventricular excitation sweeps away from it, the resultant deflection will be downward. When the electrode is in position 6 and the wave of ventricular excitation sweeps toward it, the deflection will be upward.

In summary, the ECG is a powerful tool for evaluating cardiac excitation characteristics. It must be recognized, however, that the ECG does not provide direct evidence of mechanical pumping effectiveness. For example, a leaky valve will have no direct electrocardiographic consequences but may adversely influence pumping ability of the heart.

PERSPECTIVES

With the advent of computerized imaging techniques and coronary angiography, assessment of cardiac function has come a long way from the old days of relying on ECG analysis, listening to heart sounds, and evaluation of blood pressure and vascular pulse characteristics. However, these old techniques are still useful and the skilled practitioner can obtain much useful information. It is our hope that the medical students of today will continue to develop these basic skills and, although the new techniques are quite seductive, the students will not become completely reliant upon often-expensive technology.

KEY CONCEPTS

A variety of visualization methods are available to assess cardiac mechanical function, the most common of which is echocardiography.

Ejection fraction and end-systolic pressure–volume relationships can be used for assessing cardiac contractility.

Cardiac output can be measured by applying the Fick principle (whole-body oxygen consumption) or estimated from indicator dilution or various visualization methods.

Cardiac index is equal to cardiac output normalized for body size (surface area).

The electrocardiogram is a record of the voltage changes that occur on the surface of the body as a result of the propagation of the action potential through the heart during a cardiac cycle.

There are standardized conventions used for recording electrocardiograms.

 The magnitude and direction of the net dipole formed by the wavefront of the action potential at any instant in time can be deduced from the magnitude and orientation of the electrocardiographic deflections.

 The mean electrical axis describes the orientation of the net dipole at the instant of maximum wavefront propagation during ventricular depolarization and normally falls between 0 and +90 degrees on a polar coordinate system.

 The standard 12-lead electrocardiogram is widely used to evaluate the cardiac electrical activity and consists of a combination of bipolar and unipolar records from limb electrodes and chest electrodes.

 STUDY QUESTIONS

4–1. Given the following information, calculate cardiac output and indicate if this is normal for a resting 70-kg man:

Systemic arterial blood oxygen concentration, $[O_2]_{SA} = 200 \, mL/L$

Pulmonary arterial blood oxygen concentration, $[O_2]_{PA} = 140 \, mL/L$

Total body oxygen consumption, $VO_2 = 600 \, mL/min$

4–2. If left ventricular end-diastolic volume is 150 mL and end-systolic volume is 50 mL, what is the ejection fraction? Is this "normal" for a resting adult?

4–3. A decrease in atrioventricular nodal conduction velocity will

　　a. decrease the heart rate.

　　b. increase the P-wave amplitude.

　　c. increase the PR interval.

　　d. widen the QRS complex.

　　e. increase the ST-segment duration.

4–4. The P wave on lead aVR of the normal electrocardiogram will be

　　a. an upward deflection.

　　b. a downward deflection.

　　c. not detectable.

　　d. highly variable.

4–5. If the R wave is upright and equally large on leads I and aVF, what is the mean electrical axis of the heart? Is it within the normal range? Which lead(s) will have the smallest R-wave amplitude?

4–6. What is the definition of cardiac "ejection fraction"?

    a. Stroke volume expressed as a percent of cardiac output

    b. The ratio of the end-systolic volume to the end-diastolic volume

    c. The ratio of the end-diastolic volume to the end-systolic volume

    d. The ratio of the stroke volume to the end-diastolic volume

    e. The ratio of the time spent in systole to the time spent in diastole

4–7. Electrocardiograms give information about all of the following, except

    a. atrial beating rate.

    b. site of pacemaker origination.

    c. pathway of ventricular activation.

    d. rate of AV nodal conduction.

    e. amplitude of the ventricular action potential.

4–8. If something slows the conduction pathway of the action potential through the ventricular muscle, which of the following alterations would you most likely see on the ECG?

    a. Absence of P waves

    b. Prolongation of the PR interval

    c. Prolongation of the QRS interval

    d. Shortening of the QT interval

    e. Elevation of the ST segment

Cardiac Abnormalities

5

OBJECTIVES

The student, through understanding normal cardiac function, diagnoses and appreciates the consequences of common cardiac abnormalities:

▶ *Detects common cardiac arrhythmias from the electrocardiogram, identifies their physiological bases, and describes their physiological consequences.*

▶ *Lists 4 common cardiac valve abnormalities for the left side of the heart and describes the alterations in intracardiac and arterial pressures, flow patterns, and heart sounds that accompany them.*

▶ *Identifies the consequences of similar valve abnormalities for the right side of the heart.*

Recall that effective and efficient ventricular pumping action depends on proper cardiac function in 5 basic aspects. This chapter focuses on the abnormalities in 3 of these aspects: (1) abnormal cardiac excitation and rhythmicity; (2) valvular stenosis (inadequate valve opening); and (3) valvular insufficiency (incomplete valve closure). Discussion of abnormalities in myocardial force production and cardiac filling is presented in Chapter 11. The material presented here is an introduction to the more common cardiac electrical and cardiac valve dysfunctions, with an emphasis on the primary physiological consequences of these abnormal situations.

ELECTRICAL ABNORMALITIES AND ARRHYTHMIAS

Many cardiac excitation problems can be diagnosed from the information in a single lead of an electrocardiogram (ECG). The lead II ECG traces at the top of Figures 5–1 and 5–2 are identified as normal sinus rhythms based on the following characteristics: (1) the frequency of QRS complexes is approximately 1/s, indicating a normal beating rate; (2) the shape of the QRS complex is normal for lead II and its duration is less than 120 ms, indicating rapid depolarization of the ventricles via normal conduction pathways; (3) each QRS complex is preceded by a P wave of proper configuration, indicating sinoatrial (SA) nodal origin of the excitation; (4) the PR interval is less than 200 ms, indicating proper conduction delay of the impulse propagation through the atrioventricular (AV) node; (5) the QT interval is less than half of the R-to-R interval,

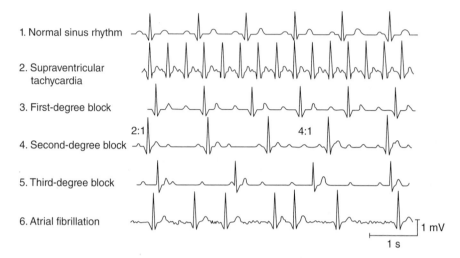

1. Normal sinus rhythm

2. Supraventricular tachycardia

3. First-degree block

4. Second-degree block
2:1
4:1

5. Third-degree block

6. Atrial fibrillation
1 mV
1 s

Figure 5–1. Supraventricular arrhythmias.

indicating normal ventricular repolarization; and (6) there are no extra P waves, indicating that no AV nodal conduction block is present. The subsequent electrocardiographic tracings in Figures 5–1 and 5–2 represent irregularities commonly found in clinical practice. Examination of each of these traces with the above characteristics in mind will aid in the differential diagnosis.

The physiological consequences of abnormal excitation and conduction in the heart depend on whether the electrical abnormality evokes a *tachycardia*, which will limit the time for cardiac filling between beats; evokes

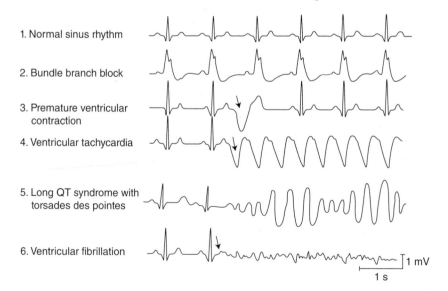

1. Normal sinus rhythm

2. Bundle branch block

3. Premature ventricular contraction

4. Ventricular tachycardia

5. Long QT syndrome with torsades des pointes

6. Ventricular fibrillation
1 mV
1 s

Figure 5–2. Ventricular arrhythmias.

a *bradycardia*, which is inadequate to support sufficient cardiac output; or decreases the coordination of myocyte contraction, which will reduce stroke volume.

Supraventricular Abnormalities

Traces 2 through 6 below the normal trace in Figure 5–1 represent typical supraventricular arrhythmias (i.e., originating in the atria or AV node). *Supraventricular tachycardia* (shown in trace 2 in Figure 5–1 and sometimes called *paroxysmal atrial tachycardia*) occurs when the atria are abnormally excited and drive the ventricles at a very rapid rate. These paroxysms often begin abruptly, last for a few minutes to a few hours, and then, just as abruptly, disappear and the heart rate (HR) reverts to normal. QRS complexes appear normal (albeit frequent) with simple paroxysmal atrial tachycardia because the ventricular conduction pathways operate normally. The P and T waves may be superimposed because of the high HR. Low blood pressure and dizziness may accompany bouts of this arrhythmia because the extremely high HR does not allow sufficient diastolic time for ventricular filling.

There are 2 mechanisms that may account for supraventricular tachycardia. First, an atrial region, often outside the SA node, may become irritable (perhaps because of local interruption in blood flow) and begin to fire rapidly to take over the pacemaker function. Such an abnormal pacemaker region is called an *ectopic focus*. Alternatively, atrial conduction may become altered so that a single wave of excitation does not die out but continually travels around some abnormal atrial conduction loop. In this case, the continual activity in the conduction loop may drive the atria and AV node at a very high frequency. This self-sustaining process is called a *reentry phenomenon* and is illustrated in Figure 5–3. This situation may develop because of abnormal repolarization and altered refractory periods in local areas of the myocardium. *Atrial flutter* is a special form of tachycardia of atrial origin in which a large reentrant pathway drives the atria at very fast rates (250–300 beats/min) and normal refractory periods of AV nodal tissue are overwhelmed. Thus, ventricular rate is often some fixed ratio of the atrial

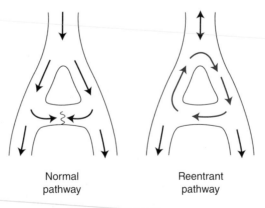

Normal
pathway

Reentrant
pathway

Figure 5–3. Normal and reentrant (circus) cardiac excitation pathways.

rate (2:1, 4:1) with frequencies often 150 to 220 beats/min. The ECG often shows a saw-tooth pattern of merged P waves with intermittent normal QRS complexes.

Conduction blocks occur at the AV node and generally represent impaired conduction through this tissue. In a *first-degree heart block* (trace 3 in Figure 5–1), the only electrical abnormality is unusually slow conduction through the AV node. This condition is detected by an abnormally long PR interval (>0.2 s). Otherwise, the ECG may be completely normal. At normal HRs, the physiological effects of the first-degree block are inconsequential. The danger, however, is that the slow conduction may deteriorate to an actual interruption of conduction.

A *second-degree heart block* (trace 4 in Figure 5–1) is said to exist when some, but not all, atrial impulses are transmitted through the AV node to the ventricle. Impulses are blocked in the AV node if the cells of the region are still in a refractory period from a previous excitation. In this situation, the primary problem is a slower-than-normal conduction through the AV nodal region and thus the second-degree block is aggravated by high atrial rates. In the second-degree block, some, but not all, P waves are accompanied by corresponding QRS complexes and T waves. Atrial rate is often faster than ventricular rate by a certain ratio (e.g., 2:1, 3:1, and 4:1). This condition may not represent a serious clinical problem if the ventricular rate is adequate to meet the pumping needs.

In a *third-degree heart block* (trace 5 in Figure 5–1), no impulses are transmitted through the AV node. In this event, some area in the ventricles—often in the common bundle or bundle branches near the exit of the AV node—assumes the pacemaker role for the ventricular tissue. Atrial rate and ventricular rate are completely independent, and P waves and QRS complexes are totally dissociated in the ECG. Ventricular rate is very likely to be slower than normal (bradycardia) and is often slow enough to impair cardiac output.

Atrial fibrillation (trace 6 in Figure 5–1) is characterized by a complete loss of the normally close synchrony of the excitation and resting phases between individual atrial cells. Cells in different areas of the atria depolarize, repolarize, and are excited again randomly. Consequently, no P waves appear in the ECG, although there may be rapid, irregular, small waves apparent throughout the diastole. The ventricular rate is often very irregular in atrial fibrillation because impulses enter the AV node from the atria at unpredictable times. Fibrillation is a self-sustaining process. The mechanisms behind it are not well understood, but impulses are thought to progress repeatedly around irregular conduction pathways (sometimes called circus pathways, which imply a reentry phenomenon as described earlier and in Figure 5–3). However, because atrial contraction often plays a minor role in ventricular filling in resting individuals, atrial fibrillation may be tolerated by some patients if ventricular rate is sufficient to maintain the cardiac output.[1]

---

[1] A real danger with atrial fibrillation lies in the tendency for blood to form clots in the atria in the absence of the normal vigorous coordinated atrial contraction. These clots can fragment and move out of the heart to lodge in small arteries throughout the systemic circulation. These emboli can have devastating effects on critical organ function. Consequently, anticoagulant therapy is strongly recommended for patients with atrial fibrillation.

Atrial flutter also represents a breakdown of the normal atrial conduction pathways but is less chaotic with much of the atrial tissue being re-excited in sync with a single rapidly reverberating circus pathway. The ECG often will look like the second-degree AV nodal block with a very rapid atrial rate (4:1 or more).

Ventricular Abnormalities

Traces 2 through 6 below the normal trace in Figure 5–2 show typical ventricular electrical abnormalities. Conduction blocks called *bundle branch blocks* or *hemiblocks* (trace 2 in Figure 5–2) can occur in either of the branches of the Purkinje system of the intraventricular septum, often as a result of a myocardial infarction. Ventricular depolarization is less synchronous than normal in the half of the heart with the nonfunctional Purkinje system. This results in a widening of the QRS complex (>0.12 s) because a longer time is required for ventricular depolarization to be completed. The direct physiological effects of bundle branch blocks are usually inconsequential.

Premature ventricular contractions (PVCs) (trace 3 in Figure 5–2) are caused by action potentials initiated by and propagated away from an ectopic focus in the ventricle. As a result, the ventricle depolarizes and contracts before it normally would. A PVC is often followed by a missed beat (called a *compensatory pause*) because the ventricular cells are still refractory when the next normal impulse emerges from the SA node. The highly abnormal ventricular depolarization pattern of a PVC produces the large-amplitude, long-duration deflections on the ECG. The shapes of the electrocardiographic records of these extra beats are highly variable and depend on the ectopic site of their origin and the depolarization pathways involved. The volume of blood ejected by the premature beat itself is smaller than normal, whereas the stroke volume of the beat following the compensatory pause is larger than normal. This is partly due to the differences in filling times and partly to an inherent phenomenon of the cardiac muscle called *postextrasystolic potentiation*. Single PVCs occur occasionally in most individuals and, although sometimes alarming to the individual experiencing them, are not dangerous. Frequent occurrence of PVCs, however, may be a signal of possible myocardial damage or perfusion problems.

Ventricular tachycardia (trace 4 in Figure 5–2) occurs when the ventricles are driven at high rates, usually by impulses originating from a ventricular ectopic focus. Ventricular tachycardia is a very serious condition. Not only is diastolic filling time limited by the rapid rate, but also the abnormal excitation pathways make ventricular contraction less synchronous and therefore less effective than normal. In addition, ventricular tachycardia often precedes ventricular fibrillation.

Prolonged QT intervals (the left side of trace 5 in Figure 5–2) are a result of delayed ventricular myocyte repolarization, which may be due to inappropriate opening of sodium channels or prolonged closure of potassium channels during the action potential plateau phase. Although the normal QT interval varies with HR, it is normally less than 40% of the cardiac cycle length (except at very high HRs). Long QT syndrome is identified when the QT interval is greater than 50%

of the cycle duration. It may be genetic in origin (mutations influencing various ion channels involved with cardiac excitability), may be acquired from several electrolyte disturbances (low blood levels of Ca^{2+}, Mg^{2+}, or K^+), or may be induced by several pharmacological agents (including some antiarrhythmic drugs). The prolongation of the myocyte refractory period, which accompanies the long QT syndrome, extends the vulnerable period during which extra stimuli can evoke tachycardia or fibrillation. Patients with long QT syndrome are predisposed to a particularly dangerous type of ventricular tachycardia called *torsades de pointes* ("twisting of points," as shown on the right side of trace 5 in Figure 5–2). This differs from the ordinary ventricular tachycardia in that the ventricular electrical complexes cyclically vary in amplitude around the baseline and can deteriorate rapidly into ventricular fibrillation.

In *ventricular fibrillation* (trace 6 in Figure 5–2), various areas of the ventricle are excited and contract asynchronously. The mechanisms are similar to those in atrial fibrillation. The ventricle is especially susceptible to fibrillation whenever a premature excitation occurs at the end of the T wave of the previous excitation, that is, when most ventricular cells are in the "hyperexcitable" or "vulnerable" period of their electrical cycle. In addition, because some cells are repolarized and some are still refractory, circus pathways can be triggered easily at this time. Because no pumping action occurs with ventricular fibrillation, the situation is fatal unless quickly corrected by *cardiac conversion*. During conversion, the artificial application of large currents to the entire heart (via paddle electrodes applied across the chest) may be effective in depolarizing all heart cells simultaneously, thus allowing a normal excitation pathway to be reestablished.

Myocardial ischemia can also cause changes in the basic ECG pattern. In addition to potential alterations in cardiac excitation and conduction described above, chronic inadequate coronary flow to the subendocardium may cause T wave inversion and ST-segment depression. A more severe interruption of coronary flow causing a transmural infarct will usually result in ST-segment elevation.

CARDIAC VALVE ABNORMALITIES

Pumping action of the heart is impaired when the valves do not function properly. Abnormal heart sounds, which often accompany cardiac valvular defects, are called *murmurs*. These sounds are caused by abnormal pressure gradients and turbulent blood flow patterns that occur during the cardiac cycle. Several techniques, ranging from simple auscultation (listening to the heart sounds) to echocardiography or cardiac catheterization, are used to obtain information about the nature and extent of these valvular malfunctions.

In general, when a valve does not open fully (i.e., is stenotic), the chamber upstream of the valve must develop more pressure during its systolic phase to achieve a given flow through the valve. This increase in "pressure" work will induce hypertrophy of cardiac muscle cells and thickening of the walls of that chamber. When a valve does not close completely (i.e., is insufficient), the regurgitant blood flow represents an additional volume that must be ejected to get sufficient forward flow out of the ventricle into the tissues. This increase in "volume" work often leads to chamber dilation but not to an increase in wall thickness.[2]

A second generality about valve abnormalities is that whenever there is an elevation in the atrial pressure because of AV valve stenosis or regurgitation, it results in higher pressures in the upstream capillary beds. If capillary hydrostatic pressures are elevated, tissue edema will ensue with consequences on the function of those upstream organs.

A brief overview of 4 of the common valve defects influencing left ventricular function is given in Figure 5–4. Note that similar stenotic and regurgitant abnormalities can occur in right ventricular valves with similar consequences on right ventricular function.

Aortic Stenosis

 Some characteristics of aortic stenosis are shown in Figure 5–4A. Normally, the aortic valve opens wide and offers a pathway of very low resistance through which blood leaves the left ventricle. If this opening is narrowed (stenotic), resistance to flow through the valve increases. A significant pressure difference between the left ventricle and the aorta may be required to eject blood through a stenotic aortic valve. As shown in Figure 5–4A, intraventricular pressures may rise to very high levels during systole, while aortic pressure rises more slowly than normal to a systolic value that is subnormal. Pulse pressure is usually low with aortic stenosis. High intraventricular pressure development is a strong stimulus for cardiac muscle cell hypertrophy, and an increase in left ventricular muscle mass invariably accompanies aortic stenosis. This tends to produce a leftward deviation of the electrical axis. (The mean electrical axis will fall in the upper right-hand quadrant as shown in Figure 4–6.) Blood being ejected through the narrowed orifice may reach very high velocities, and turbulent flow may occur as blood enters the aorta. This abnormal turbulent flow can be heard as a *systolic* (or ejection) *murmur* with a properly placed stethoscope. The primary physiological consequence of aortic stenosis is a high ventricular afterload that is caused by restriction of the outflow tract. This imposes an increased pressure workload on the left ventricle.

Mitral Stenosis

 Some characteristics of mitral stenosis are shown in Figure 5–4B. A pressure difference of more than a few millimeters of mercury across the mitral valve during diastole is distinctly abnormal and indicates the valve is stenotic. The high resistance mandates an elevated pressure difference to achieve normal flow across the valve ($\dot{Q} = \Delta P / R$). Consequently, as shown in Figure 5–4B, left atrial pressure is elevated with mitral stenosis. The high left atrial workload

---

[2] A useful analogy is to compare the hypertrophied skeletal muscles of the weightlifter (doing isometric or pressure work) to the nonhypertrophied but well-toned skeletal muscles of the long-distance runner (doing isotonic or shortening work).

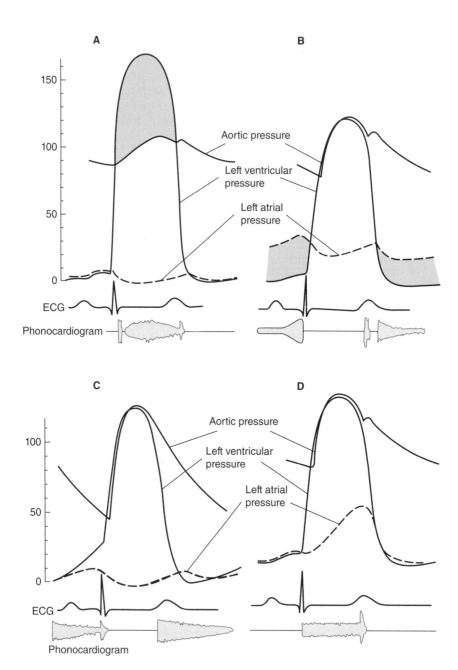

Figure 5–4. Characteristics of left ventricular valve abnormalities: (**A**) aortic stenosis; (**B**) mitral stenosis; (**C**) aortic regurgitation (insufficiency); and (**D**) mitral insufficiency.

may induce hypertrophy of the left atrial muscle. Elevated left atrial pressure is reflected into the pulmonary bed and, if high enough, causes pulmonary congestion and "shortness of breath." A *diastolic murmur* associated with turbulent flow through the stenotic mitral valve can often be heard. The primary physiological consequences of mitral stenosis are elevations in left atrial pressure and pulmonary capillary pressure. The latter can cause pulmonary edema and interference with normal gas exchange in the lungs (leading to shortness of breath).

Aortic Insufficiency

 Typical characteristics of aortic regurgitation (also known as insufficiency or incompetence) are shown in Figure 5–4C. When the leaflets of the aortic valve do not provide an adequate seal, blood regurgitates from the aorta back into the left ventricle during the diastolic period. Aortic pressure falls faster and further than normal during diastole, which causes a low diastolic pressure and a large pulse pressure. In addition, ventricular end-diastolic volume and pressure are higher than normal because of the extra blood that reenters the chamber through the incompetent aortic valve during diastole. Turbulent flow of the blood reentering the left ventricle during early diastole produces a characteristic diastolic murmur. Often the aortic valve is altered so that it is both stenotic and insufficient. In these instances, both a systolic and a diastolic murmur are present. The primary physiological consequences of aortic insufficiency are reduction in forward flow out to the tissues (if the insufficiency is severe) and increase in the volume workload of the left ventricle.

Mitral Regurgitation

 Typical characteristics of mitral regurgitation (insufficiency, incompetence) are shown in Figure 5–4D. When the mitral valve is insufficient, some blood regurgitates from the left ventricle into the left atrium during systole. A systolic murmur may accompany this abnormal flow pattern. Left atrial pressure is raised to abnormally high levels and left ventricular end-diastolic volume and pressure increase. Mitral valve *prolapse* is the most common form of mitral insufficiency in which the valve leaflets evert into the left atrium during systole. The primary physiological consequences of mitral regurgitation are somewhat similar to aortic insufficiency in that forward flow out of the left ventricle into the aorta may be compromised (if the insufficiency is severe) and there is an increase in the volume workload of the left ventricle. In addition, the elevated left atrial pressure can also lead to pulmonary effects with shortness of breath.

PERSPECTIVES

It might be useful for the student to be reminded that the heart is "simply" a pulsatile pressure-generating pump producing one-way flow through a closed hydraulic system. There are many ways that this pump can fail, and the information in this chapter just touches on the critical role of the excitation process (which sets the "speed" of the pump) and the valves (that assure forward flow). Many of the physiological consequences of abnormalities in these processes (i.e., inadequate output and lowered pressure) are easily predicted from a basic consideration of fluid dynamics.

KEY CONCEPTS

 Cardiac arrhythmias can often be detected and diagnosed from a single electro-cardiographic lead.

 Physiological consequences of abnormal excitation and conduction in the heart depend on whether the electrical abnormality limits the time for adequate cardiac filling or decreases the coordination of myocyte contractions resulting in inade-quate pressure development and ejection.

 Supraventricular arrhythmias are a result of abnormal action potential initiation at the SA node or altered propagation characteristics through the atrial tissue and the AV node.

 Tachycardias may originate either in the atria or in the ventricles and are a result of increased pacemaker automaticity, of spontaneously firing ectopic foci, or of con-tinuous circular pathways setting up a reentrant circuit.

 Abnormal conduction through the AV node results in conduction blocks which may result in bradycardia.

 Abnormal conduction pathways in the Purkinje system or in the ventricular tissue result in significant QRS alterations.

 Ventricular tachycardia and ventricular fibrillation represent severe abnormalities that are incompatible with effective cardiac pumping.

 Failure of cardiac valves to open fully (stenosis) can result in elevated upstream chamber pressure and abnormal pressure gradients, congestion in upstream vas-cular beds, chamber wall hypertrophy, turbulent forward flow across the valve, and murmurs during systole or diastole.

 Failure of cardiac valves to close completely (insufficiency, incompetence, regurgi-tation) can result in large stroke volumes, abnormal pressure pulses, congestion in upstream vascular beds, turbulent backward flow across the valve, and murmurs during systole or diastole.

5–1. You hear a systolic murmur that seems to be coming from the right side of the heart.

    a. Which valve condition(s) might be the cause of this abnormal sound?

    b. A finding of a right electrical axis deviation might support which of your possible diagnoses?

    c. Would you expect your patient to have pulmonary congestion?

5–2. Which of the following arrhythmias might result in a reduced stroke volume?

    a. Paroxysmal atrial tachycardia

    b. Ventricular tachycardia

    c. Atrial fibrillation

    d. Ventricular fibrillation

    e. Third-degree heart block

5–3. Describe the primary pressure abnormalities across the cardiac valve that are associated with

    a. aortic stenosis.

    b. mitral stenosis.

5–4. A patient has an abnormally large pulsation of the jugular vein that occurs at about the same time as S1. What is the most likely diagnosis?

5–5. What alteration in jugular venous pulsations might accompany a third-degree heart block?

5–6. Given the following data, name the abnormal valve, predict the type of murmur that might be detected, and determine whether pulmonary congestion might be present. Calculate the resistance to flow across this valve.

Aortic pressures (systolic/diastolic) = 150/100 mm Hg

Left ventricular pressures (systolic/diastolic) = 150/2 mm Hg

Left atrial pressures (systolic/diastolic) = 50/32 mm Hg

Heart rate = 60 beats/min

Stroke volume = 50 mL/beat

5–7. A 75-year-old male patient is alert with complaints of general fatigue. His heart rate = 90 beats/min and arterial pressure = 180/50 mm Hg. A diastolic murmur is present. There are no ECG abnormalities identified and mean electrical axis = 10 degrees. Cardiac catheterization indicates that LV pressure = 180/20 mm Hg and left atrial pressure = 10/3 mm Hg (as peak systolic/end-diastolic). What abnormality is most consistent with these findings?

5–8. *Evaluation of your patient's electrocardiogram shows that P waves occur at a regular rate of 90/min and QRS complexes occur at a regular rate of 37/min. Which of the following is the most likely diagnosis?*

   a. *Supraventricular tachycardia*

   b. *First-degree heart block*

   c. *Second-degree heart block*

   d. *Third-degree heart block*

   e. *Bundle branch block*

5–9. *An otherwise healthy, vigorous 74-year-old woman comes to your office with recent episodes of intermittent dizziness and weakness associated with a feeling of fluttering and/or pounding in her chest. Her blood pressure is 135/88 mm Hg and her overall pulse rate is about 80 beats/min with an irregularly irregular rhythm (i.e., no discernable pattern). What is the most likely diagnosis? What will you do next?*

The Peripheral Vascular System

6

OBJECTIVES

The student understands the basic principles of cardiovascular transport and its role in maintaining homeostasis:

▶ Identifies the factors that determine transport of substances within the vascular system and those that determine diffusion across the capillary wall.

▶ Describes how capillary wall permeability to a solute is related to the size and lipid solubility of the solute.

▶ Lists the factors that influence transcapillary fluid movement and, given data, predicts the direction of transcapillary fluid movement.

▶ Describes the lymphatic vessel system and its role in preventing fluid accumulation in the interstitial space (i.e., edema).

The student understands the physical factors that regulate blood flow through and blood volume in the various components of the vasculature:

▶ Given data, calculates the vascular resistances of networks of vessels arranged in parallel and in series.

▶ Describes differences in the blood flow velocity in the various vascular segments and how these differences are related to their total cross-sectional area.

▶ Describes laminar and turbulent flow patterns and the origin of flow sounds in the cardiovascular system.

▶ Identifies the approximate percentage of the total blood volume that is contained in the various vascular segments in the systemic circulation.

▶ Defines peripheral venous pool and central venous pool.

▶ Describes the pressure changes that occur as blood flows through a vascular bed and relates them to the vascular resistance of the various vascular segments.

▶ States how the resistance of each consecutive vascular segment contributes to an organ's overall vascular resistance and, given data, calculates the overall resistance.

▶ Defines total peripheral resistance (systemic vascular resistance) and states the relationship between it and the vascular resistance of each systemic organ.

▶ Defines vascular compliance and states how the volume–pressure curves for arteries and veins differ.

▶ Predicts what will happen to venous volume when venous smooth muscle contracts or when venous transmural pressure increases.

▶ Describes the role of arterial compliance in storing energy for blood circulation.
▶ Describes the auscultation technique for determining arterial systolic and diastolic pressures.
▶ Identifies the physical bases of the Korotkoff sounds.
▶ Indicates the relationship between arterial pressure, cardiac output, and total peripheral resistance, and predicts how arterial pressure will be altered when cardiac output and/or total peripheral resistance changes.
▶ Given arterial systolic and diastolic pressures, estimates mean arterial pressure.
▶ Indicates the relationship between pulse pressure, stroke volume, and arterial compliance, and predicts how pulse pressure will be changed by changes in stroke volume or arterial compliance.
▶ Describes how arterial compliance changes with age and how this affects arterial pulse pressure.

Recall from Chapter 1 that the primary job of the cardiovascular system is to maintain "homeostasis" within a body that contains billions of closely spaced individual cells. Homeostasis implies that every cell in the body is continually bathed in a local environment of constant composition that is optimal for cell function. In essence, the peripheral vascular system is a sophisticated irrigation system. Blood flow is continually delivering nutrients to and removing waste products from the local interstitial environment throughout the body every minute, as required.

The heart supplies the pumping power required to create flow through the system. Because of the left ventricle's action, pressure at the inlet (the aorta) of the systemic vascular network is higher than that at its outlets (the vena cavae). Everywhere within the vascular system, blood always flows passively "downhill" from higher pressure to lower pressure according to well-known physical rules. Like water flowing downhill, blood seeks to travel along the path of least resistance. Consequently, the peripheral vascular system changes the resistance of its various pathways to direct blood flow to where it is needed.

Also recall from Chapter 1 that the Fick principle governs how substances are transported by blood flow *between* the capillary bed in one organ to that in another. In this chapter, we consider first how solutes and fluid are transported between the plasma and the interstitial fluid *across* the capillary walls *within* an organ. Next, the basic equation for flow through a single vessel $\dot{Q} = \Delta P/R$ (presented in Chapter 1) is applied to the complex network of branching vessels that exist in the cardiovascular system. Then, the consequences of the elastic (balloon-like) properties of the large-diameter arteries and veins on overall cardiovascular system operation are considered. Finally, the principles behind the routine clinical measurement of arterial blood pressure are presented, along with the conclusions about overall cardiovascular function that can be made from such pressure measurements.

TRANSCAPILLARY TRANSPORT

Transcapillary Solute Diffusion

Capillaries act as efficient exchange sites where most substances cross the capillary walls simply by *passively diffusing* from regions of high concentration to regions of low concentration. There are 4 factors that determine the diffusion rate of a substance between the blood and the interstitial fluid: (1) the concentration difference; (2) the surface area for exchange; (3) the diffusion distance; and (4) the permeability of the capillary wall to the diffusing substance.[1]

Capillary beds allow huge amounts of materials to enter and leave blood because they maximize the area across which exchange can occur while minimizing the distance over which the diffusing substances must travel. Capillaries are extremely fine vessels with a *lumen* (inside) diameter of approximately 5 μm, a wall thickness of approximately 1 μm, and an average length of perhaps 0.5 mm. (For comparison, a human hair is roughly 100 μm in diameter.) Capillaries are distributed in incredible numbers in organs and communicate intimately with all regions of the interstitial space. It is estimated that there are approximately 10^{10} capillaries in the systemic organs with a collective surface area of approximately 100 m^2. That is roughly the area of one player's side of a single tennis court. Recall from Chapter 1 that no cell is more than approximately 10 μm (less than 1/10th the thickness of paper) from a capillary. Diffusion is a tremendously powerful mechanism for material exchange when operating over such a short distance and through such a large area. We are far from being able to duplicate—in an artificial lung or kidney, for example—the favorable geometry for diffusional exchange that exists in our own tissues.

As illustrated in Figure 6–1, the capillary wall itself consists of only a single thickness of endothelial cells joined to form a tube. The ease with which a particular solute crosses the capillary wall is expressed in a parameter called its capillary *permeability*. Permeability takes into account all the factors (diffusion coefficient, diffusion distance, and surface area)—except concentration difference—that affect the rate at which a solute crosses the capillary wall.

Careful experimental studies on how rapidly different substances cross capillary walls indicate that 2 fundamentally distinct pathways exist for transcapillary exchange. Lipid-soluble substances, such as the gases oxygen and carbon dioxide, cross the capillary wall easily. Because lipid endothelial cell plasma membranes are not a significant diffusion barrier for lipid-soluble substances, transcapillary movement of these substances can occur through the *entire* capillary surface area.

The capillary permeability to small polar particles such as sodium and potassium ions is approximately 10,000-fold less than that for oxygen. Nevertheless, the capillary permeability to small ions is several orders of magnitude higher than the

---

[1] These factors are combined in an equation (Fick's first law of diffusion) that describes the rate of diffusion ($\dot{X}_d$) of a substance X across a barrier: $\dot{X}_d = DA(\Delta[X]/\Delta L)$ where D, A, $\Delta[X]$, and ΔL represent the diffusion coefficient, surface area, concentration difference, and diffusion distance, respectively.

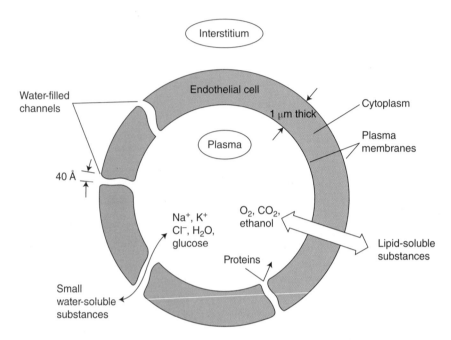

Figure 6–1. Pathways for transcapillary solute diffusion.

permeability that would be expected if the ions were forced to move through the lipid plasma membranes. It is, therefore, postulated that capillaries are somehow perforated at intervals with water-filled channels or *pores*.[2] Calculations from diffusion data indicate that the collective cross-sectional area of the pores relative to the total capillary surface area varies greatly between capillaries in different organs. Brain capillaries appear to be very tight (have few pores), whereas capillaries in the kidney and fluid-producing glands are much more leaky. On an average, however, pores constitute only a very small fraction of total capillary surface area—perhaps 0.01%. This area is, nevertheless, sufficient to allow very rapid equilibration of small water-soluble substances between the plasma and interstitial fluids of most organs. Thus, the concentrations of inorganic ions measured in a plasma sample can be taken to indicate their concentrations throughout the entire extracellular space.

An effective maximum diameter of approximately 40 Å has been assigned to individual pores because substances with molecular diameters larger than this essentially do not cross capillary walls.[3] Thus, albumin and other proteins in the plasma are normally confined to the plasma space.

---

[2] Pores as such are not readily apparent in electron micrographs of capillary endothelial cells. Most believe the pores are either clefts in the junctions between endothelial cells or perhaps specialized channels through the membrane.

[3] The precise mechanism responsible for this size selectivity remains controversial. It may stem from the actual physical dimensions of the "pores," or it may represent the filtering properties of a fiber matrix that either covers or fills the pores.

Endothelial Cells

In addition to forming capillaries, a layer of endothelial cells lines the entire cardiovascular system—including the heart chambers and valves. Because of their ubiquitous and intimate contact with blood, endothelial cells have evolved to serve many functions other than acting as a barrier to transcapillary solute and water exchange. These functions can include

1. enzymatic conversion of some circulating hormones from inactive to active forms,
2. producing substances that lead to blood clot formation and the stemming of bleeding in the event of tissue injury,
3. playing key roles in angiogenesis and remodeling of the vasculature with tissue growth and adaptation, and
4. producing vasoactive substances that can act on the smooth muscle cells of muscular arterioles to influence their diameter.

Transcapillary Fluid Movement

In addition to providing a diffusion pathway for small charged molecules, the water-filled channels that traverse capillary walls permit fluid flow through the capillary wall. A family of specialized transmembrane proteins, aquaporins, form the water-filled channels in many endothelial cells throughout the vasculature. They play important roles in regulating water permeability through this barrier, particularly in vascular beds that are involved in fluid transport such as the kidneys and gastrointestinal tract organs. Net shifts of fluid between the blood and the interstitial compartments are important for a host of physiological functions, including the maintenance of circulating blood volume, intestinal fluid absorption, tissue edema formation, and saliva, sweat, and urine production. Net fluid movement out of capillaries is referred to as *filtration*, and fluid movement into capillaries is called *reabsorption.*

Fluid flows through transcapillary channels in response to pressure differences between the interstitial and intracapillary fluids according to the basic flow equation. However, both *hydrostatic* and *osmotic pressures* influence transcapillary fluid movement. The fact that intravascular hydrostatic pressure provides the driving force for causing blood flow *along* vessels has been discussed previously. For example, the hydrostatic pressure inside capillaries, P_c, is approximately 25 mm Hg and is the driving force that causes blood to return to the right side of the heart from the capillaries of systemic organs. In addition, however, the 25 mm Hg hydrostatic intracapillary pressure tends to cause fluid to flow through the transcapillary pores into the interstitium where the hydrostatic pressure (P_i) is near or below 0 mm Hg. Thus, there is normally a large hydrostatic pressure difference favoring fluid filtration across the capillary wall. Our entire plasma volume would soon be in the interstitium if there were not some counteracting force tending to draw fluid into the capillaries. The balancing force is an osmotic pressure that arises from the fact that plasma has a higher protein concentration than does interstitial fluid.

Recall that water always tends to move from regions of low to regions of high total solute concentration in establishing osmotic equilibrium. Also, recall that osmotic forces are quantitatively expressed in terms of osmotic pressure. The osmotic pressure of a given solution is defined as the hydrostatic pressure necessary to prevent osmotic water movement into the test solution when it is exposed to pure water across a membrane permeable only to water. The total osmotic pressure of a solution is proportional to the total concentration of individual solute *particles* in the solution.[4] Plasma, for example, has a total osmotic pressure of approximately 5000 mm Hg—nearly all of which is attributable to dissolved mineral salts such as NaCl and KCl. As discussed, the capillary permeability to small ions is very high. Their concentrations in plasma and interstitial fluid are very nearly equal and, consequently, they do not affect transcapillary fluid movement.

There is, however, a small but important difference in the osmotic pressures of plasma and interstitial fluid that is due to the presence of albumin and other large proteins in the plasma, which are normally absent from the interstitial fluid. A special term, *oncotic pressure* (or *colloid osmotic pressure*), is used to denote the portion of a solution's total osmotic pressure that is due to particles that do not move freely across capillaries. Because of the plasma proteins, the oncotic pressure of plasma (π_c) is approximately 25 mm Hg. Because of the absence of proteins, the oncotic pressure of the interstitial fluid (π_i) is near 0 mm Hg. Thus, there is normally a large osmotic force for fluid reabsorption into capillaries that counteracts the tendency for intracapillary hydrostatic pressure to drive fluid out of capillaries. The forces that influence transcapillary fluid movement are summarized on the left side of Figure 6–2.[5]

The relationship among the factors that influence transcapillary fluid movement, known as the *Starling hypothesis*,[6] can be expressed by the equation:

$$\text{Net filtration rate} = K[(P_c - P_i)] - (\pi_c - \pi_i)]$$

where P_c = the hydrostatic pressure of intracapillary fluid
π_c = the oncotic pressure of intracapillary fluid
P_i and π_i = the same quantities for interstitial fluid
K = a constant expressing how readily fluid can move across capillaries (essentially the reciprocal of the resistance to fluid flow through the capillary wall).

Fluid balance within a tissue (the absence of net transcapillary water movement) occurs when the bracketed term in this equation is zero. This equilibrium

---

[4] The word "particles" in this sentence is very important to notice. For example, the "normal saline" solution used in medical practice is 150 mM NaCl. However, normal saline actually contains 300 mOsm/L of dissolved particles because NaCl completely dissociates into Na^+ and Cl^- ions in water.

[5] The preceding is a simplified description of the effect of plasma proteins on transcapillary fluid movement. A more thorough analysis would include some additional factors (called Gibbs–Donnan effects) caused by the fact that proteins in solution carry multiple electrical charges. These nuances do not change the basic fact that plasma proteins create an osmotic force favoring fluid reabsorption across capillary walls.

[6] After the British physiologist Ernest Starling (1866–1927).

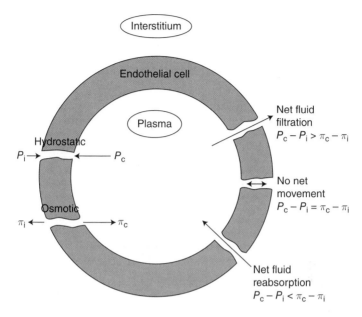

Figure 6–2. Factors influencing transcapillary fluid movement.

may be upset by alterations in any of the 4 pressure terms. The pressure imbalances that cause capillary filtration and reabsorption are indicated on the right side of Figure 6–2.

In most tissues, rapid net filtration of fluid is abnormal and causes tissue swelling as a result of excess fluid in the interstitial space (edema). For example, a substance called *histamine* is often released in damaged tissue. One of its actions is to increase capillary permeability to the extent that proteins leak into the interstitium. Net filtration and edema accompany histamine release, in part, because the oncotic pressure difference $(\pi_c - \pi_i)$ is reduced.

Transcapillary fluid filtration is not always detrimental. For example, fluid-producing organs such as salivary glands and kidneys utilize high intracapillary hydrostatic pressure to produce continual net filtration. Moreover, in certain abnormal situations, such as severe loss of blood volume through hemorrhage, the net fluid reabsorption accompanying diminished intracapillary hydrostatic pressure helps restore the volume of circulating fluid.

The Lymphatic System

Despite the extremely low capillary permeability to proteins, these molecules and other large particles, such as long-chain fatty acids and bacteria, do slowly find their way into the interstitial space. If such particles are allowed to accumulate in the interstitial space, filtration forces will ultimately exceed reabsorption forces and edema would result. The lymphatic vessel network represents a flow pathway that normally operates to guard against such edema. It does so in 2 synergistic ways. First, it is a pathway for returning excess interstitial fluid to the plasma space. Second, it automatically removes colloid particles from the interstitium. The latter effect lowers interstitial colloid osmotic pressure and thus reduces the tendency for fluid filtration from blood plasma to the interstitium.

The lymphatic system begins in the tissues with blind-ended lymphatic capillaries that are roughly equivalent in size to, but much less numerous than, regular capillaries. These capillaries are very porous and easily collect large particles accompanied by interstitial fluid. This fluid, called *lymph*, moves through the converging lymphatic vessels, is filtered through lymph nodes where bacteria and particulate matter are removed, and ultimately reenters the circulatory system near the point where the peripheral venous blood enters the right heart.

Flow of lymph from the tissues toward the entry point into the circulatory system is promoted by 2 factors: (1) increases in tissue interstitial pressure (due to fluid accumulation or due to movement of surrounding tissue) and (2) contractions of the lymphatic vessels themselves. Valves located in these vessels also prevent backward flow.

Roughly 2.5 L of lymphatic fluid enters the cardiovascular system each day. In the steady state, this indicates a total body *net* transcapillary fluid filtration rate of 2.5 L/day. When compared with the total amount of blood that circulates each day (approximately 7000 L), this may seem like an insignificant amount of net capillary fluid leakage. However, lymphatic blockage is a very serious problem and is accompanied by severe tissue swelling. Thus, the lymphatics play a critical role in keeping the interstitial protein concentration low and in removing excess capillary filtrate from the tissues.

RESISTANCE AND FLOW IN NETWORKS OF VESSELS

In Chapter 1, it was asserted that the basic flow equation ($\dot{Q} = \Delta P / R$) may be applied to networks of tubes and to individual tubes. The reason is that any network of resistances, however complex, can always be reduced to a single "equivalent" resistor that relates the total flow through the network to the pressure difference across the network. Of course, one way of finding the overall resistance of a network is to perform an experiment to see how much flow goes through it for a given pressure difference between its inlet and outlet. Another approach to finding the overall resistance of a network is to calculate it from knowledge of the resistances of the individual elements in the network and how they are connected. When one looks at the overall design of the body's vascular system as illustrated in Figure 1–8, one sees 2 patterns: (1) the arterial, arteriolar, capillary, and venous segments are connected in *series* (one after the other); and (2) within each segment, there are many vessels arranged in *parallel* (beside each other). So, to even begin comprehending what happens within such a complex network, one must first understand the basic physics involved in series and parallel combinations of resistance elements.

Vessels in Series

When vessels with individual resistances R_1, R_2, ..., R_n are connected in series, the overall resistance of the network is the sum of the individual resistances, as indicated by the following formula:

$$R_s = R_1 + R_2 + \cdots + R_n$$

Figure 6–3A shows an example of 3 vessels connected *in series* between some region where the pressure is P_i and another region with a lower pressure P_o, so that the total pressure difference across the network, ΔP, is equal to $P_i - P_o$. By the series resistance equation, the total resistance across this network (R_s) is equal to $R_1 + R_2 + R_3$. By the basic flow equation, the flow through the network $(\dot{Q})$ is equal to $\Delta P/R_s$. It should be intuitively obvious that $\dot{Q}$ is also the flow (volume/time) through each of the elements in the series, as indicated in Figure 6–3B.

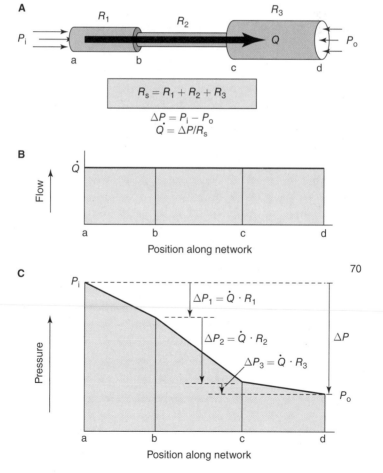

Figure 6–3. Series resistance network.

(Fluid particles may move with different velocities (distance/time) in different elements of a series network, but the volume that passes through each element in a minute must be identical.)

As shown in Figure 6–3C, a portion of the total pressure drop across the network occurs within each element of the series. The pressure drop across any element in the series can be calculated by applying the basic flow equation to *that* element, for example, $\Delta P_1 = \dot{Q}\ R_1$. Note that the largest portion of the overall pressure drop will occur across the element in the series with the largest resistance to flow (R_2 in Figure 6–3).

One implication of the series resistance equation is that elements with the highest relative resistance to flow contribute more to the network's overall resistance than do elements with relatively low resistance. Therefore, high-resistance elements are inherently in an advantageous position to be able to control the overall resistance of the network and, therefore, the flow through it. As we shall see shortly, the arteriolar network normally presents the largest portion of the overall resistance to blood flow through organs. Thus, it is not surprising that changes in arteriolar diameter are the primary mechanism that the body uses to regulate organ blood flow.

Vessels in Parallel

As indicated in Figure 6–4, when several tubes with individual resistances R_1, R_2, ..., R_n are brought together to form a *parallel* network of vessels, one can calculate a single overall resistance for the parallel network R_p according to the following formula:

$$\frac{1}{R_p} = \frac{1}{R_1} + \frac{1}{R_2} + \cdots + \frac{1}{R_n}$$

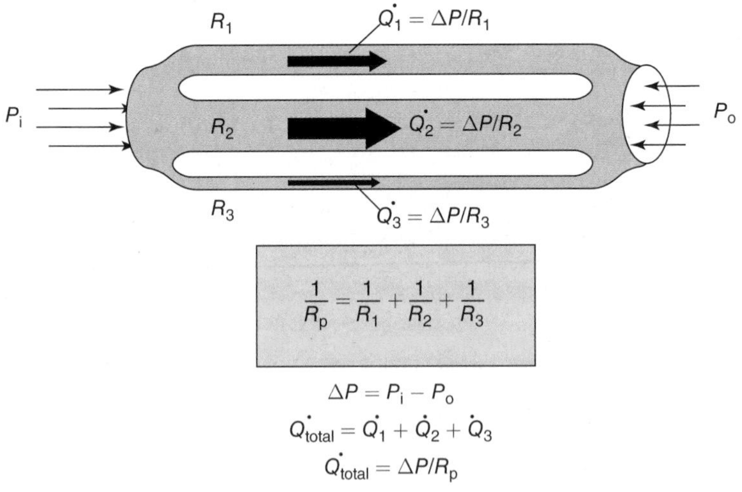

$$\dot{Q}_1 = \Delta P/R_1$$
$$\dot{Q}_2 = \Delta P/R_2$$
$$\dot{Q}_3 = \Delta P/R_3$$

$$\frac{1}{R_p} = \frac{1}{R_1} + \frac{1}{R_2} + \frac{1}{R_3}$$

$$\Delta P = P_i - P_o$$
$$\dot{Q}_{total} = \dot{Q}_1 + \dot{Q}_2 + \dot{Q}_3$$
$$\dot{Q}_{total} = \Delta P/R_p$$

Figure 6–4. Parallel resistance network.

The total flow through a parallel network is determined by $\Delta P/R_p$. As the preceding equation implies, the overall effective resistance of any parallel network will always be less than that of any of the elements in the network. (In the special case where the individual elements that form the network have identical resistances R_x, the overall resistance of the network is equal to the resistance of an individual element divided by the number (n) of parallel elements in the network: $R_p = R_x/n$.) In general, the more parallel elements that occur in the network, the lower the overall resistance of the network. Thus, for example, a capillary bed that consists of many individual capillary vessels in parallel can have a very low overall resistance to flow even though the resistance of a single capillary is relatively high.

The series and parallel resistance equations may be used alternately to analyze resistance networks of great complexity. For example, any or all the series resistances shown in Figure 6–3 could represent the calculated overall resistance of many vessels arranged in parallel.

NORMAL CONDITIONS IN THE PERIPHERAL VASCULATURE

From uncountable anatomical and physiological studies, a clear picture has developed about what conditions normally exist within the peripheral vasculature. The major points are illustrated in traces of Figure 6–5. Each is discussed separately below.

Peripheral Blood Flow Velocities

The top trace in Figure 6–5 shows the differences in blood flow velocity (distance/time) that normally exist within various segments of the peripheral vasculature. But how can these differences exist when the flow (volume/time) through all the consecutive segments must be equal? (Recall that when cardiac output is 5 L/min, 5 L/min must also be passing through the aorta, arterioles, capillaries, and veins.) The answer is that the total cross-sectional area through which the cardiac output is flowing varies greatly between different segments of the peripheral vasculature (see Figure 1–8). Therefore, for the same through-flow, blood must travel with greater velocity through regions with smaller cross-sectional area.

Blood normally flows through all vessels in the cardiovascular system in an orderly streamlined manner called *laminar flow*. With laminar flow, there is a parabolic velocity profile across the tube, as shown on the left side of Figure 6–6. Velocity is fastest along the central axis of the tube and falls to zero at the wall. The concentric layers of fluid with different velocities slip smoothly over one another. Little mixing occurs between fluid layers so that individual particles move in straight streamlines parallel to the axis of the flow. Laminar flow is very efficient because little energy is wasted on anything but producing forward fluid motion.

Because blood is a viscous fluid, its movement through a vessel exerts a *shear stress* on the walls of the vessel. This is a force that wants to drag the inside surface (the endothelial cell layer) of the vessel along with the flow. With laminar flow, the shear stress on the wall of a vessel is proportional to the rate of flow through it.

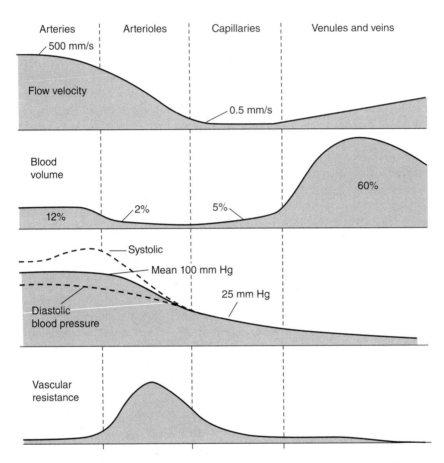

Figure 6–5. Flow velocities, blood volumes, blood pressures, and vascular resistances in the peripheral vasculature from aorta to right atrium.

The endothelial cells that line a vessel can sense (and respond to) changes in the rate of blood flow through the vessel by detecting changes in the shear stress on them. Shear stress may also be an important factor in certain pathological situations. For example, atherosclerotic plaques tend to form preferentially near branches of large arteries where, for complex hemodynamic reasons beyond the scope of this text, high shear stresses exist.

When blood is forced to move with too high a velocity through a narrow opening, the normal laminar flow pattern may break down into the *turbulent flow* pattern shown in the center of Figure 6–6. With turbulent flow, there is much internal mixing and friction. When the flow within a vessel is turbulent, the vessel's resistance to flow is significantly higher than that predicted from the Poiseuille equation given in Chapter 1. Turbulent flow also generates sound, which can be heard with a stethoscope. Cardiac murmurs, for example, are manifestations of turbulent flow patterns generated by cardiac valves that do not

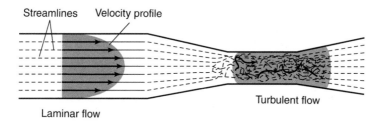

Figure 6–6. Laminar and turbulent flow patterns.

open fully when they are supposed to be open or leak backward when they are supposed to be closed. Detection of sounds from peripheral arteries (*bruits*) is also abnormal. They represent significant pathological reduction of a large vessel's cross-sectional area. Commonly, this is due to an atherosclerotic plaque encroaching on the vessel's lumen. As shown in Figure 6–5, the flow velocities in arterioles, capillaries, and veins are relatively low. Turbulent flow does not occur normally in these vessels. Thus, the presence of a bruit *always* indicates pathology in a large artery.

Peripheral Blood Volumes

The second trace in Figure 6–5 shows the approximate percentage of the total circulating blood volume that is contained in the different vascular regions of the systemic organs at any instant of time. (Approximately 20% of the total volume is contained in the pulmonary system and the heart chambers and is not accounted for in this figure.)

 Note that most of the circulating blood is contained within the veins of the systemic organs. This diffuse but large blood reservoir is often referred to as the *peripheral venous pool*. A second but smaller reservoir of venous blood (not explicitly indicated in Figure 6–5) is called the *central venous pool* and is contained in the great veins of the thorax and the right atrium. When peripheral veins constrict, blood is displaced from the peripheral venous pool and enters the central pool. An increase in the central venous volume, and thus central venous pressure, enhances cardiac filling. That augments stroke volume according to the Frank–Starling law of the heart. The important message is that peripheral veins can act to influence cardiac output. This is an extremely important mechanism of cardiovascular regulation and will be discussed in much greater detail in Chapter 8.

Peripheral Blood Pressures

Blood pressure decreases in the consecutive vascular segments with the pattern shown in the third trace in Figure 6–5. Recall from Figure 3–1 that aortic pressure fluctuates between a systolic value and a diastolic value with each heartbeat, and the same is true throughout the arterial system. (For complex hemodynamic reasons, the difference between systolic and diastolic pressures increases with distance from the heart in the large arteries.[7]) The average pressure in the arch of the aorta, however, is approximately 100 mm Hg, and this *mean arterial pressure* falls by only a small amount within the arterial system.

A large pressure drop occurs in the arterioles, where the pulsatile nature of the pressure also nearly disappears. The average capillary pressure is approximately 25 mm Hg. Pressure continues to decrease in the venules and veins as blood returns to the right heart. The central venous pressure (which is the filling pressure for the right side of the heart) is normally very close to 0 mm Hg.

Peripheral Vascular Resistances

The bottom trace in Figure 6–5 indicates the relative resistance to flow that exists in each of the consecutive vascular regions. Recall from Chapter 1 that resistance, pressure difference, and flow are related by the basic flow equation $\dot{Q} = \Delta P / R$. Because the flow $(\dot{Q})$ must be the same through each of the consecutive regions indicated in Figure 6–5, the pressure drop that occurs across each of these regions is a direct reflection of the resistance to flow within that region (see Figure 6–3). Thus, the large pressure drop occurring as blood moves through arterioles indicates that arterioles present a large resistance to flow. The mean pressure drops very little in arteries because they have very little resistance to flow. Similarly, the modest pressure drop that exists across capillaries reflects the fact that the capillary bed has a modest resistance to flow when compared with that of the arteriolar bed. (Recall from Figure 6–4 that the capillary bed can have a low resistance to flow because it is a parallel network of a very large number of individual capillaries.) Although the converging nature of vessels on the venous side of the circulation decreases the collective total cross-sectional area for blood flow, the overall venous resistance is very low. This is because of the large number and large individual diameters of the major veins and the very compliant nature of the venous vessel walls (as will be discussed in a subsequent section). These conditions greatly reduce the energy cost of getting blood back to the heart.

Blood flow through many individual organs can vary over a 10-fold or greater range. Because mean arterial pressure is a relatively stable cardiovascular variable, large changes in an organ's blood flow are achieved by changes in its overall vascular resistance to blood flow. The consecutive vascular segments are arranged in series within an organ, and the overall vascular resistance of the organ must equal the sum of the resistances of its consecutive vascular segments:

$$R_{organ} = R_{arteries} + R_{arterioles} + R_{capillaries} + R_{venules} + R_{veins}$$

---

[7] A rigorous analysis of the dynamics of pulsatile fluid flow in tapered, branching, elastic tubes is required to explain such behavior. Pressure does not increase simultaneously throughout the arterial system with the onset of cardiac ejection. Rather, the pressure increase begins at the root of the aorta and travels outward from there. When this rapidly moving pressure wave encounters obstacles such as vessel bifurcations, reflected waves are generated, which travel back toward the heart. These reflected waves can summate with and reinforce the oncoming wave in a manner somewhat analogous to the progressive cresting of surface waves as they impinge on a beach.

Because arterioles have such a large vascular resistance in comparison to the other vascular segments, the overall vascular resistance of any organ is determined to a very large extent by the resistance of its arterioles. Arteriolar resistance is, of course, strongly influenced by arteriolar diameter. Thus, the blood flow through an organ is primarily regulated by adjustments in the internal diameter of arterioles caused by contraction or relaxation of their muscular arteriolar walls.

When the arterioles of an organ change diameter, not only does the flow to the organ change but the way the pressures drop within the organ is also modified. The effects of arteriolar dilation and constriction on the pressure profile within a vascular bed are illustrated in Figure 6–7. Arteriolar constriction causes a greater pressure drop across the arterioles, and this tends to increase the arterial pressure while it decreases the pressure in capillaries and veins. (The arterioles function somewhat like a dam; closing a dam's gates decreases the flow while increasing the level of the reservoir behind it and decreasing the level of its outflow stream.) Conversely, increased organ blood flow caused by arteriolar dilation is accompanied by decreased arterial pressure and increased capillary pressure. Because of the changes in capillary hydrostatic pressure, arteriolar constriction tends to cause transcapillary fluid reabsorption, whereas arteriolar dilation tends to promote transcapillary fluid filtration.

Total Peripheral Resistance

The overall resistance to flow through the entire systemic circulation is called the *total peripheral resistance (TPR)*. Because the systemic organs are generally

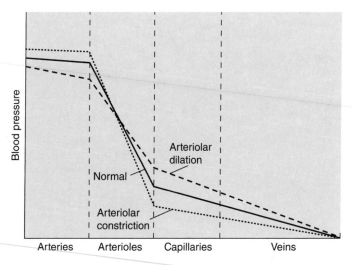

Figure 6–7. Effect of changes in arteriolar resistance on vascular pressures.

arranged in parallel (Figure 1–2), the vascular resistance of each organ contributes to the TPR according to the following parallel resistance equation:

$$\frac{1}{\text{TPR}} = \frac{1}{R_{\text{organ}_1}} + \frac{1}{R_{\text{organ}_2}} + \cdots + \frac{1}{R_{\text{organ}_n}}$$

As discussed later in this chapter, the TPR is an important determinant of arterial blood pressure.

Elastic Properties of Arteries and Veins

As indicated earlier, arteries and veins contribute only a small portion to the overall resistance to flow through a vascular bed. Therefore, changes in their diameters have no significant effect on the blood flow through systemic organs. The elastic behavior of arteries and veins is, however, very important to overall cardiovascular function because they can act as reservoirs and store substantial amounts of blood. Arteries or veins behave more like balloons with one pressure throughout rather than as resistive pipes with a flow-related pressure difference from end to end. Thus, we often think of an "arterial compartment" and a "venous compartment," each with an internal pressure that is related to the volume of blood within it at any instant and how elastic (stretchy) its walls are.

The elastic nature of a vascular region is characterized by a parameter called *compliance* (C) that describes how much its volume changes (ΔV) in response to a given change in distending pressure (ΔP): $C = \Delta V / \Delta P$. Distending pressure is the difference between the internal and external pressures on the vascular walls.

The volume–pressure curves for the systemic arterial and venous compartments are shown in Figure 6–8. It is immediately apparent from the disparate

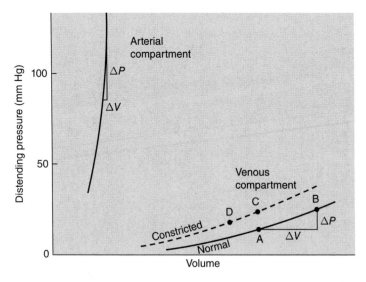

Figure 6–8. Volume–pressure curves of arterial and venous compartments.

slopes of the curves in this figure that the elastic properties of arteries and veins are very different. For the arterial compartment, the $\Delta V/\Delta P$ measured near a normal operating pressure of 100 mm Hg indicates a compliance of approximately 2 mL/mm Hg. By contrast, the venous pool has a compliance of more than 100 mL/mm Hg near its normal operating pressure of 5 to 10 mm Hg.

Because veins are so compliant, even small changes in peripheral venous pressure can cause a significant amount of the circulating blood volume to shift into or out of the peripheral venous pool. Standing upright, for example, increases venous pressure in the lower extremities, distends the compliant veins, and promotes blood accumulation (pooling) in these vessels, as might be represented by a shift from point A to point B in Figure 6–8. Fortunately, this process can be counteracted by active venous constriction. The dashed line in Figure 6–8 shows the venous volume–pressure relationship that exists when veins are constricted by activation of venous smooth muscle. In constricted veins, volume may be normal (point C) or even below normal (point D) despite higher-than-normal venous pressure. Peripheral venous constriction tends to increase peripheral venous pressure and shift blood out of the peripheral venous compartment.

The elasticity of arteries allows them to act as a blood reservoir on a beat-to-beat basis. Arteries play an important role in converting the pulsatile flow output of the heart into a steady flow of blood through the vascular beds of systemic organs. During the early rapid phase of cardiac ejection, the arterial volume increases because blood is entering the aorta more rapidly than it is passing into systemic arterioles. Thus, part of the work the heart does in ejecting blood goes to stretching the elastic walls of arteries. Toward the end of systole and throughout diastole, arterial volume decreases because the flow out of arteries exceeds flow into the aorta. Previously stretched arterial walls recoil to shorter lengths and in the process give up their stored potential energy. This reconverted energy is what does the work of propelling blood through the peripheral vascular beds during diastole. If the arteries were rigid tubes that could not store energy by expanding elastically, arterial pressure would immediately fall to zero with the termination of each cardiac ejection.

MEASUREMENT OF ARTERIAL PRESSURE

Recall that the systemic arterial pressure fluctuates with each heart cycle between a diastolic value (P_D) and a higher systolic value (P_S). Obtaining estimates of an individual's systolic and diastolic pressures is one of the most routine diagnostic techniques available to the physician. The basic principles of the *auscultation* technique used to measure blood pressure are described here with the aid of Figure 6–9.

An inflatable cuff is wrapped around the upper arm, and a device, such as a mercury manometer, is attached to monitor the pressure within the cuff. The cuff is initially inflated with air to a pressure ($\approx 175 - 200$ mm Hg) that is well above normal systolic values. This pressure is transmitted from the flexible cuff into the

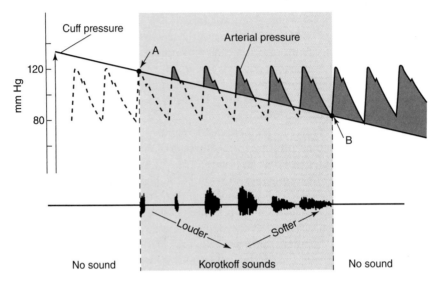

Figure 6–9. Blood pressure measurement by auscultation. Point **A** indicates systolic pressure and point **B** indicates diastolic pressure.

upper arm tissues, where it causes all blood vessels to collapse. No blood flows into (or out of) the forearm if the cuff pressure is higher than the systolic arterial pressure. After the initial inflation, air is allowed to gradually "bleed" from the cuff so that the pressure within it falls slowly and steadily through the range of arterial pressure fluctuations. The moment the cuff pressure falls below the peak systolic arterial pressure, some blood is able to pass through the arteries beneath the cuff during the systolic phase of the cycle. This flow is intermittent and occurs only over a brief period of each heart cycle. Moreover, because it occurs through partially collapsed vessels beneath the cuff, the flow is turbulent rather than laminar. The intermittent periods of flow beneath the cuff produce tapping sounds, which can be detected with a stethoscope placed over the radial artery at the elbow. As indicated in Figure 6–9, sounds of varying character, known collectively as *Korotkoff sounds*, are heard whenever the cuff pressure is between the systolic and diastolic aortic pressures.

Because there is no blood flow and no sound when cuff pressure is higher than systolic arterial pressure, *the highest cuff pressure at which tapping sounds are heard is taken as the systolic arterial pressure.* When the cuff pressure falls below the diastolic pressure, blood flows through the vessels beneath the cuff without periodic interruption and again no sound is detected over the radial artery. *The cuff pressure at which the sounds become muffled or disappear is taken as the diastolic arterial pressure.* The Korotkoff sounds are more distinct when the cuff pressure is near the systolic arterial pressure than when it is near the diastolic pressure. Thus, consistency in determining diastolic pressure by auscultation requires concentration and experience.

DETERMINANTS OF ARTERIAL PRESSURE

Mean Arterial Pressure

 Mean arterial pressure is a critically important cardiovascular variable because it is the average effective pressure that drives blood through the systemic organs. One of the most fundamental equations of cardiovascular physiology is that which indicates how mean arterial pressure $(\bar{P}_A)$ is related to cardiac output (CO) and total peripheral resistance (TPR):

$$\bar{P}_A = CO \times TPR$$

This equation is simply a rearrangement of the basic flow equation ($\dot{Q} = \Delta P / R$) applied to the entire systemic circulation with the single assumption that central venous pressure is approximately zero so that $\Delta P = \bar{P}_A$. Note that mean arterial pressure is influenced both by the heart (via cardiac output) and by the peripheral vasculature (via TPR). *All changes in mean arterial pressure result from changes in either cardiac output or total peripheral resistance.*

Calculating the true value of mean arterial pressure requires mathematically averaging the arterial pressure waveform over one or more complete heart cycles. Most often, however, we know from auscultation only the systolic and diastolic pressures, yet wish to make some estimate of the mean arterial pressure. Mean arterial pressure necessarily falls between the systolic and diastolic pressures. A useful rule of thumb is that mean arterial pressure $(\bar{P}_A)$ is approximately equal to diastolic pressure (P_D) plus one-third of the difference between systolic and diastolic pressures $(P_S - P_D)$:

$$\bar{P}_A \doteq P_D + \frac{1}{3}(P_S - P_D)$$

Arterial Pulse Pressure

The *arterial pulse pressure* (P_p) is defined simply as systolic pressure minus diastolic pressure:

$$P_p = (P_S - P_D)$$

To be able to use pulse pressure to deduce something about how the cardiovascular system is operating, one must do more than just define it. It is important to understand what *determines* pulse pressure; that is, what causes it to be what it is and what can cause it to change. In a previous section of this chapter, there was a brief discussion about how, as a consequence of the compliance of the arterial vessels, arterial pressure increases as arterial blood volume is expanded during cardiac ejection. The magnitude of the pressure increase (ΔP) caused by an increase in arterial volume depends on how large the volume change (ΔV) is and on how compliant (C_A) the arterial compartment is: $\Delta P = \Delta V / C_A$. If, for the moment, the fact that some blood leaves the arterial compartment *during* cardiac ejection is neglected, then the increase in arterial volume during each heartbeat is equal to the stroke volume (SV).

 Thus, pulse pressure is, to a first approximation, equal to stroke volume divided by arterial compliance:

$$P_P \simeq \frac{SV}{C_A}$$

Arterial pulse pressure is approximately 40 mm Hg in a normal resting young adult because stroke volume is approximately 80 mL and arterial compliance is approximately 2 mL/mm Hg. Pulse pressure tends to increase with age in adults because of a decrease in arterial compliance ("hardening of the arteries"). Arterial volume–pressure curves for a 20-year-old and a 70-year-old are shown in Figure 6–10. The decrease in arterial compliance with age is indicated by the steeper curve for the 70-year-old (more ΔP for a given ΔV) than for the 20-year-old. Thus, a 70-year-old will necessarily have a larger pulse pressure for a given stroke volume than a 20-year-old. As indicated in Figure 6–10, the decrease in arterial compliance is sufficient to cause increased pulse pressure even though stroke volume tends to decrease with age.

Figure 6–10 also illustrates the fact that arterial blood volume and mean arterial pressure tend to increase with age. The increase in *mean* arterial pressure is *not* caused by the decreased arterial compliance because compliance changes do not

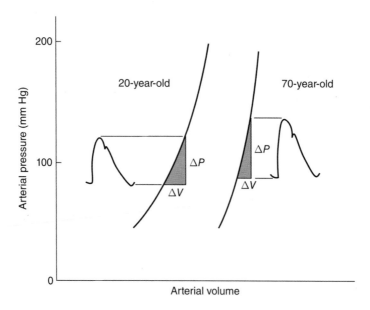

Figure 6–10. Observed effects of aging on the pressure–volume relationship of arteries. Also indicated are normal age-related changes in stroke volume (ΔV) and arterial pressures.

directly influence either cardiac output or TPR, which are the *sole determinants* of $\overline{P}_A$. Mean arterial pressure tends to increase with age because of an age-dependent increase in TPR, which is controlled primarily by arterioles, not arteries.

Arterial compliance also decreases with increasing mean arterial pressure, as evidenced by the curvature of the volume–pressure relationships shown in Figure 6–10. Otherwise, arterial compliance is a relatively stable parameter. Thus, most acute changes in arterial pulse pressure are the result of changes in stroke volume.

The preceding equation for pulse pressure is a much-simplified description of some very complex hemodynamic processes. It correctly identifies stroke volume and arterial compliance as the major determinants of arterial pulse pressure but assumes that no blood leaves the aorta during systolic ejection. Obviously, this is not strictly correct. Furthermore, close examination of Figure 3–1 will reveal that peak systolic pressure is reached even before cardiac ejection is complete. It is, therefore, not surprising that several factors other than arterial compliance and stroke volume have minor influences on pulse pressure. For example, because the arteries have viscous properties and elastic characteristics, faster cardiac ejection caused by increased myocardial contractility tends to increase pulse pressure somewhat even if stroke volume remains constant. Changes in TPR, however, have *little or no effect on pulse pressure*, because a change in TPR causes parallel changes in both systolic and diastolic pressures.

A common misconception in cardiovascular physiology is that the systolic pressure alone or the diastolic pressure alone indicates the status of a specific cardiovascular variable. For example, high diastolic pressure is often taken to indicate high TPR. This is not necessarily so because high diastolic pressure can exist with normal (or even reduced) TPR if the heart rate (HR) and cardiac output are high. Systolic *and* diastolic pressures are both influenced by the HR, stroke volume, TPR, and C_A. The student should not attempt to interpret systolic and diastolic pressure values independently. Interpretation is much more straightforward when the focus is on mean arterial pressure ($\overline{P}_A = CO \times TPR$) and arterial pulse pressure ($P_p \doteq SV/C_A$). (See study questions 6–13 and 6–14.)

PERSPECTIVES

Proper operation of the vasculature is equally important to proper operation of the heart for normal cardiovascular function. The elegant design of branching and converging vessels with parallel supply of blood flow to individual organs make this network an incredibly efficient system for adjusting flow to match changing metabolic needs. Severe compromise of the material transport system occurs when the compliance characteristics of the large vessels are altered, control of arteriolar resistance is inappropriate, or density of the microcirculation is inadequate. Once again we would like to draw attention to Appendix C in which many of the most important relationships for both vascular and cardiac function are summarized.

KEY CONCEPTS

Within the cardiovascular system, convection is used to transport substances between capillary beds, and diffusion is used to transport substances between blood and tissue.

Water may move out of (filtration) or into (reabsorption) capillaries depending on the net balance of hydrostatic and osmotic forces across capillary walls.

Plasma proteins are responsible for the major osmotic force across capillary walls.

Lymphatic vessels serve to remove excess filtrate from tissues and keep interstitial protein concentration low.

Vascular beds are complex networks of vessels arranged in series and in parallel.

The velocity of blood flow is inversely proportional to the total cross-sectional area of the vascular segment and is slowest in capillaries.

Turbulent blood flow is abnormal and makes noise (murmurs and bruits).

Veins contain most of the total blood volume.

Arterioles contribute most to the resistance to flow through organs.

Arteriolar constriction tends to reduce flow through an organ, reduce capillary hydrostatic pressure, and promote transcapillary fluid reabsorption within the organ.

Venous constriction is important for cardiac filling and the ability to cope with blood loss.

Because arteries are elastic, the intermittent flow from the heart is converted to continuous flow through capillaries.

Mean systemic arterial pressure is determined by the product of cardiac output and total peripheral resistance.

Changes in arterial pulse pressure reflect changes in stroke volume and/or the compliance of the arterial space.

STUDY QUESTIONS

6–1. Determine the direction of transcapillary fluid movement ($\dot{F}$) within a tissue, given the following data:

capillary hydrostatic pressure, $P_c = 28$ mm Hg

plasma oncotic pressure, $\pi_c = 24$ mm Hg

tissue hydrostatic pressure, $P_i = -4$ mm Hg

tissue oncotic pressure, $\pi_i = 0$ mm Hg

6–2. Which of the following conditions favor edema formation?

a. Lymphatic blockage

b. Thrombophlebitis (venous clot)

c. Decreased plasma protein concentration

d. Greatly increased capillary pore size

6–3. Assume that three vessels with identical dimensions are combined into a network of one vessel followed by a parallel combination of the other two and that a pressure P_i is applied to the inlet of the first vessel, while a lower pressure P_o exists at the outlet of the parallel pair.

a. Find the overall resistance of the network R_n if the resistance of each vessel is equal to R_e.

b. Is the pressure P_j at the central junction of the network closer to P_i or P_o?

6–4. Given the following data, calculate an individual's total peripheral resistance (TPR):

Mean arterial pressure, $\bar{P}_A = 100$ mm Hg

Central venous pressure, $P_{CV} = 0$ mm Hg

Cardiac output, $= 6$ L/min

6-5. TPR is always greater than the resistance to flow through any of the systemic organs. True or false?

6-6. If the resistance to flow through the kidneys increases and the resistance to flow through other systemic organs remains constant, TPR will increase. True or false?

6-7. Constriction of arterioles in an organ promotes reabsorption of interstitial fluid from that organ. True or false?

6-8. Chronic elevation of arterial pressure requires that either cardiac output or TPR (or both) be chronically elevated. True or false?

6-9. Whenever cardiac output is increased, mean arterial pressure must also be increased. True or false?

6-10. Acute rapid increases in arterial pulse pressure usually result from increases in stroke volume. True or false?

6-11. An increase in TPR increases diastolic pressure (P_D) more than systolic pressure (P_S). True or false?

6-12. Estimate the mean arterial pressure when the measured arterial pressure is 110/70 mm Hg.

6-13. At rest, the patient has a pulse rate of 70 beats/min and an arterial blood pressure of 119/80 mm Hg. During exercise on a treadmill, pulse rate is 140 beats/min and blood pressure is 135/90 mm Hg. Use this information to estimate the exercise-related changes in the following variables:

stroke volume

cardiac output

total peripheral resistance (TPR)

6-14. Which of the following is consistent with a normal mean arterial pressure but an abnormally high arterial pulse pressure?

a. Low stroke volume

b. High heart rate

c. Decreased total peripheral resistance

d. Increased arterial stiffness

e. Aortic valve stenosis

Vascular Control

OBJECTIVES

The student understands the general mechanisms involved in local vascular control:

▶ Identifies the major ways in which smooth muscle differs anatomically and functionally from striated muscle.

▶ Lists the steps leading to cross-bridge cycling in smooth muscle.

▶ Lists the major ion channels involved in the regulation of membrane potential in smooth muscle.

▶ Describes the processes of electromechanical and pharmacomechanical coupling in smooth muscle.

▶ Defines basal tone.

▶ Lists several substances potentially involved in local metabolic control.

▶ States the local metabolic vasodilator hypothesis.

▶ Describes how vascular tone may be influenced by endothelin, prostaglandins, histamine, and bradykinin.

▶ Describes the myogenic response of blood vessels.

▶ Defines active and reactive hyperemia and indicates a possible mechanism for each.

▶ Defines autoregulation of blood flow and briefly describes the metabolic, myogenic, and tissue pressure theories of autoregulation.

▶ Defines neurogenic tone of vascular muscle and describes how sympathetic neural influences can alter it.

▶ Describes how vascular tone is influenced by circulating catecholamines, vasopressin, and angiotensin II.

▶ Lists the major influences on venous diameters.

▶ Describes how control of flow differs between organs with strong local metabolic control of arteriolar tone and organs with strong neurogenic control of arteriolar tone.

The student knows the dominant mechanisms of flow and blood volume control in the major body organs:

▶ States the relative importance of local metabolic and neural control of coronary blood flow.

▶ Defines systolic compression and indicates its importance to blood flow in the endocardial and epicardial regions of the right and left ventricular walls.

▶ *Describes the unique features and major mechanisms of flow and blood volume control in each of the following systemic organs: skeletal muscle, brain, splanchnic organs, kidney, and skin.*

▶ *Explains why mean pulmonary arterial pressure is lower than mean systemic arterial pressure.*

▶ *Describes how pulmonary vascular control differs from that in systemic organs.*

Because the body's metabolic needs are continually changing, the cardio-vascular system must continually adjust the diameter of its vessels. The purposes of these vascular changes are (1) to efficiently distribute the cardiac output among tissues with different current needs (the job of arterioles) and (2) to regulate the distribution of blood volume and cardiac filling (the function of veins). In this chapter, we discuss our current understanding of how this is accomplished.

VASCULAR SMOOTH MUSCLE

Although long-term adaptations in vascular diameters may depend on remodeling of both the active (i.e., smooth muscle) and passive (i.e., structural, connective tissue) components of the vascular wall, short-term vascular diameter adjustments are made by regulating the contractile activity of vascular smooth muscle cells. These contractile cells are present in the walls of all vessels except capillaries. The task of the vascular smooth muscle is unique, because to maintain a certain vessel diameter in the face of the continual distending pressure of the blood within it, the vascular smooth muscle must be able to sustain active tension for prolonged periods.

There are many functional characteristics that distinguish smooth muscle from either skeletal or cardiac muscle. For example, when compared with these other muscle types, smooth muscle cells

1. contract and relax much more slowly;
2. can change their contractile activity as a result of either action potentials or changes in resting membrane potential;
3. can change their contractile activity in the absence of any changes in membrane potential;
4. can maintain tension for prolonged periods at low energy cost; and
5. can be activated by stretch.

Vascular smooth muscle cells are small (approximately 5×50 μm) spindle-shaped cells, usually arranged circumferentially or at small helical angles in muscular blood vessel walls. In many, but not all, vessels, adjacent smooth muscle cells are electrically connected by gap junctions similar to those found in the myocardium.

Contractile Processes

Just as in other muscle types, smooth muscle force development and shortening are thought to be the result of cross-bridge interaction between thick and thin contractile filaments composed of myosin and actin, respectively. In smooth muscle, however, these filaments are not arranged in regular, repeating sarcomere units. Consequently, "smooth" muscle cells lack the microscopically visible striations, characteristic of skeletal and cardiac muscle cells. The actin filaments in smooth muscle are much longer than those in striated muscle. Many of these actin filaments attach to the inner surface of the cell at structures called *dense bands*. In the interior of the cell, actin filaments do not attach to Z lines but rather anchor to small transverse structures called *dense bodies* that are themselves tethered to the surface membrane by cable-like *intermediate filaments*. Myosin filaments are interspersed between the smooth muscle actin filaments but in a more haphazard fashion than the regular interweaving pattern of striated muscle. In striated muscle, the contractile filaments are invariably aligned with the long axis of the cell, whereas in smooth muscle, many contractile filaments travel obliquely or even transversely to the long axis of the cell. Despite the absence of organized sarcomeres, changes in smooth muscle length affect its ability to actively develop tension. That is, smooth muscle exhibits a "length–tension relationship" analogous to that observed in striated muscle (see Figure 2–8). Similar to striated muscle, the strength of the cross-bridge interaction between myosin and actin filaments in smooth muscle is controlled primarily by changes in the intracellular free Ca^{2+} level, which range from approximately 10^{-8} M in the relaxed muscle to 10^{-5} M during maximal contraction. However, the sequence of steps linking an increased free Ca^{2+} concentration to contractile filament interaction is different in smooth muscle than in striated muscle. In the smooth muscle:

1. Intracellular free Ca^{2+} first forms a complex with the calcium-binding protein *calmodulin*.
2. The Ca^{2+}–calmodulin complex then activates a phosphorylating enzyme called *myosin light-chain kinase* (MLC kinase).
3. This enzyme allows the phosphorylation by adenosine triphosphate (ATP) of the light-chain protein that is a portion of the cross-bridge head of myosin (MLC).
4. MLC phosphorylation enables cross-bridge formation and cycling during which energy from ATP is utilized for tension development and shortening.

Smooth muscle is also unique in that once tension is developed, it can be maintained at very low energy costs, that is, without the need to continually split ATP in cross-bridge cycling. The mechanisms responsible are still somewhat unclear but presumably involve very slowly cycling or even noncycling cross-bridges. This is often referred to as the *latch state* and may involve light-chain dephosphorylation of attached cross-bridges.

By mechanisms that are yet incompletely understood, it is apparent that vascular smooth muscle contractile activity is regulated not only by changes in intracellular free Ca^{2+} levels but also by changes in the Ca^{2+} *sensitivity* of the contractile machinery. Thus, the contractile state of vascular smooth muscle may sometimes change in the absence of changes in intracellular free Ca^{2+} levels. The variable Ca^{2+} sensitivity of the activation of smooth muscle contractile apparatus may be due to the modifiable activity of another enzyme, *myosin phosphatase*, that facilitates a reaction that involves the phosphorylated MLC as a reactant. For example, factors that increase the intracellular concentrations of cyclic nucleotides often lead to relaxation of the vascular smooth muscle. Thus, the *net* state of phosphorylation of the MLC (and thus presumably contractile strength) depends on a balance between the effects of the Ca^{2+}-dependent enzyme MLC kinase, and the Ca^{2+}-independent enzyme MLC phosphatase.[1]

Membrane Potentials

Smooth muscle cells have resting membrane potentials ranging from -40 to -65 mV and are generally less negative than those in striated muscle. As in all cells, the resting membrane potential of the smooth muscle is determined largely by the cell permeability to potassium. Many types of K^+ channels have been identified in smooth muscle. The one that seems to be predominantly responsible for determining the resting membrane potential is termed an *inward rectifying-type* K^+ channel. There are also *ATP-dependent* K^+ channels that are closed when cellular ATP levels are normal but open if ATP levels fall. Such channels have been proposed to be important in matching organ blood flow to the metabolic state of the tissue.

Smooth muscle cells regularly have action potentials only in certain vessels. When they do occur, smooth muscle action potentials are initiated primarily by inward Ca^{2+} current and are developed slowly like the "slow-type" cardiac action potentials (see Figure 2–2C and D). As in the heart, this inward (depolarizing) Ca^{2+} current flows through a *voltage-operated channel* (VOC) for Ca^{2+}; this type of channel is one of several types of calcium channels present in the smooth muscle. The repolarization phase of the action potential occurs primarily by an outward flux of potassium ions through both *delayed* K^+ channels and *calcium-activated* K^+ channels.

Many types of ion channels in addition to those mentioned have been identified in vascular smooth muscle, but in most cases, their exact role in cardiovascular function remains obscure. For example, there appear to be nonselective, stretch-sensitive cation channels that may be involved in the response of smooth

---

[1] It is very important when thinking about biological processes to keep in mind that ANY "enzyme" is simply a chemical catalyst. As such, enzymes do not *cause* reactions to happen; rather, they *let* reactions happen faster than they would in their absence. That is, catalysts do not determine the direction in which chemical reactions proceed. With or without catalysts, chemical reactions ALWAYS relentlessly proceed only in the direction of chemical equilibrium. The "case in point" example here is that, although the Ca^{2+} activation of MLC kinase may well facilitate a reaction that would result in phosphorylated MLC as a product, it is naïve to think that Ca^{2+} removal from the intracellular space (and therefore lowered MLC kinase activity) would in itself reverse the process. The absence of a catalyst cannot make a reaction proceed backward! Moreover, it is equally erroneous to conceive there could be different catalysts for a given chemical reaction that could make it proceed in opposite directions. Ergo, MLC kinase, and MLC phosphatase must facilitate distinctly different chemical reactions.

muscle to stretch. The reader should note, however, that many of the important ion channels in vascular smooth muscle are also important in heart muscle (see Table 2–1).

Electromechanical versus Pharmacomechanical Coupling

In smooth muscle, changes in intracellular free Ca^{2+} levels can occur both with *and* without changes in membrane potential. The processes involved are called *electromechanical coupling* and *pharmacomechanical coupling*, respectively, and are illustrated in Figure 7–1.

Electromechanical coupling, shown in the left half of Figure 7–1, occurs because the smooth muscle surface membrane contains VOCs for calcium (the same VOCs that are involved in action potential generation). Membrane depolarization increases the open-state probability of these channels and thus leads to smooth muscle cell contraction and vessel constriction. Conversely, membrane hyperpolarization leads to smooth muscle relaxation and vessel dilation. Because the VOCs for Ca^{2+} are partially activated by the low resting membrane potential of the vascular smooth muscle, changes in resting potential can alter the resting calcium influx rate and therefore the basal contractile state.

With pharmacomechanical coupling, chemical agents (e.g., released neurotransmitters) can induce smooth muscle contraction without changing membrane potential. As illustrated on the right side of Figure 7–1, the combination of a

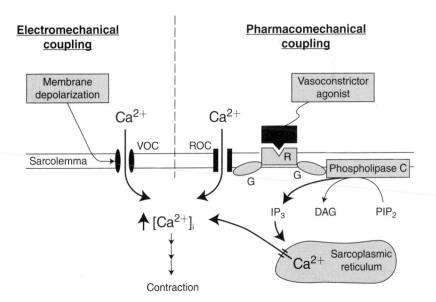

Figure 7–1. General mechanisms for activation of the vascular smooth muscle. VOC, voltage-operated Ca^{2+} channel; ROC, receptor-operated Ca^{2+} channel; R, agonist-specific receptor; G, GTP-binding protein; PIP_2, phosphatidylinositol biphosphate; IP_3, inositol triphosphate; DAG, diacylglycerol.

vasoconstrictor agonist (such as norepinephrine) with a specific membrane-bound receptor (such as an α_1-adrenergic receptor) initiates events that cause intracellular free Ca^{2+} levels to increase by 2 mechanisms. One, the activated receptor may open surface membrane *receptor-operated channels* for Ca^{2+} that allow Ca^{2+} influx from the extracellular fluid. Two, the activated receptor may induce the formation of an intracellular "second messenger," inositol trisphosphate (IP_3), which opens specific channels that release Ca^{2+} from the intracellular sarcoplasmic reticulum stores. In both processes, the activated receptor first stimulates specific guanosine triphosphate-binding proteins (GTP-binding proteins or *G proteins*). Such receptor-associated G proteins seem to represent a general first step through which most membrane receptors operate to initiate their particular cascade of events that ultimately lead to specific cellular responses.

The reader should *not* conclude from Figure 7–1 that all vasoactive chemical agents (chemical agents that cause vascular effects) produce their actions on the smooth muscle without changing membrane potential. In fact, most vasoactive chemical agents do cause changes in membrane potential because their receptors can be linked, by G proteins or other means, to ion channels of many kinds. However, often these effects in membrane potential are rather small.

In addition to the well-established signaling pathways shown in Figure 7–1, there is substantial evidence that purely mechanical influences on blood vessels such as wall tension and shear stress can influence vascular tone. Such influences could act directly through alterations in the mechanical forces on cytoskeletal and contractile proteins.

Not shown in Figure 7–1 are the processes that remove Ca^{2+} from the cytoplasm of the vascular smooth muscle, although they are important as well in determining the free cytosolic Ca^{2+} levels. As in cardiac cells (see Figure 2–7), smooth muscle cells actively pump calcium into the sarcoplasmic reticulum and outward across the sarcolemma. Calcium is also transported out of the cell via the sodium/calcium exchanger.

Mechanisms for Relaxation

Hyperpolarization of the cell membrane is one mechanism for causing smooth muscle relaxation and vessel dilation. In addition, however, there are at least 2 general mechanisms that certain chemical vasodilator agents can cause smooth muscle relaxation by pharmacomechanical means. In Figure 7–1, the specific receptor for a chemical vasoconstrictor agent is shown linked by a specific G protein to phospholipase C. In an analogous manner, other specific receptors may be linked by other specific G proteins to other enzymes that produce second messengers other than IP_3. An example is the β_2-adrenergic receptor[2] that is present in arterioles of the skeletal muscle and liver. β_2-Receptors are not innervated but can sometimes be activated by elevated levels of circulating *epinephrine*. The β_2-receptor is linked

---

[2] Vascular β-receptors are designated β_2-receptors and are pharmacologically distinct from the β_1-receptors found on cardiac cells.

by a particular G protein (G_s) to adenylate cyclase. Adenylate cyclase catalyzes the conversion of ATP to cyclic adenosine monophosphate (cAMP). Increased intracellular levels of cAMP cause the activation of protein kinase A, a phosphorylating enzyme that in turn causes phosphorylation of proteins at many sites. The overall result is stimulation of Ca^{2+} efflux, membrane hyperpolarization, and decreased contractile machinery sensitivity to Ca^{2+}—all of which act synergistically to cause vasodilation. In addition to epinephrine, histamine and vasoactive intestinal peptide are other vasodilator substances that act through the cAMP pathway.

In addition to cAMP, cyclic guanosine monophosphate (cGMP) is an important intracellular second messenger that causes vascular smooth muscle relaxation. Nitric oxide is an important vasodilator substance that operates via the cGMP pathway. Nitric oxide can be produced by endothelial cells and by nitrates, a clinically important class of vasodilator drugs. Nitric oxide is gaseous and easily diffuses into smooth muscle cells, where it activates the enzyme guanylyl cyclase that causes cGMP formation.

CONTROL OF ARTERIOLAR TONE

Vascular tone is a term commonly used to characterize the general contractile state of a vessel or a vascular region. The "vascular tone" of a region can be taken as an indication of the "level of activation" of the individual smooth muscle cells in that region. As described in Chapter 6, the blood flow through any organ is determined largely by its vascular resistance, which is dependent primarily on the diameter of its arterioles. Consequently, an organ's flow is controlled by factors that influence the arteriolar smooth muscle tone.

Basal Tone

Arterioles remain in a state of partial constriction even when all external influences on them are removed; hence, they are said to have a degree of *basal tone* (sometimes referred to as *intrinsic tone*). The understanding of the mechanism is incomplete; however, basal arteriolar tone may reflect the fact that smooth muscle cells inherently and actively resist being stretched as they continually are in pressurized arterioles. Another hypothesis is that the basal tone of arterioles is the result of a tonic production of local vasoconstrictor substances by the endothelial cells that line their inner surface. In any case, this basal tone establishes a baseline of partial arteriolar constriction from which the external influences on arterioles exert their dilating or constricting effects. These influences can be separated into 3 categories: local influences, neural influences, and hormonal influences.

Local Influences on Arterioles

METABOLIC INFLUENCES

The arterioles that control flow through a given organ lie within the organ tissue itself. Thus, arterioles and the smooth muscle in their walls are exposed to the chemical composition of the interstitial fluid of the organ

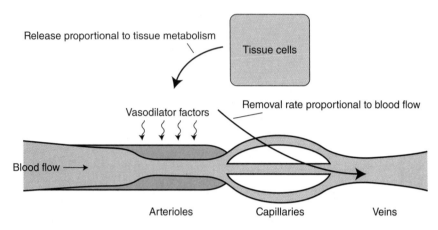

Figure 7-2. Local metabolic vasodilator hypothesis.

they serve. The interstitial concentrations of many substances reflect the balance between the metabolic activity of the tissue and its blood supply. Interstitial oxygen levels, for example, fall whenever the tissue cells are using oxygen faster than it is being supplied to the tissue by blood flow. Conversely, interstitial oxygen levels rise whenever excess oxygen is being delivered to a tissue from the blood. In nearly all vascular beds, exposure to low oxygen reduces arteriolar tone and causes vasodilation, whereas high oxygen levels cause arteriolar vasoconstriction.[3] Thus, a local feedback mechanism exists that automatically operates on arterioles to regulate a tissue's blood flow in accordance with its metabolic needs. Whenever blood flow and oxygen delivery fall below a tissue's oxygen demand, the oxygen levels around arterioles fall, the arterioles dilate, and the blood flow through the organ appropriately increases.

Many substances in addition to oxygen are present within tissues and can affect the tone of the vascular smooth muscle. When the metabolic rate of skeletal muscle is increased by exercise, tissue levels of oxygen decrease, but those of carbon dioxide, H^+, and K^+ increase. Muscle tissue osmolarity also increases during exercise. All these chemical alterations cause arteriolar dilation. In addition, with increased metabolic activity or oxygen deprivation, cells in many tissues may release *adenosine*, which is an extremely potent vasodilator agent.

At present, it is not known which of these (and possibly other) metabolically related chemical alterations within tissues are most important in the local metabolic control of blood flow. It appears likely that arteriolar tone depends on the combined action of many factors.

For conceptual purposes, Figure 7-2 summarizes current understanding of local metabolic control. Vasodilator factors enter the interstitial space from the tissue cells at a rate proportional to tissue metabolism. These vasodilator factors are removed from the tissue at a rate proportional to blood flow. Whenever tissue

---

[3] An important exception to this rule occurs in the pulmonary circulation and is discussed later in this chapter.

metabolism is proceeding at a rate for which the blood flow is inadequate, the interstitial vasodilator factor concentrations automatically build up and cause the arterioles to dilate. This, of course, causes blood flow to increase. The process continues until blood flow has risen sufficiently to appropriately match the tissue metabolic rate and prevent further accumulation of vasodilator factors. The same system also operates to reduce blood flow when it is higher than required by the tissue's metabolic activity, because this situation causes a reduction in the interstitial concentrations of metabolic vasodilator factors.

Local metabolic mechanisms represent by far the most important means of local flow control. By these mechanisms, individual organs can regulate their own flow in accordance with their specific metabolic needs.

As indicated below, several other types of local influences on blood vessels have been identified. However, many of these represent fine-tuning mechanisms and many are important only in certain, usually pathological, situations.

LOCAL INFLUENCES FROM ENDOTHELIAL CELLS

Endothelial cells cover the entire inner surface of the cardiovascular system. A large number of studies have shown that blood vessels respond very differently to certain vascular influences when their endothelial lining is missing. Acetylcholine, for example, causes vasodilation of intact vessels but causes vasoconstriction of vessels stripped of their endothelial lining. These studies suggest that endothelial cells can actively participate in the control of arteriolar diameter by producing local chemicals that affect the tone of the surrounding smooth muscle cells. In the case of the vasodilator effect of infusing acetylcholine through intact vessels, the vasodilator influence produced by endothelial cells has been identified as nitric oxide. Nitric oxide is produced within endothelial cells from the amino acid, l-arginine, by the action of an enzyme, nitric oxide synthase. Nitric oxide synthase is activated by a rise in the intracellular level of the Ca^{2+}. Nitric oxide is a small lipid-soluble molecule that, once formed, easily diffuses into adjacent smooth muscle cells where it causes relaxation by stimulating cGMP production as mentioned previously.

Acetylcholine and several other agents (including bradykinin, vasoactive intestinal peptide, and substance P) stimulate endothelial cell nitric oxide production because their receptors on endothelial cells are linked to receptor-operated Ca^{2+} channels. Probably more importantly from a physiological standpoint, flow-related shear stresses on endothelial cells stimulate their nitric oxide production presumably because stretch-sensitive channels for Ca^{2+} are activated. Such flow-related endothelial cell nitric oxide production may explain why, for example, exercise and increased blood flow through muscles of the lower leg can cause dilation of the blood-supplying femoral artery at points far upstream of the exercising muscle itself.

Agents that block nitric oxide production by inhibiting nitric oxide synthase cause significant increases in the vascular resistances of most organs. For this reason, it is believed that endothelial cells are normally always producing some nitric oxide that is importantly involved, along with other factors, in reducing the normal resting tone of arterioles throughout the body.

Endothelial cells have also been shown to produce several other locally acting vasoactive agents, including the vasodilators "endothelial-derived hyperpolarizing factor," prostacyclin and the vasoconstrictor *endothelin*. Endothelin in particular is the topic of intense current research. It has the greatest vasoconstrictor potency of any known substance and appears to have many other biological effects as well. Much recent evidence suggests that endothelin may play important roles in such important overall body processes such as salt handling and blood pressure regulation.

One general unresolved issue with the concept that arteriolar tone (and therefore local nutrient blood flow) is regulated by factors produced by *arteriolar* endothelial cells is how these cells could sense what the metabolic needs of the downstream tissue are. This is because the endothelial cells lining arterioles are exposed to arterial blood whose composition is constant regardless of flow rate or what is happening downstream. One hypothesis is that there exists some sort of communication system between vascular endothelial cells. That way, endothelial cells in capillaries or venules could telegraph upstream information about whether the blood flow is indeed adequate.

OTHER LOCAL CHEMICAL INFLUENCES

In addition to local metabolic influences on vascular tone, many specific locally produced and locally reacting chemical substances have been identified that have vascular effects and therefore could be important in local vascular regulation in certain instances. In most cases, however, definite information about the relative importance of these substances in cardiovascular regulation is lacking. This is due to the difficulty in studying small blood vessel regulation.

Prostaglandins and *thromboxane* are a group of several chemically related products of the cyclooxygenase pathway of arachidonic acid metabolism. Certain prostaglandins are potent vasodilators, whereas others are potent vasoconstrictors. Despite the vasoactive potency of the prostaglandins and the fact that most tissues (including endothelial cells and vascular smooth muscle cells) are capable of synthesizing prostaglandins, it has not been demonstrated convincingly that prostaglandins play a crucial role in *normal* vascular control. It is clear, however, that vasodilator prostaglandins are involved in inflammatory responses. Consequently, inhibitors of prostaglandin synthesis, such as aspirin, are effective anti-inflammatory drugs. Prostaglandins produced by platelets and endothelial cells are important in the hemostatic (flow stopping, antibleeding) vasoconstrictor and platelet-aggregating responses to vascular injury. Hence, aspirin is often prescribed to reduce the tendency for blood clotting—especially in patients with potential coronary flow limitations. Arachidonic acid metabolites produced via the lipoxygenase system (e.g., *leukotrienes*) also have vasoactive properties and may influence blood flow and vascular permeability during inflammatory processes.

Histamine is synthesized and stored in high concentrations in secretory granules of tissue mast cells and circulating basophils. When released, histamine produces arteriolar vasodilation (via the cAMP pathway) and increases vascular permeability, which leads to edema formation and local tissue swelling. Histamine increases vascular permeability by causing separations in the junctions between the endothelial cells that line the vascular system. Histamine release is classically associated with *antigen–antibody reactions* in various allergic and immune responses. Many drugs and physical or chemical insults that damage tissue also cause histamine release. Histamine can stimulate sensory nerve endings to cause itching and pain sensations. Although clearly important in many pathological situations, it seems unlikely that histamine participates in normal cardiovascular regulation.

Bradykinin is a small polypeptide that has approximately 10 times the vasodilator potency of histamine on a molar basis. It also acts to increase capillary permeability by opening the junctions between endothelial cells. Bradykinin is formed from certain plasma globulin substrates by the action of an enzyme, *kallikrein*, and is subsequently rapidly degraded into inactive fragments by various tissue kinases. Like histamine, bradykinin is thought to be involved in the vascular responses associated with tissue injury and immune reactions. It also stimulates nociceptive nerves and may thus be involved in the pain associated with tissue injury.

TRANSMURAL PRESSURE

The passive elastic mechanical properties of arteries and veins and how changes in transmural pressure affect their diameters are discussed in Chapter 6. The effect of transmural pressure on arteriolar diameter is more complex because arterioles respond both *passively* and *actively* to changes in transmural pressure. For example, a sudden increase in the internal pressure within an arteriole produces (1) first an initial slight passive mechanical distention (slight because arterioles are relatively thick-walled and muscular), and (2) then an active constriction that, within seconds, may completely reverse the initial distention. A sudden decrease in transmural pressure elicits essentially the opposite response, that is, an immediate passive decrease in diameter followed shortly by a decrease in active tone, which returns the arteriolar diameter to near that which existed before the pressure change. The active phase of such behavior is referred to as a *myogenic response*, because it seems to originate within the smooth muscle itself. The precise mechanism of the myogenic response is unknown; however, stretch-sensitive ion channels on arteriolar vascular smooth muscle cells are likely candidates for involvement.

All arterioles have some normal distending pressure that they are probably actively responding to. Therefore, the myogenic mechanism is likely to be a fundamentally important factor in determining the basal tone of arterioles everywhere. Also, for obvious reasons and as soon discussed, the myogenic response is potentially involved in the vascular reaction to any cardiovascular disturbance that involves a change in arteriolar transmural pressure.

FLOW RESPONSES CAUSED BY LOCAL MECHANISMS

Whatever the mechanisms involved, Figures 7–3 and 7–4 illustrate typical flow responses caused by *local* mechanisms within organs. Similar results were observed during experiments on most *isolated* organs. Because the organs were isolated, it

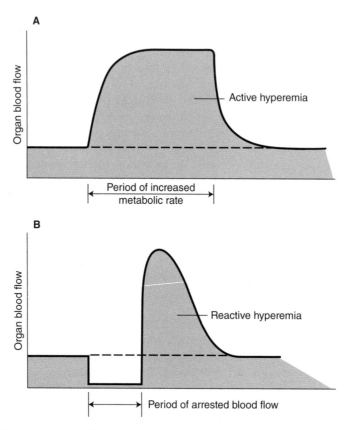

Figure 7–3. Organ blood flow responses caused by local mechanisms: **(A)** active hyperemia **(B)** reactive hyperemia.

is presumed that such responses reflect *only* the operation of local influences on arterioles. That is, these responses do not involve *global* influences on arterioles like changes in sympathetic nerve activity or blood levels of circulating vasoactive substances.

Active Hyperemia—In organs with a highly variable metabolic rate, such as skeletal and cardiac muscles, the blood flow closely follows the tissue's metabolic rate. For example, skeletal muscle blood flow increases within seconds of the onset of muscle exercise and returns to control values shortly after exercise ceases. This phenomenon, which is illustrated in Figure 7–3A, is known as *exercise* or *active hyperemia* (*hyperemia* means high flow). It should be clear how active hyperemia could result from the local metabolic vasodilator feedback on the arteriolar smooth muscle. As alluded to previously, once initiated by local metabolic influences on small resistance vessels, endothelial flow-dependent mechanisms may assist in propagating the vasodilation to larger vessels upstream, which helps promote the delivery of blood to the exercising muscle.

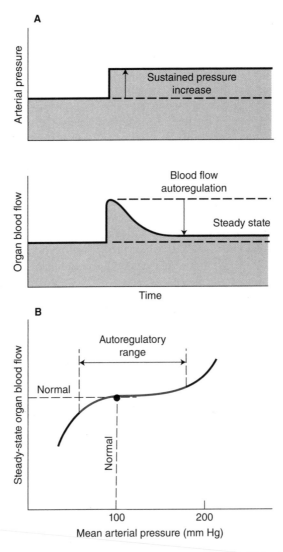

Figure 7-4. Autoregulation of organ blood flow. **(A)** With sustained increases in arterial pressure, arteriolar resistance increases returning organ blood flow to its steady state to prevent over-perfusion. **(B)** Autoregulation helps to maintain steady-state blood flow over a higher than normal range of pressures, thus preventing downstream damage.

The onset of the active hyperemia response in Figure 7–3A illustrates that organs actively resist being *under*-perfused for their current metabolic rate by decreasing their arteriolar resistance. Moreover, the offset of the response in Figure 7–3A illustrates that organs resist being *over*-perfused by increasing their arteriolar resistance. The bottom line is that organs inherently tend to regulate their own blood flow to only that which they themselves currently require. If all organs simultaneously do this, the collective result is that the heart does not have to pump any more blood flow (i.e., cardiac output) than is needed to maintain overall body homeostasis. Thus, the local mechanisms of arteriolar control inherently tend to minimize the work that the heart must do in any situation.

Reactive Hyperemia—In this case, the higher-than-normal blood flow occurs transiently after the removal of any restriction that has caused a period of lower-than-normal blood flow and is sometimes referred to as *post-occlusion hyperemia*. The phenomenon is illustrated in Figure 7–3B. For example, flow through an extremity is higher than normal for a period after a tourniquet is removed from the extremity. Both local metabolic and myogenic mechanisms may be involved in producing reactive hyperemia. The magnitude and duration of reactive hyperemia depend on the duration and severity of the occlusion and the metabolic rate of the tissue. These findings are best explained by an interstitial accumulation of metabolic vasodilator substances during the period of flow restriction. However, unexpectedly large flow increases can follow arterial occlusions lasting only 1 or 2 seconds. These may be explained best by a myogenic dilation response to the reduced intravascular pressure and decreased stretch of the arteriolar walls that exists during the period of occlusion.

Autoregulation—Except when displaying active and reactive hyperemia, nearly all organs tend to keep their blood flow constant despite variations in arterial pressure—that is, they *autoregulate* their blood flow. As shown in Figure 7–4A, an abrupt increase in arterial pressure is normally accompanied by an initial abrupt increase in organ blood flow that then gradually returns toward normal despite the sustained elevation in arterial pressure. The initial rise in flow with increased pressure is expected from the basic flow equation ($\dot{Q} = \Delta P/R$). The subsequent return of flow toward the normal level is caused by a gradual increase in active arteriolar tone and resistance to blood flow. Ultimately, a new steady state is reached with only slightly elevated blood flow because the increased driving pressure is counteracted by a higher-than-normal vascular resistance. As with the phenomenon of reactive hyperemia, blood flow autoregulation may be caused by both local metabolic feedback mechanisms and myogenic mechanisms. The arteriolar vasoconstriction responsible for the autoregulatory response shown in Figure 7–4A, for example, may be partially due to (1) a "washout" of metabolic vasodilator factors from the interstitium by the excessive initial blood flow and (2) a myogenic increase in arteriolar tone stimulated by the increase in stretching forces that the increase in pressure imposes on the vessel walls. There is also a *tissue pressure hypothesis* of blood flow autoregulation for which it is assumed that an abrupt increase in arterial pressure causes transcapillary fluid filtration and thus leads to a gradual increase in interstitial fluid volume and pressure. Presumably, the increase in extravascular pressure would cause a decrease in vessel diameter by simple compression. This mechanism might be especially important in organs such as the kidney and brain whose volumes are constrained by external structures.

Although not illustrated in Figure 7–4A, autoregulatory mechanisms operate in the opposite direction in response to a decrease in arterial pressure below the normal value. One important general consequence of local autoregulatory mechanisms is that the steady-state blood flow in many organs tends to remain near the normal value over quite a wide range of arterial pressure. This is illustrated in the graph in Figure 7–4B. As discussed later, the inherent ability of certain organs to maintain adequate blood flow despite lower-than-normal arterial pressure is of considerable importance in situations such as shock from blood loss.

The phenomenon of autoregulation again illustrates that local mechanisms act to prevent under- or over-perfusion of individual organs whatever the situation.

Neural Influences on Arterioles

SYMPATHETIC VASOCONSTRICTOR NERVES

These neural fibers innervate arterioles in all systemic organs and provide by far the most important means of *reflex* control of the vasculature. Sympathetic vasoconstrictor nerves are the backbone of the system for controlling total peripheral resistance and are thus essential participants in global cardiovascular tasks such as regulating arterial blood pressure.

Sympathetic vasoconstrictor nerves release norepinephrine from their terminal structures in amounts generally proportional to their action potential frequency. Norepinephrine causes an increase in the tone of arterioles after combining with an α_1-*adrenergic receptor* on smooth muscle cells. Norepinephrine appears to increase vascular tone primarily by pharmacomechanical means. The mechanism involves G-protein linkage of α-adrenergic receptors to phospholipase C and subsequent Ca^{2+} release from intracellular stores by the action of the second messenger IP_3, as illustrated on the right side of Figure 7–1.

Sympathetic vasoconstrictor nerves normally have a continual or *tonic firing activity*. This tonic activity of sympathetic vasoconstrictor nerves makes the normal contractile tone of arterioles considerably greater than their basal tone. The additional component of vascular tone is called *neurogenic tone*. When the firing rate of sympathetic vasoconstrictor nerves is increased above normal, arterioles constrict and cause organ blood flow to fall below normal. Conversely, vasodilation and increased organ blood flow can be caused by sympathetic vasoconstrictor nerves if their normal tonic activity level is reduced. Thus, an organ's blood flow can either be reduced below normal or increased above normal by changes in the sympathetic vasoconstrictor fiber firing rate.

OTHER NEURAL INFLUENCES

Blood vessels, as a general rule, do not receive innervation from the parasympathetic division of the autonomic nervous system. However, *parasympathetic vasodilator nerves*, which release *acetylcholine*, are present in the vessels of the brain and the heart, but their influence on arteriolar tone in these organs appears to be inconsequential. Parasympathetic vasodilator nerves are also present in the vessels of the salivary glands, pancreas, and gastric mucosa where they have important influences on secretion and motility. In the external genitalia, they are responsible for the vasodilation of inflow vessels responsible for promoting secretion and erection.

Hormonal Influences on Arterioles

Under normal circumstances, short-term hormonal influences on blood vessels are generally thought to be of minor consequence in comparison to the local metabolic and neural influences. However, it should be emphasized that the understanding of how the cardiovascular system operates in many situations is incomplete. Thus, the hormones discussed in the following sections may play more important roles in cardiovascular regulation than is now appreciated.

CIRCULATING CATECHOLAMINES

During activation of the sympathetic nervous system, the adrenal glands release the catecholamines *epinephrine* and *norepinephrine* into the bloodstream. Under normal circumstances, the blood levels of these agents are probably not high enough to cause significant cardiovascular effects. However, circulating catecholamines may have cardiovascular effects in situations (such as vigorous exercise or hemorrhagic shock) that involve high activity of the sympathetic nervous system. In general, the cardiovascular effects of high levels of circulating catecholamines parallel the direct effects of sympathetic activation, which have already been discussed; both epinephrine and norepinephrine can activate cardiac β_1-adrenergic receptors to increase the heart rate and myocardial contractility and can activate vascular α-receptors to cause vasoconstriction. Recall that in addition to the α_1-receptors that mediate vasoconstriction, arterioles in a few organs also possess β_2-adrenergic receptors that mediate vasodilation. Because vascular β_2-receptors are more sensitive to epinephrine than are vascular α_1-receptors, moderately elevated levels of circulating epinephrine can cause vasodilation, whereas higher levels cause α_1-receptor-mediated vasoconstriction. Vascular β_2-receptors are not innervated and therefore are not activated by norepinephrine, released from sympathetic vasoconstrictor nerves. The physiological importance of these vascular β_2-receptors is unclear because adrenal epinephrine release occurs during periods of increased sympathetic activity when arterioles would simultaneously be undergoing direct neurogenic vasoconstriction. Again, under normal circumstances, circulating catecholamines are not an important factor in cardiovascular regulation.

VASOPRESSIN

This polypeptide hormone, also known as antidiuretic hormone (or ADH), plays an important role in extracellular fluid homeostasis and is released into the bloodstream from the posterior pituitary gland in response to low blood volume and/ or high extracellular fluid osmolarity. Vasopressin acts on collecting ducts in the kidneys to decrease renal excretion of water. Its role in body fluid balance has some very important indirect influences on cardiovascular function, which is discussed in more detail in Chapter 9. Vasopressin, however, is also a potent arteriolar vasoconstrictor. Although it is not thought to be significantly involved in normal vascular control, direct vascular constriction from abnormally high levels of vasopressin may be important in the response to certain disturbances such as severe blood loss through hemorrhage.

ANGIOTENSIN II

 Angiotensin II is a circulating polypeptide that regulates aldosterone release from the adrenal cortex as part of the system for controlling body's sodium balance. This system, discussed in greater detail in Chapter 9, is very important in blood volume regulation. Angiotensin II is also a very potent vasoconstrictor agent. Although it should not be viewed as a normal regulator of arteriolar tone, direct vasoconstriction from angiotensin II seems to be an important component of the general cardiovascular response to severe blood loss. There is also strong evidence suggesting that direct vascular actions of angiotensin II may be involved in intrarenal mechanisms for controlling kidney function. In addition, angiotensin II may be partially responsible for the abnormal vasoconstriction that accompanies many forms of hypertension. Again, it should be emphasized that knowledge of many pathological situations—including hypertension—is incomplete. These situations may well involve vascular influences that are not yet recognized.

CONTROL OF VENOUS TONE

Before considering the details of the control of venous tone, recall that venules and veins play a much different role in the cardiovascular system than do arterioles. Arterioles are the inflow valves that control the rate of nutritive blood flow through organs and individual regions within them. Appropriately, arterioles are usually strongly influenced by the current local metabolic needs of the region in which they reside, whereas veins are not. Veins do, however, collectively regulate the distribution of available blood volume between the peripheral and central venous compartments. Recall that central blood volume (and therefore pressure) has a marked influence on stroke volume and cardiac output. Consequently, when one considers what *peripheral* veins are doing, one should be thinking primarily about what the effects will be on *central* venous pressure and cardiac output.

 Veins contain the vascular smooth muscle that is influenced by many things that influence the vascular smooth muscle of arterioles. Constriction of the veins (venoconstriction) is largely mediated through activity of the sympathetic nerves that innervate them. As in arterioles, these sympathetic nerves release norepinephrine, which interacts with α_1-receptors and produces an increase in venous tone and a decrease in vessel diameter. There are, however, several functionally important differences between veins and arterioles. Compared with arterioles, veins normally have little basal tone. Thus, veins are normally in a dilated state. One important consequence of the lack of basal venous tone is that vasodilator metabolites that may accumulate in the tissue have little effect on veins.

Because of their thin walls, veins are much more susceptible to physical influences than are arterioles. The large effect of internal venous pressure on venous diameter was discussed in Chapter 6 and is evident in the pooling of blood in the veins of the lower extremities that occurs during prolonged standing (as discussed further in Chapter 10).

Often external compressional forces are an important determinant of venous volume. This is especially true of veins in the skeletal muscle. Very high pressures are developed inside skeletal muscle tissue during contraction and cause venous vessels to collapse. Because veins and venules have one-way valves, the blood displaced from veins during skeletal muscle contraction is forced in the forward direction toward the right side of the heart. In fact, rhythmic skeletal muscle contractions may produce a considerable pumping action, often called the *skeletal muscle pump*, which helps return blood to the heart during exercise.

SUMMARY OF PRIMARY VASCULAR CONTROL MECHANISMS

As is apparent from the previous discussion, vessels are subject to a wide variety of influences, and special influences and/or situations often apply to particular organs. Certain general factors, however, dominate the primary control of the peripheral vasculature when it is viewed from the standpoint of overall cardiovascular system function; these influences are summarized in Figure 7–5. Basal tone, local metabolic vasodilator factors, and sympathetic vasoconstrictor nerves acting through α_1-receptors are the major factors controlling arteriolar tone and, therefore, the blood flow rate through peripheral organs. Sympathetic vasoconstrictor nerves, internal pressure, and external compressional forces are the most important influences on venous diameter and therefore on peripheral–central distribution of blood volume.

   As evident in the remaining sections of this chapter, many details of vascular control vary from organs to organs. However, regarding flow control, most organs

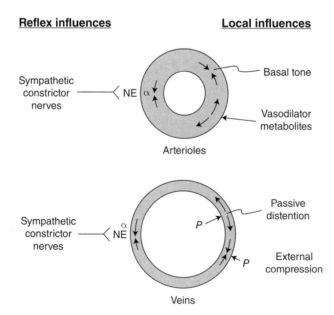

Figure 7–5. Primary influences on arterioles (top) and veins (bottom). Neural influences (left) mediated by norepinephrine (NE) acting on alpha-adrenergic receptors (a) and local influences (right) mediated by metabolites and transmural pressure (P) changes.

can be placed somewhere in a spectrum that ranges from almost total dominance by local metabolic mechanisms to almost total dominance by sympathetic vasoconstrictor nerves.

The flow in organs such as the brain, heart muscle, and skeletal muscle is very strongly controlled by local metabolic control, whereas the flow in the kidneys, skin, and splanchnic organs is very strongly controlled by sympathetic nerve activity. Consequently, some organs are automatically forced to participate in overall cardiovascular reflex responses to a greater extent than are other organs. The overall plan seems to be that, in cardiovascular emergency, flow to the brain and heart will be preserved at the expense of everything else if need be.

VASCULAR CONTROL IN SPECIFIC ORGANS

The general types of vascular influences outlined previously in this chapter have different relative importance in different organs. In the following sections, we consider how blood flow control differs between some major organs. Such differences obviously influence what determines the blood flow through the organ in question. But it is well to keep in perspective that all organs are part of the overall, hydraulically interconnected cardiovascular system. What happens in any single organ ultimately has ramifications throughout the entire system. In the following lists of the vascular characteristics of specific organs, we attempt to address both local and global issues by identifying the important and sometimes unique factors that control flow in major organs or organ systems.

Coronary Blood Flow

1. The major right and left coronary arteries that serve the heart tissue are the first vessels to branch off the aorta. Thus, *the driving force for myocardial blood flow is the systemic arterial pressure, just as it is for other systemic organs.* Most of the blood that flows through the myocardial tissue returns to the right atrium by way of a large cardiac vein called the *coronary sinus.*

2. *Coronary blood flow is controlled primarily by local metabolic mechanisms.* Flow responds rapidly and accurately to changes in metabolic demands, which are reflected by myocardial oxygen consumption. In a resting individual, the myocardium extracts 70% to 75% of the oxygen in the blood that passes through it. Because of this high extraction rate, coronary sinus blood normally has a lower oxygen content than blood at any other place in the cardiovascular system.

3. Because myocardial oxygen extraction cannot increase significantly from its high resting value, *increases in myocardial oxygen consumption must be accompanied by appropriate increases in coronary blood flow.*

4. The issue of which metabolic vasodilator factors play the dominant role in modulating the tone of coronary arterioles is still not fully resolved although adenosine, hydrogen ions, and nitric oxide have all been found to participate.

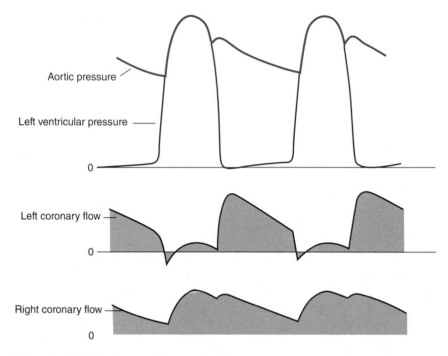

Figure 7-6. Phasic flows in the left and right coronary arteries in relation to aortic and left ventricular pressures.

5. *Large forces and/or pressures are generated within the myocardial tissue during cardiac muscle contraction.* Intramyocardial forces press on the outside of coronary vessels and cause them to collapse during systole. Because of this *systolic compression* of all vessels, coronary vascular resistance is greatly increased during systole. The result, at least for much of the left ventricular myocardium, is that coronary flow is lower during systole than during diastole, even though systemic arterial pressure (i.e., coronary perfusion pressure) is highest during systole. This is illustrated in the left coronary artery flow trace shown in Figure 7-6. Systolic compression has much less effect on flow through the right ventricular myocardium, as is evident from the right coronary artery flow trace in Figure 7-6. This is because the peak systolic intraventricular pressure is much lower for the right heart than for the left heart, and the systolic compressional forces in the right ventricular wall are correspondingly less than those in the left ventricular wall.

6. *Systolic compressional forces on coronary vessels are greater in the subendocardial (inside) layers of the left ventricular wall than in the subepicardial layers.*[4] Thus, the flow to the subendocardial layers of the left ventricle is impeded more than

---

[4] Consider that the endocardial surface of the left ventricle is exposed to intraventricular pressure ($\simeq$ 120 mm Hg during systole), whereas the epicardial surface is exposed only to intrathoracic pressure ($\simeq$ 0 mm Hg).

the flow to the subepicardial layers by systolic compression. Normally, the subendocardial region of the myocardium can make up for the lack of flow during systole by a high flow in the diastolic interval. However, when coronary blood flow is limited—for example, by coronary disease and stenosis—the subendocardial layers of the left ventricle are often the first regions of the heart to have difficulty maintaining a flow sufficient for their metabolic needs. *Myocardial infarcts* (areas of tissue damaged by insufficient blood flow) occur most frequently in the subendocardial layers of the left ventricle.

7. *Coronary arterioles are densely innervated with sympathetic vasoconstrictor fibers, yet when the activity of the sympathetic nervous system increases, the coronary arterioles normally vasodilate rather than vasoconstrict.* This is because an increase in sympathetic tone increases myocardial oxygen consumption by increasing the heart rate and contractility. The increased local metabolic vasodilator influence apparently outweighs the concurrent vasoconstrictor influence of an increase in the activity of sympathetic vasoconstrictor fibers that terminate on coronary arterioles. It has been experimentally demonstrated that a given increase in cardiac sympathetic nerve activity causes a greater increase in coronary blood flow after the direct vasoconstrictor influence of sympathetic nerves on coronary vessels has been eliminated with α-receptor-blocking agents. However, sympathetic vasoconstrictor nerves do not normally appear to influence coronary flow enough to affect the mechanical performance of normal hearts.

Skeletal Muscle Blood Flow

1. *Because of the large total mass of the skeletal muscle, blood flow through this "organ" is an important factor in overall cardiovascular hemodynamics.* Collectively, the skeletal muscles constitute 40% to 45% of body weight—more than any other single body organ. Even at rest, approximately 15% of the cardiac output goes to skeletal muscle, and during strenuous exercise, the skeletal muscle may receive more than 80% of the cardiac output.

2. *Resting skeletal muscle has a high level of intrinsic vascular tone.* Because of this high tone of the smooth muscle in resistance vessels of resting skeletal muscles, the blood flow per gram of tissue is quite low when compared with that of other organs such as the kidneys. However, resting skeletal muscle blood flow is still substantially above that required to sustain its metabolic needs. Resting skeletal muscles normally extract only 25% to 30% of the oxygen delivered to them in arterial blood. Thus, changes in the activity of sympathetic vasoconstrictor fibers can reduce resting muscle blood flow without seriously compromising resting tissue metabolic processes.

3. *Local metabolic control of arteriolar tone is the most important influence on blood flow through exercising muscle.* A particularly important characteristic of skeletal muscle is its very wide range of metabolic rates. During heavy exercise, the oxygen consumption rate of and oxygen extraction by skeletal muscle tissue can reach the high values typical of the myocardium.

In most respects, the factors that control blood flow to exercising muscle are similar to those that control coronary blood flow. Local metabolic control of arteriolar tone is very strong in exercising skeletal muscle, and muscle oxygen consumption is the most important determinant of its blood flow. Blood flow in the skeletal muscle can increase 20-fold during a bout of strenuous exercise.

4. *Alterations in sympathetic neural activity can alter nonexercising skeletal muscle blood flow.* For example, maximum sympathetic discharge rates can decrease blood flow in a resting muscle to less than one-fourth its normal value, and conversely, if all neurogenic tone is removed, resting skeletal muscle blood flow may double. This is a modest increase in flow compared with what can occur in an exercising skeletal muscle. Nonetheless, because of the large mass of tissue involved, changes in the vascular resistance of resting skeletal muscle brought about by changes in sympathetic activity are very important in the overall reflex regulation of arterial pressure.

5. *Alterations in sympathetic neural activity can influence exercising skeletal muscle blood flow.* As will be discussed in Chapter 10, the cardiovascular response to muscle exercise involves a general increase in sympathetic activity. This of course reduces flow to susceptible organs including nonexercising muscles. In exercising muscles, the increased sympathetic vasoconstrictor nerve activity is not evident as outright vasoconstriction but does limit the degree of metabolic vasodilation. One important function that this seemingly counterproductive process may serve is that of preventing an excessive reduction in total peripheral resistance during exercise. Indeed, if arterioles in most of the skeletal muscles in the body were allowed to dilate to their maximum capacity simultaneously, total peripheral resistance would be so low that the heart could not possibly supply enough cardiac output to maintain arterial pressure.

6. *Rhythmic contractions of exercising skeletal muscle can increase venous return.* As in the heart, muscle contraction produces large compressional forces within the tissue, which can collapse vessels and impede blood flow. Strong, sustained (tetanic) skeletal muscle contractions may stop muscle blood flow. Approximately 10% of the total blood volume is normally contained within the veins of the skeletal muscle, and during rhythmic exercise, the "skeletal muscle pump" is very effective in displacing blood from skeletal muscle veins. Valves in the veins prevent reverse flow back into the muscles. Blood displacement from the skeletal muscle into the central venous pool is an important factor in the hemodynamics of strenuous whole body exercise.

7. *Veins in skeletal muscle can constrict in response to increased sympathetic* activity. However, veins in skeletal muscle are rather sparsely innervated with sympathetic vasoconstrictor fibers, and the rather small volume of blood that can be mobilized from the skeletal muscle by sympathetic nerve activation is probably not of much significance to total body hemodynamics. This is in sharp contrast to the large displacement of blood from exercising muscle by the muscle pump mechanism. (This will be discussed in more detail when postural reflexes are considered in Chapter 10.)

Cerebral Blood Flow

1. *Interruption of cerebral blood flow for more than a few seconds leads to unconsciousness and brain damage within a very short period.* One rule of overall cardiovascular system function is that, in *all* situations, measures are taken that are appropriate to preserve adequate blood flow to the brain. This is normally accomplished by very rapid reflex adjustments in cardiac output and total peripheral resistance designed to keep mean arterial pressure constant (discussed in more detail in Chapters 9 and 10).

2. *Cerebral blood flow is regulated almost entirely by local mechanisms.* The brain as a whole has a nearly constant rate of metabolism that, on a per gram basis, is nearly as high as that of myocardial tissue. Flow through the cerebrum is autoregulated very strongly and is little affected by changes in arterial pressure unless it falls below approximately 60 mm Hg. When arterial pressure decreases below 60 mm Hg, brain blood flow decreases proportionately. It is presently unresolved whether metabolic mechanisms or myogenic mechanisms or both are involved in the phenomenon of cerebral autoregulation. Despite the relative constancy of the overall brain blood flow, blood flow to discrete regions is not constant but closely follows the local neuronal activity. The mechanisms responsible for this strong local control of cerebral blood flow are yet undefined, but H^+, K^+, oxygen, and adenosine seem most likely to be involved.

3. The "neurovascular unit" is a unique structural and functional feature of the cerebral circulation. Complex roles are played by closely associated/adjoined endothelial cells, basement membranes, pericytes, astrocytes, and neurons to influence capillary function and local flow. These structures are collectively referred to as the "neurovascular unit" and crosstalk among the components accounts for localized functional hyperemia. Abnormalities in the ability of these elements to coordinate local blood flow may contribute to many pathological states.

4. *The "blood–brain barrier" refers to the tightly connected vascular endothelial cells that severely restrict transcapillary movement of all polar and many other substances.*[5] Because of this blood–brain barrier, the extracellular space of the brain represents a special fluid compartment in which the chemical composition is regulated separately from that in the plasma and general body extracellular fluid compartment. The extracellular compartment of the brain encompasses both interstitial fluid and *cerebrospinal fluid* (CSF), which surrounds the brain and the spinal cord and fills the brain ventricles. The CSF is formed from plasma by selective secretion (not simple filtration) by specialized tissues, the *choroid plexus*, located within the brain ventricles. These processes regulate the chemical composition of the CSF. The interstitial fluid of

---

[5] Brain capillaries have a special carrier system for glucose and present no barrier to oxygen and carbon dioxide diffusion. Thus, the blood–brain barrier does not restrict nutrient supply to the brain tissue.

the brain takes on the chemical composition of CSF through free diffusional exchange.

The blood–brain barrier serves to protect the cerebral cells from ionic disturbances in the plasma. Also, by exclusion and/or endothelial cell metabolism, it prevents many circulating hormones (and drugs) from influencing the parenchymal cells of the brain and the vascular smooth muscle cells in brain vessels.

5. *Cerebral blood flow decreases whenever arterial blood P_{CO_2} falls below normal.* Conversely, cerebral blood flow increases whenever the partial pressure of carbon dioxide (P_{CO_2}) is raised above normal in the arterial blood. This is the normal situation in most tissues, but it plays out importantly when it happens in the brain. For example, the dizziness, confusion, and even fainting that can occur when a person hyperventilates (and "blows off" CO_2) are a direct result of cerebral vasoconstriction. It appears that cerebral arterioles respond not to changes in P_{CO_2} but to changes in the extracellular H^+ concentration (i.e., pH) caused by changes in P_{CO_2}. Cerebral arterioles also vasodilate whenever the partial pressure of oxygen (P_{O_2}) in arterial blood falls significantly below normal values. However, higher-than-normal arterial blood P_{O_2}, such as that caused by pure oxygen inhalation, produces little decrease in cerebral blood flow.

6. *Sympathetic and parasympathetic neural influences on cerebral blood flow are minimal.* Although cerebral vessels receive both sympathetic vasoconstrictor and parasympathetic vasodilator fiber innervation, cerebral blood flow is influenced very little by changes in the autonomic activity under normal circumstances. Sympathetic vasoconstrictor responses may, however, be important in protecting cerebral vessels from excessive passive distention following large, abrupt increases in arterial pressure.

7. Although many organs can tolerate some level of edema (the accumulation of excess extracellular fluid), *edema in the brain represents a crisis.* Cerebral edema increases intracranial pressure, which must be promptly relieved to avoid brain damage. Special mechanisms involving various specific ion channels and transporters precisely regulate the transport of solute and water across astrocytes and the endothelial barrier. These mechanisms contribute to normal maintenance of intracellular and extracellular fluid balance.

Splanchnic Blood Flow

1. *Because of the high blood flow* through *and the high blood volume* in *the splanchnic bed, its vascular control importantly influences overall cardiovascular hemodynamics.* Several abdominal organs, including the gastrointestinal (GI) tract, spleen, pancreas, and liver, are collectively supplied with what is called the *splanchnic blood flow.* Splanchnic blood flow is supplied to these abdominal organs through many arteries, but it all ultimately passes through the liver and returns to the inferior vena cava through the hepatic veins. The organs of the splanchnic region receive approximately 25% of the resting cardiac output and

contain more than 20% of the circulating blood volume. Thus, adjustments in either the blood flow or the blood volume of this region have extremely important effects on the cardiovascular system.

2. *Sympathetic neural activity plays an important role in vascular control of the splanchnic circulation.* Collectively, the splanchnic organs have a relatively high blood flow and extract only 15% to 20% of the oxygen delivered to them in the arterial blood. The arteries and veins of all the organs involved in the splanchnic circulation are richly innervated with sympathetic vasoconstrictor nerves. Maximal activation of sympathetic vasoconstrictor nerves can produce an 80% reduction in flow to the splanchnic region and cause a large shift of blood from the splanchnic organs to the central venous pool. In humans, a large fraction of the blood mobilized from the splanchnic circulation during periods of sympathetic activation comes from the constriction of veins in the liver. In many other species, the spleen acts as a major reservoir from which blood is mobilized by sympathetically mediated contraction of the smooth muscle located in the outer capsule of the organ.

3. *Local metabolic activity associated with gastrointestinal motility, secretion, and absorption is associated with local increases in splanchnic blood flow.* There is great diversity of vascular structure and function among individual organs and even regions within organs in the splanchnic region. The mechanisms of vascular control in specific areas of the splanchnic region are not well understood but are likely to be quite varied. Nonetheless, because most splanchnic organs are involved in the digestion and absorption of food from the GI tract, overall splanchnic blood flow increases after food ingestion. *Parasympathetic neural activity* is involved in many of these GI functions, so it is indirectly involved in increasing splanchnic blood flow. A large meal can elicit a 30% to 100% increase in splanchnic flow, but individual organs in the splanchnic region probably have higher percentage increases in flow at certain times because they are involved sequentially in the digestion–absorption process.

4. The GI circulation plays an important role in maintaining the barrier functions and defense mechanisms of the GI mucosa. Prolonged ischemia can lead to damage of the epithelial/mucosal barrier and *septicemia* (infection caused by micro-organisms and toxins circulating in the blood). Reperfusion may lead to tissue damage and produce inflammatory responses.

Renal Blood Flow

1. *Renal blood flow plays a critical role in the kidney's main long-term job of regulating the body's water balance and therefore circulating blood volume.* However, acute adjustments in renal blood flow also have important short-term hemodynamic consequences. The kidneys normally receive approximately 20% of the cardiac output of a resting individual. This flow can be reduced to practically zero during strong sympathetic activation. Thus, the control of renal blood

flow is important to overall cardiovascular function and will be discussed in more detail in Chapter 9.

2. *Renal blood flow is strongly influenced by sympathetic neural stimulation.* Alterations in sympathetic neural activity can have marked effects on total renal blood flow by altering the neurogenic tone of renal resistance vessels. In fact, extreme situations involving intense and prolonged sympathetic vasoconstrictor activity (as may accompany severe blood loss) can lead to dramatic reduction in renal blood flow, permanent kidney damage, and renal failure.

3. *Local metabolic mechanisms may influence local vascular tone, but physiological mechanisms are not clear.* It has long been known that experimentally *isolated* kidneys (i.e., kidneys deprived of their normal sympathetic input) autoregulate their flow quite strongly. The mechanism responsible for this phenomenon has not been definitively established, but myogenic, tissue pressure, and metabolic mechanisms may all be involved. The real question is what purpose such a strong local mechanism plays in the intact organism where it seems to be largely overridden by reflex mechanisms. In an intact individual, renal blood flow is not constant but is highly variable, depending on the prevailing level of sympathetic vasoconstrictor nerve activity.

4. Although the details of the unique structural components of the renal vasculature are not included in this text, it should be pointed out that the kidney has an elegant, localized mechanism called tubuloglomerular feedback that is largely responsible for (a) adjusting local renal blood flow in response to changes in sodium concentration in the blood and (b) regulating filtration of fluid out of the blood in the presence of altered arterial pressure. This mechanism sets into action changes in the renin–aldosterone–angiotensin system that will be discussed more fully in Chapter 9.

Cutaneous Blood Flow

1. *One of the major physiological roles of skin blood flow is to help regulate body temperature.* The metabolic activity of body cells produces heat, which must be lost for the body temperature to remain constant. The skin is the primary site of exchange of body heat with the external environment. Alterations in cutaneous blood flow in response to various metabolic states and environmental conditions provide the primary mechanism responsible for temperature homeostasis. (Other mechanisms such as shivering, sweating, and panting also participate in body temperature regulation under more extreme conditions.)

2. *Decreases in body temperature decrease skin blood flow and vice versa.* Cutaneous blood flow, which is approximately 6% of resting cardiac output, can decrease to about one-twentieth of its normal value when heat is to be retained (e.g., in a cold environment, during the development stages of a fever). In contrast, cutaneous blood flow can increase up to 7 times its normal value when heat is to be lost (e.g., in a hot environment, accompanying a high metabolic rate, after a fever "breaks").

3. *Structural adaptations of the cutaneous vascular beds promote heat loss or heat conservation.* The anatomic interconnections between microvessels in the skin are highly specialized and extremely complex. An extensive system of interconnected veins called the *venous plexus* normally contains the largest fraction of cutaneous blood volume, which, in individuals with lightly pigmented skin, gives the skin a reddish hue. To a large extent, heat transfer from the blood takes place across the large surface area of the venous plexus. The venous plexus is richly innervated with sympathetic vasoconstrictor nerves. When these fibers are activated, blood is displaced from the venous plexus, and this helps reduce heat loss and also lightens the skin color. Because the skin is one of the largest body organs, venous constriction can shift a considerable amount of blood into the central venous pool.

4. *Reflex sympathetic neural activity has important but complex influences on skin blood flow.* Cutaneous resistance vessels are richly innervated with sympathetic vasoconstrictor nerves, and because these fibers have a normal tonic activity, cutaneous resistance vessels normally have a high degree of neurogenic tone. When body temperature rises above normal, skin blood flow is increased by reflex mechanisms. In certain areas (such as the hands, ears, and nose), vasodilation appears to result entirely from the withdrawal of sympathetic vasoconstrictor tone. In other areas (such as the forearm, forehead, chin, neck, and chest), the cutaneous vasodilation that occurs with body heating greatly exceeds that which occurs with just the removal of sympathetic vasoconstrictor tone. This "active" vasodilation is closely linked to the onset of sweating in these areas. The sweat glands in human cutaneous tissue involved in thermoregulation are innervated by *cholinergic sympathetic fibers* that release acetylcholine. Activation of these nerves elicits sweating *and* an associated marked cutaneous vasodilation. The exact mechanism for this sweating-related cutaneous vasodilation remains unclear because it is not abolished by agents that block acetylcholine's vascular effects. It has long been thought that it was caused by local bradykinin formation secondary to the process of sweat gland activation. Newer evidence suggests that the cholinergic sympathetic nerves to sweat glands may release not only acetylcholine but also other vasodilator transmitters. Although these special sympathetic nerves are very important to temperature regulation, they do not participate in the normal, moment-to-moment regulation of the cardiovascular system.

5. *Cutaneous vessels respond to changes in local skin temperature.* In general, local cooling leads to local vasoconstriction and local heating causes local vasodilation. The mechanisms for this are unknown. If the hand is placed in ice water, there is initially a nearly complete cessation of hand blood flow accompanied by intense pain. After some minutes, hand blood flow begins to rise to reach values greatly more than the normal value, hand temperature increases, and the pain disappears. This phenomenon is referred to as *cold-induced vasodilation.* With continued immersion, hand blood flow cycles every few minutes between periods of essentially no flow and periods of hyperemia.

The mechanism responsible for cold vasodilation remains unknown, but it has been suggested that norepinephrine may lose its ability to constrict vessels when their temperature approaches 0°C. Cold-induced vasodilation apparently serves to protect exposed tissues from cold damage.

6. *Cutaneous vessels respond to local damage with observable responses.* Tissue damage from burns, ultraviolet radiation, cold injury, caustic chemicals, and mechanical trauma produces reactions in skin blood flow. A classical reaction called the *triple response* is evoked after vigorously stroking the skin with a blunt point. The first component of the triple response is a *red line* that develops along the direct path of the abrasion in approximately 15 seconds. Shortly thereafter, an irregular *red flare* appears that extends approximately 2 cm on either side of the red line. Finally, after a minute or two, a *wheal* appears along the line of the injury. The mechanisms involved in the triple response are not well understood, but it seems likely that histamine release from damaged cells is at least partially responsible for the dilation evidenced by the red line and the subsequent edema formation of the wheal. The red flare seems to involve nerves in some sort of a local *axon reflex*, because it can be evoked immediately after cutaneous nerves are sectioned but not after the peripheral portions of the sectioned nerves degenerate.

Pulmonary Blood Flow

1. *Pulmonary blood flow equals cardiac output.* Except for very transient adjustments, the rate of blood flow through the lungs is necessarily equal to cardiac output of the left ventricle in all circumstances. When cardiac output to the systemic circulation increases 3-fold during exercise, for example, pulmonary blood flow must also increase 3-fold.

2. *Pulmonary vascular resistance is about one-seventh of total systemic vascular resistance.* Pulmonary vessels do offer some vascular resistance. Although the level of pulmonary vascular resistance does not usually influence the pulmonary flow rate, it is important because it is one of the determinants of pulmonary arterial pressure ($\Delta P = \dot{Q}R$). Recall that mean *pulmonary* arterial pressure is approximately 13 mm Hg, whereas mean *systemic* arterial pressure is approximately 100 mm Hg. The reason for the difference in pulmonary and systemic arterial pressures is not that the right side of the heart is weaker than the left side of the heart, but rather that pulmonary vascular resistance is inherently much lower than systemic total peripheral resistance. The pulmonary bed has a low resistance because it has relatively large vessels throughout.

3. *Pulmonary arteries and arterioles are less muscular and more compliant than systemic arteries and arterioles.* When pulmonary arterial pressure increases, the pulmonary arteries and arterioles become larger in diameter. Thus, an increase in pulmonary arterial pressure *decreases* pulmonary vascular resistance. This phenomenon is important because it tends to limit the increase in pulmonary arterial pressure that occurs with increases in cardiac output.

4. *Pulmonary arterioles constrict in response to local alveolar hypoxia.* One of the most unique active responses in pulmonary vasculature is *hypoxic vasoconstriction* of pulmonary arterioles in response to low oxygen levels within alveoli. (*Note*: This is a local response to *alveolar* hypoxia, not to low levels of oxygen in the blood—that is, hypoxemia.) This is exactly opposite to the vasodilation that occurs in systemic arterioles in response to low tissue Po_2. The mechanisms that cause this unusual response in pulmonary vessels are unclear but may be dependent on a direct oxygen sensing by the pulmonary arterial smooth muscle cells (i.e., local alveolar hypoxia inhibits a vascular smooth muscle cell potassium channel, which induces depolarization allowing calcium influx and initiating contraction and local vasoconstriction). Current evidence also suggests that local endothelin production or prostaglandin synthesis may be involved in pulmonary hypoxic vasoconstriction. Whatever the mechanism, hypoxic vasoconstriction is essential to efficient lung gas exchange because it diverts blood flow away from areas of the lung that are poorly ventilated or collapsed. Consequently, the best-ventilated areas of the lung also receive the most blood flow. As a consequence of hypoxic arteriolar vasoconstriction, general hypoxia (such as that encountered at high altitude) causes an increase in pulmonary vascular resistance and pulmonary arterial hypertension.

5. *Autonomic nerves play no major role in the control of pulmonary vascular activity.* Both pulmonary arteries and veins receive sympathetic vasoconstrictor fiber innervation, but reflex influences on pulmonary vessels appear to be much less important than the physical and local hypoxic influences. Pulmonary veins serve a blood reservoir function for the cardiovascular system, and sympathetic vasoconstriction of pulmonary veins may be important in mobilizing this blood during periods of general cardiovascular stress.

6. *Low capillary hydrostatic pressure promotes fluid reabsorption and prevents fluid accumulation in pulmonary airways.* A consequence of the low mean pulmonary arterial pressure is the low pulmonary capillary hydrostatic pressure of approximately 8 mm Hg (compared with approximately 25 mm Hg in systemic capillaries). Because the plasma oncotic pressure in lung capillaries is near 25 mm Hg, as it is in all capillaries, it is likely that the transcapillary forces in the lungs strongly favor continual fluid reabsorption. This cannot be the complete story, however, because the lungs, like other tissues, continually produce some lymph, and some net capillary filtration is required to produce lymphatic fluid. This filtration is possible despite the unusually low pulmonary capillary hydrostatic pressure because pulmonary interstitial fluid has an unusually high protein concentration and thus oncotic pressure.

PERSPECTIVES

As should be evident from the broad overview attempted in this chapter, vascular control is indeed a very complex issue. Our current understanding of many of the factors involved is still quite "fuzzy" at best. For openers, we do not understand how vascular smooth muscle itself works, and we understand how striated muscles work. If that were not enough, smooth muscle operation seems to be potentially influenced by vastly more chemical and mechanical factors than does that of striated muscle. Because of recent advances in cellular and molecular biology, we are now beginning to understand the intricate multiple molecular steps through which some of these pathways act to influence operation of vascular smooth muscle cells. This, of course, has been a stimulus to the pharmaceutical industry to develop drugs that can block (or enhance) this pathway or that. But knowing the mechanism through which a particular influence acts really does nothing to answer the basic issues a practicing physician must face. For example: Do multiple influences just add or do they interact in complex ways? Is the mix of influences importantly different between organs or even within an organ? Is there some adaptation to an influence so that its effect diminishes over time? How is blood flow controlled in transplanted organs? There is much that we do not understand.

KEY CONCEPTS

Continual adjustments of vascular diameter are required to properly distribute the cardiac output to the various systemic tissues (the role of arterioles) and maintain adequate cardiac filling (the role of veins).

Vascular adjustments are made by changes in the tone of the vascular smooth muscle.

The vascular smooth muscle has many unique properties that make it sensitive to a wide array of local and reflex stimuli and capable of maintaining tone for long periods.

The tone of arterioles, but not veins, can be strongly influenced by local vasodilator factors produced by local tissue metabolism.

In abnormal situations (such as tissue injury or severe blood volume depletion), certain local factors such as histamine and bradykinin, and hormonal factors such as vasopressin and angiotensin have significant vascular influences.

Sympathetic vasoconstrictor nerves provide the primary reflex mechanisms for regulating both arteriolar and venous tones.

Sympathetic vasoconstrictor nerves release norepinephrine, which interacts with α_1-adrenergic receptors on the vascular smooth muscle to induce vasoconstriction.

The relative importance of local metabolic versus reflex sympathetic control of arteriolar tone (and therefore blood flow) varies from organs to organs.

In some organs (such as the brain, heart muscle, and exercising skeletal muscle), blood flow normally closely follows metabolic rate because of local metabolic influences on arterioles.

In other organs (such as skin and kidneys), blood flow is normally regulated more by sympathetic nerves than by local metabolic conditions.

Special unique features of the pulmonary circulation include hypoxic vasoconstriction (that diverts blood from underventilated areas) and low capillary hydrostatic pressure (that keeps the lungs dry).

STUDY QUESTIONS

7–1. *Which of the following would increase blood flow through a skeletal muscle?*

    a. An increase in tissue P_{CO_2}

    b. An increase in tissue adenosine

    c. The presence of α-receptor-blocking drugs

    d. Sympathetic activation

7–2. *Autoregulation of blood flow implies that arterial pressure is adjusted by local mechanisms to ensure constant flow through an organ. True or false?*

7–3. *Coronary blood flow will normally increase when*

    a. arterial pressure increases.

    b. the heart rate increases.

    c. sympathetic activity increases.

7–4. *The arterioles of skeletal muscle would have little or no tone in the absence of normal sympathetic vasoconstrictor fiber activity. True or false?*

7–5. *A person who breathes rapidly and deeply gets dizzy. Why?*

7–6. *A patient complains of severe leg pains after walking a short distance. The pains disappear after the patient rests. (This symptom is called intermittent claudication.) What might be the problem?*

7–7. *How would a stenotic aortic valve influence coronary blood flow?*

7–8. *Vascular smooth muscle differs from cardiac muscle in that it*

    a. contains no actin molecules.

    b. can be directly activated in the absence of action potentials.

    c. is unresponsive to changes in intracellular calcium levels.

    d. is unresponsive to changes in membrane potentials.

    e. is unresponsive to changes in muscle length.

7-9. Arteriolar constriction tends to do which of the following?
  a. Decrease total peripheral resistance
  b. Decrease mean arterial pressure
  c. Decrease capillary hydrostatic pressure
  d. Increase transcapillary fluid filtration
  e. Increase blood flow through the capillary bed

7-10. When an organ responds to an increase in metabolic activity with a decrease in its arteriolar resistance, this is known as
  a. active hyperemia.
  b. reactive hyperemia.
  c. autoregulation of blood flow.
  d. flow-dependent vasodilation.
  e. metabolic vasoconstriction.

7-11. In which of the following organs does reduced P_{O_2} cause arteriolar vasoconstriction?
  a. Lungs
  b. Skin
  c. Skeletal muscle
  d. Brain
  e. None of the above

7-12. Coronary blood flow occurs mostly during diastole. True or false?

Hemodynamic Interactions 8

OBJECTIVES

The student understands how central venous pressure can be used to assess circulatory status and how venous return, cardiac output, and central venous pressure are interrelated:

▶ *Describes the overall arrangement of the systemic circulation and identifies the primary functional properties of each of its major components.*

▶ *Defines mean circulatory filling pressure and states the primary factors that determine it.*

▶ *Defines venous return and explains how it is distinguished from cardiac output.*

▶ *States the reason why cardiac output and venous return must be equal in the steady state.*

▶ *Lists the factors that control venous return.*

▶ *Describes the relationship between central venous pressure and venous return and draws the normal venous return curve.*

▶ *Defines peripheral venous pressure.*

▶ *Lists the factors that determine peripheral venous pressure.*

▶ *Predicts the shifts in the venous return curve that occur with altered blood volume and altered venous tone.*

▶ *Describes how the output of the left heart pump is matched to that of the right heart pump.*

▶ *Draws the normal venous return and cardiac output curves on a graph and describes the significance of the point of curve intersection.*

▶ *Predicts how normal venous return, cardiac output, and central venous pressure will be altered with any given combination of changes in cardiac sympathetic tone, peripheral venous sympathetic tone, or circulating blood volume.*

▶ *Identifies possible conditions that result in abnormally high or low central venous pressure.*

In previous chapters, we have primarily described how individual components in the cardiovascular system work. That is, we have tried to establish their fundamental individual "rules of operation." (For example, a basic rule for the heart is $CO = SV \times HR$, and a basic rule for any vessel is $\dot{Q} = \Delta P/R$.) Such individual rules must be obeyed in all situations including those that exist within the intact cardiovascular system. However, in the intact cardiovascular system, the individual components are interconnected. An abnormal operation of any one component necessarily causes "ripple-effect" changes throughout the entire system that may seem abnormal. Such interactions are the subject of this chapter. They are of special importance to the clinician who must be able to distinguish between primary abnormalities and secondary consequences.

KEY SYSTEM COMPONENTS

As illustrated in Figure 8–1, the cardiovascular system is a closed hydraulic circuit that includes the heart, arteries, arterioles, capillaries, and veins.[1] The venous side of this system is often conceptually separated into 2 different compartments: (1) a large and diverse peripheral section (the peripheral venous compartment) and (2) a smaller intrathoracic section that includes the vena cavae and the right atrium (the central venous compartment). Each of the segments of this circuit has a distinctly different role to play in the overall operation of the system because of inherent differences in anatomical volume, resistance to flow, and compliance that are summarized in Table 8–1.

Note especially the surprisingly high ventricular diastolic compliance of 24 mL/mm Hg in Table 8–1. This value indicates how exquisitely sensitive the ventricular end-diastolic volume (and therefore stroke volume and cardiac output) is to small changes in cardiac filling pressure (i.e., central venous pressure). In all physiological and pathological situations, cardiac filling pressure is a crucial factor that determines how well the cardiovascular system will be operating.

Mean Circulatory Filling Pressure

Imagine the heart arrested in diastole with no flow around the circuit shown in Figure 8–1. It will take a certain amount of blood just to fill the anatomical space contained by the systemic system without stretching any of its walls or developing any internal pressure. This amount is 3.56 L, as indicated by the total systemic circuit volume (V_0) in Table 8–1. Normally, however, the systemic circuit contains approximately 4.5 L of blood and is thus somewhat inflated. From the total systemic circuit compliance (C) given in Table 8–1, one can see that an extra 1000 mL of blood would result in an internal pressure of approximately 7 mm Hg (i.e., 1000 mL/140 mL/mm Hg). This theoretical pressure is called the *mean circulatory filling pressure* and is the actual pressure that would exist throughout the system in the absence of flow. The 2 major variables that affect mean circulatory filling pressure are the circulating blood volume and the state of the peripheral venous vessel tone. In the latter case, look at Figure 8–1 and imagine how constriction of the vessels of the large venous compartment (increasing venous tone) will significantly increase pressure throughout the system. In contrast, squeezing on arterioles (increasing arteriolar tone) will have a negligible effect on mean circulatory filling pressure because arterioles contain so

---

[1] The pulmonary circuit is not included in Figure 8–1 because it does not influence the major points to be discussed in this chapter. The primary leap of faith in this omission is that, because of the Starling law of the heart, changes in the end-diastolic volume of the *right* ventricle cause equal changes in the end-diastolic volume of the *left* ventricle.

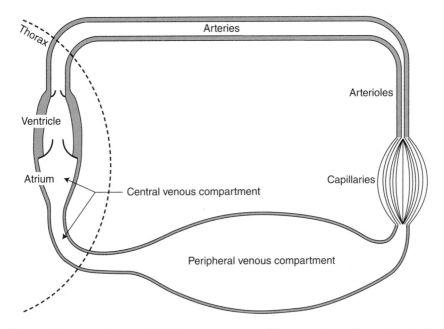

Figure 8–1. Major functionally distinct components of the systemic cardiovascular circuit.

little blood in any state. The other major components of the system (arteries and capillaries) do not actively change their volume.

Flow-Induced Distribution of Blood Volume and Pressure

The presence of flow around the circuit does not change the total volume of blood in the system or the mean circulatory filling pressure. The flow caused by cardiac pumping action does, however, tend to shift some of the blood volume from the

Table 8–1. Typical Properties of the Major Components of the Systemic Cardiovascular Circuit*

Compartment	V_0 (mL)	C (mL/mm Hg)	R (mm Hg/L/min)
Left ventricle in diastole	30	24	0
Arteries	600	2	1
Arterioles	100	0	13
Capillaries	250	0	5
Peripheral venous compartment	2500	110	1
Central venous compartment	80	4	0
Entire circuit	3560	140	20

C, compliance of compartment; R, resistance to flow through compartment; V_0, anatomical volume of compartment at zero pressure.
*Values are for a normal, young, resting 70-kg adult.

venous side of the circuit to the arterial side. This causes pressures on the arterial side to rise above the mean circulatory pressure, whereas pressures on the venous side fall below it. Because veins are approximately 50 times more compliant than arteries (Table 8–1), the flow-induced decrease in venous pressure is only approximately 1/50th as large as the accompanying increase in arterial pressure. Thus, flow or no flow, pressure in the peripheral venous compartment is normally quite close to the mean circulatory filling pressure.

CENTRAL VENOUS PRESSURE: AN INDICATOR OF CIRCULATORY STATUS

The cardiovascular system must adjust its operation continually to meet changing metabolic demands of the body. Because the cardiovascular system is a closed hydraulic loop, adjustments in any one part of the circuit will have pressure, flow, and volume effects throughout the circuit. Because of the critical influence of cardiac filling on cardiovascular function, the remainder of this chapter focuses on the factors that determine the pressure in the central venous compartment. In addition, the way in which measures of central venous pressure can provide clinically useful information about the state of the circulatory system is discussed.

The central venous compartment corresponds roughly to the volume enclosed by the right atrium and the great veins in the thorax. Blood *leaves* the central venous compartment by entering the right ventricle at a rate that is equal to the cardiac output. *Venous return*, in contrast, is by definition the rate at which blood returns to the thorax from the peripheral vascular beds and is thus the rate at which blood *enters* the central venous compartment. The important distinction between venous return *to* the central venous compartment and cardiac output *from* the central venous compartment is illustrated in Figure 8–2.

In any stable situation, venous return must equal cardiac output or blood would gradually accumulate in either the central venous compartment or the

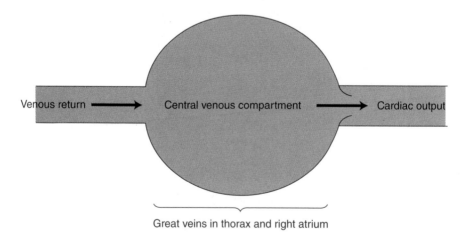

Great veins in thorax and right atrium

Figure 8–2. Distinction between cardiac output and venous return.

peripheral vasculature. However, there are often temporary differences between cardiac output and venous return. Whenever such differences exist, the volume of the central venous compartment must be changing. Because the central venous compartment is enclosed by elastic tissues, any change in central venous volume produces a corresponding change in central venous pressure.

As discussed in Chapter 3, the central venous pressure (i.e., cardiac filling pressure) has an extremely important *positive* influence on stroke volume, and therefore, cardiac output (the Starling law of the heart). As argued later, central venous pressure has an equally important *negative* effect on venous return. Thus, central venous pressure is always automatically driven to a value that makes cardiac output equal to venous return. The factors that determine central venous pressure in any given situation are discussed in the following section.

Influence of Central Venous Pressure on Venous Return

The important factors involved in the process of venous return can be summarized as shown in Figure 8–3A. Basically, venous return is blood flow from the peripheral venous compartment to the central venous compartment through converging vessels. Anatomically, the peripheral venous compartment is scattered throughout the systemic organs, but functionally, it can be viewed as a single vascular space that has a particular pressure (P_{PV}) at any instant of time. The normal operating pressure in the peripheral venous compartment is usually very close to the mean circulatory filling pressure. Moreover, the same factors that influence mean circulatory filling pressure have essentially equal influences on peripheral venous pressure. Thus, "peripheral venous pressure" can be viewed as essentially equivalent to "mean circulatory filling pressure." The blood flow rate between the peripheral venous compartment and the central venous compartment is governed by the basic flow equation ($\dot{Q} = \Delta P/R$), where ΔP is the pressure drop between the peripheral and central venous compartments and R is the small resistance associated with the peripheral veins. In the example in Figure 8–3, peripheral venous pressure is assumed to be 7 mm Hg. Thus, there will be no venous return when the central venous pressure (P_{CV}) is also 7 mm Hg, as shown in Figure 8–3B.

If the peripheral venous pressure remains at 7 mm Hg, decreasing central venous pressure will increase the pressure drop across the venous resistance and consequently cause an elevation in venous return. This relationship is summarized by the *venous function curve*, which shows how venous return increases as central venous pressure drops.[2] If central venous pressure reaches very low values and falls below the intrathoracic pressure, the veins in the thorax are compressed, which therefore tends to limit venous return. In the

---

[2] The slope of the venous function curve is determined by the value of the venous vascular resistance. Lowering the venous vascular resistance would tend to raise the venous function curve and make it steeper because more venous return would result for a given difference between P_{PV} and P_{CV}. However, if P_{PV} is 7 mm Hg, venous return will be 0 L/min when $P_{CV} = 7$ mm Hg at any level of venous vascular resistance ($\dot{Q} = \Delta P/R$). We have chosen to ignore the complicating issue of changes in venous vascular resistance because they do not affect the general conclusions to be drawn from the discussion of venous function curves.

A

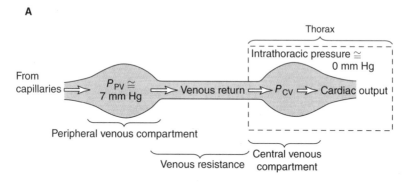

B

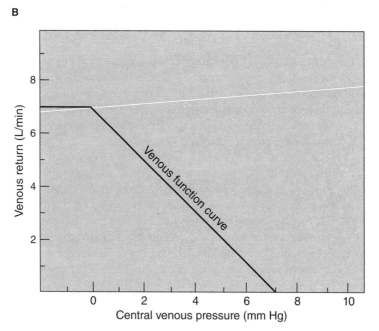

Figure 8–3. (**A**) Factors influencing venous return and (**B**) the venous function curve.

example in Figure 8–3, intrathoracic pressure is taken to be 0 mm Hg and the flat portion of the venous function curve indicates that lowering central venous pressure below 0 mm Hg produces no additional increase in venous return.

Just as a cardiac function curve shows how central venous pressure influences cardiac output, *a venous function curve shows how central venous pressure influences venous return.*[3]

---

[3] Graphic relationships are almost invariably plotted with the *independent* variable on the horizontal axis (abscissa) and the *dependent* variable on the vertical axis (ordinate) and they *must* be read in that sense. For example, Figure 8–3B says that increasing central venous pressure tends to cause decreased venous return. Figure 8–3B *does not* imply that increasing venous return will tend to lower central venous pressure.

Influence of Peripheral Venous Pressure on Venous Return

As can be deduced from Figure 8–3A, it is the pressure difference between the peripheral and central venous compartments that determines venous return. Therefore, an increase in peripheral venous pressure can be just as effective in increasing venous return as a drop in central venous pressure.

The 2 ways in which peripheral venous pressure can change were discussed in Chapter 6. First, because veins are elastic vessels, changes in the *volume* of blood contained within the peripheral veins alter the peripheral venous pressure. Moreover, because the veins are much more compliant than any other vascular segment, changes in circulating blood volume produce larger changes in the volume of blood in the veins than in any other vascular segment. For example, blood loss by hemorrhage or loss of body fluids through severe sweating, vomiting, or diarrhea decreases circulating blood volume and significantly reduces the volume of blood contained in the veins and thus decreases the peripheral venous pressure. Conversely, transfusion, fluid retention by the kidney, or transcapillary fluid reabsorption increase circulating blood volume and venous blood volume. Whenever circulating blood volume increases, so does peripheral venous pressure.

Recall from Chapter 7 that the second way that peripheral venous pressure can be altered is through changes in venous tone produced by increasing or decreasing the activity of sympathetic vasoconstrictor nerves supplying the venous smooth muscle. Peripheral venous pressure increases whenever the activity of sympathetic vasoconstrictor fibers in veins increases. In addition, an increase in any force compressing veins from the outside has the same effect on the pressure inside veins as an increase in venous tone. Thus, such things as muscle exercise and wearing elastic stockings tend to elevate peripheral venous pressure.

Whenever peripheral venous pressure is altered, the relationship between central venous pressure and venous return is also altered. For example, whenever peripheral venous pressure is elevated by increase in blood volume or by sympathetic stimulation, the venous function curve shifts upward and to the right (Figure 8–4). This phenomenon can be most easily understood by focusing first on the central venous pressure at which there will be no venous return. If peripheral venous pressure is 7 mm Hg, then venous return will be 0 L/min when central venous pressure is 7 mm Hg. If peripheral venous pressure is increased to 10 mm Hg, then considerable venous return will occur when central venous pressure is 7 mm Hg, and venous return will stop only when central venous pressure is raised to 10 mm Hg. Thus, increasing peripheral venous pressure shifts the whole venous function curve upward and to the right. By similar logic, decreased peripheral venous pressure caused by blood loss or decreased sympathetic vasoconstriction of peripheral veins shifts the venous function curve downward and to the left (Figure 8–4).

Determination of Cardiac Output and Venous Return by Central Venous Pressure

The significance of the fact that central venous pressure simultaneously affects both cardiac output and venous return can be best seen by plotting the cardiac

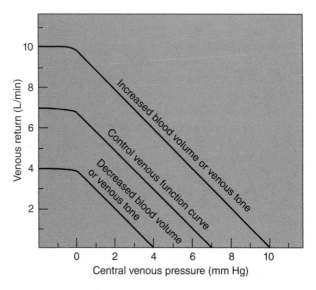

Figure 8–4. Effect of changes in blood volume and venous tone on venous function curves.

function curve and the venous function curve on the same graph, as shown in Figure 8–5.

Central venous pressure, as defined earlier, is the filling pressure of the right heart. Strictly speaking, this pressure directly affects only the stroke volume and output of the *right* heart pump. In most contexts, however, "cardiac output" implies

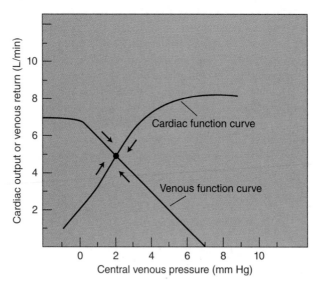

Figure 8–5. Interaction of cardiac output and venous return through central venous pressure.

the output of the *left* heart pump. How is it then, as we have previously implied, that central venous pressure (the filling pressure of the right side of the heart) profoundly affects the output of the left side of the heart? The short answer is that in the steady state, the right and left sides of the heart have equal outputs. (Because the right and left sides of the heart always beat with identical rates, this implies that their stroke volumes must be equal in the steady state.) The proper answer is that changes in central venous pressure automatically cause essentially parallel changes in the filling pressure of the left side of the heart (i.e., in left atrial pressure). Consider, for example, the following sequence of consequences that a small step increase in central venous pressure has on a heart that previously was in a steady state:

1. Increased central venous pressure.
2. Increased right ventricular stroke volume via the Starling law of the heart.
3. Increased output of the right side of the heart.
4. The right side of the heart output temporarily exceeds that of the left side of the heart.
5. As long as this imbalance exists, blood accumulates in the pulmonary vasculature and raises pulmonary venous and left atrial pressures.
6. Increased left atrial pressure increases left ventricular stroke volume via the Starling law.
7. Very quickly, a new steady state will be reached when left atrial pressure has risen sufficiently to make left ventricular stroke volume exactly equal to the increased right ventricular stroke volume.

The major conclusion here is that left atrial pressure will automatically change in the correct direction to match left ventricular stroke volume to the current right ventricular stroke volume. Consequently, it is usually an acceptable simplification to say that central venous pressure affects cardiac output as if the heart consisted only of a single pump.

Note that in Figure 8–5, cardiac output and venous return are equal (at 5 L/min) *only* when the central venous pressure is 2 mm Hg. If central venous pressure were to decrease to 0 mm Hg for any reason, cardiac output would fall (to 2 L/min) and venous return would increase (to 7 L/min). With a venous return of 7 L/min and a cardiac output of 2 L/min, the volume of the central venous compartment would necessarily increase, and this would produce a progressively increasing central venous pressure. In this manner, central venous pressure would return to the original level (2 mm Hg) in a very short time. Moreover, if central venous pressure were to increase from 2 to 4 mm Hg for any reason, venous return would decrease (to 3 L/min) and cardiac output would increase (to 7 L/min). This would quickly reduce the volume of blood in the central venous pool, and the central venous pressure would soon fall back to the original level. *The cardiovascular system automatically adjusts to operate at the point where the cardiac and venous function curves intersect.*

 Central venous pressure is always inherently driven to the value that makes cardiac output and venous return equal. Cardiac output and venous return always stabilize at the level where the cardiac function and venous function curves intersect.

To fulfill its homeostatic role in the body, the cardiovascular system must be able to alter its cardiac output. Recall from Chapter 3 that cardiac output is affected by more than just cardiac filling pressure and that at any moment the heart may be operating on any one of several cardiac function curves, depending on the existing level of cardiac sympathetic tone. The family of possible cardiac function curves may be plotted along with the family of possible venous function curves, as shown in Figure 8–6. At a particular moment, the existing influences on the heart dictate the cardiac function curve on which it is operating, and similarly, the existing influences on peripheral venous pressure dictate the particular venous function curve that applies. Thus, the influences on the heart and on the peripheral vasculature determine where the cardiac and venous function curves intersect and thus what the central venous pressure and cardiac output (and venous return) are in the steady state. In the intact cardiovascular system, cardiac output can rise only when the point of intersection of the cardiac and venous function curves is raised. *All changes in cardiac output are caused by either a shift in the cardiac function curve, a shift in the venous function curve, or both.*

The cardiac function and venous function curves are useful for understanding the complex interactions that occur in the intact cardiovascular system. With the help of Figure 8–7, let us consider, for example, what happens to the cardiovascular system when there is a significant loss of blood (hemorrhage). Assume that before the hemorrhage, sympathetic activity to the heart and peripheral vessels is normal, as is the blood volume. Therefore, cardiac output is related to central venous pressure, as indicated by the "normal" cardiac function curve in Figure 8–7.

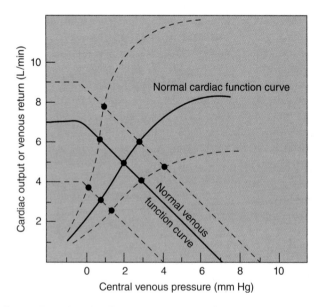

Figure 8–6. Families of cardiac function and venous function curves. Intersection points indicate equilibrium values for cardiac output, venous return, and central venous pressure under various conditions.

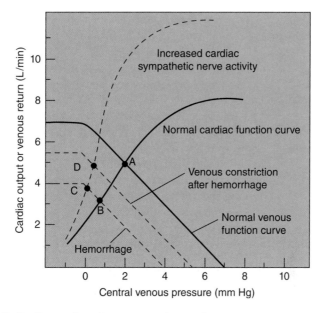

Figure 8–7. Cardiovascular adjustments to hemorrhage.

In addition, venous return is determined by central venous pressure, as indicated by the "normal" venous function curve shown. The normal cardiac and venous function curves intersect at point A, so cardiac output is 5 L/min and central venous pressure is 2 mm Hg in the normal state. When blood volume decreases because of hemorrhage, the peripheral venous pressure falls, and the venous function curve is shifted to the left. In the absence of any cardiovascular responses, the cardio-vascular system must switch its operation to point B because this is now the point at which the cardiac function curve and the new venous function curve inter-sect. This automatically occurs because, at the moment of blood loss, the venous function curve is shifted to the left and venous return falls below cardiac output at the central venous pressure of 2 mm Hg. This is what leads to the fall in the central venous compartment's volume and pressure that causes the shift in opera-tion from point A to point B. Note by comparing points A and B in Figure 8–7 that blood loss itself lowers cardiac output and central venous pressure by shifting the venous function curve. In going from point A to point B, cardiac output falls solely because of decreased filling pressure and the Starling law of the heart.

Subnormal cardiac output evokes cardiovascular compensatory mechanisms to bring cardiac output back to more normal levels. One of these compensatory mechanisms is an increase in the activity of cardiac sympathetic nerves, which, as discussed in Chapter 3, shifts the heart's operation to a cardiac function curve that is higher than normal. The effect of increasing cardiac sympathetic activity is illustrated by a shift in cardiovascular operation from point B to point C. The increased cardiac sympathetic nerve activity increases cardiac output (from 3 to 4 L/min) but causes a further decrease in central venous pressure. This drop in central venous pressure occurs because points B and C lie on the same venous function curve. *Cardiac* sympathetic nerves do not affect the venous function curve.[4]

An additional compensatory mechanism evoked by blood loss is increased activity of the sympathetic nerves leading to veins. Recall that this raises peripheral venous pressure and causes a rightward shift of the venous function curve. Therefore, increased sympathetic activity to veins tends to shift the venous function curve, originally lowered by blood loss, back toward normal. Because of the increased peripheral venous tone and the shift to a more normal venous function curve, the cardiovascular operation shifts from point C to point D in Figure 8–7. Thus, peripheral venous constriction increases cardiac output by raising central venous pressure and moving the heart's operation upward along a fixed cardiac function curve. It must be pointed out that separating the response to hemorrhage into distinct, progressive steps (i.e., A to B to C to D) is only a conceptualization for appreciating the individual effects of the different processes involved. In reality, the reflex venous and cardiac responses occur simultaneously and so quickly that they will easily keep up with the blood loss as it occurs. Thus, the actual course of a patient's net response to hemorrhage would follow nearly a straight line from point A to point D.

In summary, point D illustrates that near-normal cardiac output can be sustained in the face of blood loss by the combined effect of peripheral and cardiac adjustments. Hemorrhage is only one of an almost infinite variety of disturbances to the cardiovascular system. Plots such as those shown in Figure 8–7 are very useful for understanding the many disturbances to the cardiovascular system and the ways in which they may be compensated.

Clinical Implications of Abnormal Central Venous Pressures

Although, in the clinical situation, there is no way to determine the position of either cardiac function or venous function curves, important information about the patient's circulatory status can be obtained from measures of central venous pressure. From what has been presented in this chapter, it is possible to conclude that a patient with *abnormally high* central venous pressure must have a depressed cardiac function curve, a right-shifted venous function curve, or both. As will be discussed in Chapter 11, very high central venous pressures are a hallmark of patients with congestive heart failure because they have the combination of dysfunctional heart muscle (depressed cardiac function curve) *and* excessive fluid volume (right-shifted venous function curve).[5] *Abnormally low* central venous pressures, on the other hand, could theoretically be caused by either an elevated cardiac function curve or a left-shifted venous function curve. The clinical reality is that abnormally low central venous pressures are

---

[4] Venous return is higher at point C than at point B, but the venous function *curve* has not shifted.

[5] One notable exception to the conclusion that high central venous pressure implies either depressed cardiac function or excess fluid volume is the example of *cardiac tamponade*. In this case, fluid accumulating in the pericardial sac prevents adequate filling of the ventricles and central venous pressure rises.

almost always the result of a left shift of the venous function curve, caused by either low blood volume or lack of venous tone.

Rough estimates of a patient's central venous pressure can be obtained quite easily by observing the external jugular veins. Because the force of gravity tends to keep veins in the head and neck collapsed when an individual is in an upright position, there should be no distention (or retrograde pulsations from atrial contractions) in these neck veins. Conversely, when an individual is fully recumbent, the neck veins should be full and pulsations should be easily detected. If a healthy individual is placed in a semi-recumbent position so that the external jugular veins are positioned at ~7 cm above the right atrium, the point between the collapsed venous segment and the filled segment can usually be visualized.[6] Abnormally high central venous pressures will be associated with neck vein distention at a higher level (perhaps even when the patient is upright).

Because of its diagnostic value in critical care situations, central venous pressure is often monitored continuously via a catheter that is inserted in a peripheral vein and advanced centrally until its tip is in the central venous compartment (i.e., near or in the right atrium). In some situations, it is desirable to assess *left atrial* pressure, which is the filling pressure for the left side of the heart. This is commonly done with a specialized flow-directed venous catheter that uses a small inflatable balloon at its tip to drag it with the blood flow through the right ventricle and pulmonic valve into the pulmonary artery. The balloon is then deflated, and the cannula is advanced further until it wedges into a terminal branch of the pulmonary vasculature. The *pulmonary wedge pressure* recorded at this junction provides a useful estimate of left atrial pressure.

PERSPECTIVES

The junction of the venous side of the circulation with the heart is a critical site of functional integration between the heart and the vasculature. As previously stated, flow through the circulation depends upon the pressure difference across the circulation and the vascular resistance. A primary determinant of the arterial pressure is the cardiac output. The 2 determinants of the cardiac output are the heart rate and the stroke volume. A major determinant of the stroke volume is ventricular filling, which, as described in this chapter, is a function of the central venous pressure. Thus, we come back to strongly emphasize the original statement in this chapter that a change in any one variable will have ripple effects throughout the system, and the alert clinician will have to discern the primary disturbances from secondary consequences.

---

[6] The astute reader will note that 7-cm H_2O is equal to approximately 5 mm Hg. This is significantly higher than the 2-mm Hg central venous pressure we have used for argument elsewhere in this text. As will be discussed in Chapter 10, gravity causes body position-dependent shifts of blood volume between the peripheral and central venous pools. Thus, central venous pressure is normally higher in the recumbent than in the upright position.

KEY CONCEPTS

Mean circulatory filling pressure is a theoretical measure of pressure in the systemic circuit when flow is stopped and is influenced primarily by blood volume and peripheral venous tone.

Central venous pressure has a negative influence on venous return that can be illustrated graphically as a venous function curve.

Peripheral venous pressure has a positive influence on venous return and can be elevated by increased blood volume and/or increased venous tone.

Because of its opposing influences on cardiac output and venous return, central venous pressure automatically assumes a value that makes cardiac output and venous return equal.

Central venous pressure gives clinically relevant information about circulatory status.

Central venous pressure can be estimated noninvasively by noting the fullness of a patient's jugular veins.

STUDY QUESTIONS

8–1. Which of the following will decrease the mean circulatory filling pressure?

a. Increased circulating blood volume

b. Decreased arteriolar tone

c. Increased venous tone

8–2. What determines central venous pressure?

8–3. According to the Starling law, cardiac output always decreases when central venous pressure decreases. True or false?

8–4. In a steady state, venous return will be greater than cardiac output when

a. peripheral venous pressure is higher than normal.

b. blood volume is higher than normal.

c. cardiac sympathetic nerve activity is lower than normal.

8–5. What approaches might a physician logically pursue to lower a patient's cardiac preload?

8–6. In a severely dehydrated patient, you might expect to find

  a. a depressed cardiac function curve.

  b. an increased mean circulatory filling pressure.

  c. an increased central venous pressure.

  d. distended jugular veins.

  e. decreased cardiac output.

8–7. If you gave a blood transfusion to a patient who had recently experienced a severe hemorrhage, you would expect

  a. to expand arterial volume.

  b. To expand venous volume.

  c. to decrease central venous pressure.

  d. to decrease the mean circulatory filling pressure.

  e. to reduce cardiac output.

8–8. Which of the following would directly (by themselves in the absence of any compensatory responses) tend to decrease central venous (cardiac filling) pressure?

  a. Increased sympathetic nerve activity to only the heart

  b. Increased parasympathetic nerve activity to only the heart

  c. Increased blood volume

  d. Decreased total peripheral resistance

  e. Immersion in water up to the waist

Regulation of Arterial Pressure

9

OBJECTIVES

The student understands the primary mechanisms involved in the short-term regulation of arterial pressure:

▶ *Identifies the sensory receptors, afferent pathways, central integrating centers, efferent pathways, and effector organs that participate in the arterial baroreceptor reflex.*

▶ *States the location of the arterial baroreceptors and describes their operation.*

▶ *Describes how changes in the afferent input from arterial baroreceptors influence the activity of the sympathetic and parasympathetic preganglionic fibers.*

▶ *Diagrams the chain of events that are initiated by the arterial baroreceptor reflex to compensate for a change in arterial pressure.*

▶ *Describes how inputs to the medullary cardiovascular center from cardiopulmonary baroreceptors, arterial and central chemoreceptors, receptors in skeletal muscle, the cerebral cortex, and the hypothalamus influence sympathetic activity, parasympathetic activity, and mean arterial pressure.*

▶ *Describes and indicates the mechanisms involved in the Bezold–Jarisch reflex, the cerebral ischemic response, the Cushing reflex, the alerting reaction, blushing, vasovagal syncope, the dive reflex, and the cardiovascular responses to emotion and pain.*

The student comprehends the role of the kidney in long-term arterial pressure regulation:

▶ *Describes baroreceptor adaptation.*

▶ *Describes the influence of changes in body fluid volume on arterial pressure and diagrams the steps involved in this process.*

▶ *Indicates the mechanisms whereby altered arterial pressure alters glomerular filtration rate and renal tubular function to influence urinary output.*

▶ *Describes how mean arterial pressure is adjusted in the long term to that which causes fluid output rate to equal fluid intake rate.*

Arterial pressure is an important variable in the cardiovascular system because it is the driving force that causes blood circulation in the first place. With zero arterial pressure, there would be no flow through any organ and, at the other extreme, with high arterial pressure, there is an excessive workload on the heart and potential injury of arterial vessels.

Consequently, multiple mechanisms exist for regulating mean arterial pressure (MAP) to a normal value of about 100 mm Hg.

Despite the clinical importance of a person's arterial pressure, it is best remembered that the single most important requirement for proper operation of the cardiovascular system is to provide adequate perfusion of all tissues in the body at all times. At the local level, this is accomplished by regulating *local* vascular resistance to adjust blood flow to meet local metabolic needs. Because of the parallel arrangement of blood flow to body organs, the system-wide consequence of these individual changes in local vascular resistances is a change in *total* peripheral resistance (TPR). (For example, when a person is exercising strenuously, TPR is roughly one-third that at rest.) For MAP to stay constant, the heart must respond to changes in TPR by making reciprocal changes in cardiac output (CO) via adjustments in its heart rate (HR) and stroke volume (SV) (CO = HR × SV). Thus, how well arterial pressure is regulated depends primarily on how well the heart reacts to changes in TPR.

Because MAP = CO × TPR, system-wide adjustments in TPR are sometimes initiated to participate in the regulation of MAP. Indeed, such adjustments are very important in pathological situations like blood loss, wherein the capacity of the heart to produce CO is compromised. Looking at the big picture, it seems to make little sense to restrict organ blood flow (via increased TPR) to create adequate arterial pressure when the sole purpose of the system is to produce adequate organ blood flow. In fact, to prevent damage of susceptible organs, the body initiates various mechanisms involving changes in blood volume (which will influence cardiac output) to adjust for long-term regulation of arterial pressure.

Arterial pressure is continuously monitored by various sensors located within the body. Whenever arterial pressure varies from normal, multiple reflex responses are initiated, which cause the adjustments in cardiac output, and TPR needed to return arterial pressure to its normal value. In the short term (seconds to minutes), these adjustments are brought about by changes in the activity of the autonomic nerves leading to the heart and peripheral vessels. In the long term (hours to days), other mechanisms such as blood volume adjustments involving renal mechanisms for fluid regulation play an increasingly important role in the control of arterial pressure. The short- and long-term regulations of arterial pressure are discussed in this chapter.

SHORT-TERM REGULATION OF ARTERIAL PRESSURE

Arterial Baroreceptor Reflex

  The *arterial baroreceptor reflex* is the single most important mechanism providing short-term regulation of arterial pressure. Recall that the usual components of a reflex pathway include sensory receptors, afferent pathways, integrating centers in the central nervous system (CNS), efferent pathways, and effector organs. As shown in Figure 9–1, the efferent pathways of the arterial baroreceptor reflex are the cardiovascular sympathetic and cardiac parasympathetic nerves. The effector organs are the heart and peripheral blood vessels.

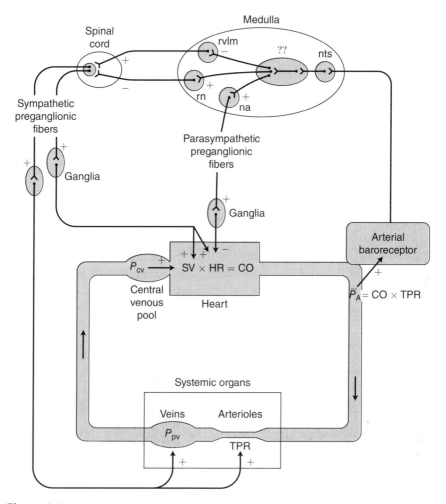

Figure 9–1. Components of the arterial baroreceptor reflex pathway. nts, nucleus tractus solitarius; rvlm, rostral ventrolateral medullary group; rn, raphé nucleus; na, nucleus ambiguus; ??, incompletely mapped integration pathways that may also involve structures outside the medulla.

Efferent Pathways

Previous chapters have discussed many actions of the sympathetic and parasympathetic nerves leading to the heart and blood vessels. For both systems, *postganglionic fibers*, whose cell bodies are in ganglia outside the CNS, form the terminal link to the heart and vessels. The influences of these post-ganglionic fibers on key cardiovascular variables are summarized in Figure 9–1.

The activity of the terminal postganglionic fibers of the autonomic nervous system is determined by the activity of *preganglionic fibers* whose cell bodies lie within the CNS. In the sympathetic pathways, the cell bodies of the preganglionic fibers are located within the spinal cord. These preganglionic neurons have spontaneous activity that is modulated by excitatory and inhibitory inputs, which arise from centers in the brainstem and descend in distinct *excitatory* and *inhibitory* spinal pathways. In the parasympathetic system, the cell bodies of the preganglionic fibers are located within the brainstem. Their spontaneous activity is modulated by inputs from adjacent centers in the brainstem.

AFFERENT PATHWAYS

Sensory receptors, called *arterial baroreceptors*, are found in abundance in the walls of the aorta and carotid arteries. Major concentrations of these receptors are found near the arch of the aorta (the *aortic baroreceptors*) and at the bifurcation of the common carotid artery into the internal and external carotid arteries on either side of the neck (the *carotid sinus baroreceptors*). The receptors themselves are mechanoreceptors that sense arterial pressure indirectly from the degree of stretch of the elastic arterial walls. In general, *increased stretch causes an increased action potential generation rate by the arterial baroreceptors.* Baroreceptors sense not only absolute stretch but also the rate of change of stretch. For this reason, both the MAP and the arterial pulse pressure affect baroreceptor firing rate, as indicated in Figure 9–2. The dashed curve in Figure 9–2 shows how baroreceptor firing rate is affected by different levels of a steady arterial pressure. The solid curve in Figure 9–2 indicates how baroreceptor firing rate is affected by the mean value of a pulsatile arterial pressure. Note that in the presence of pulsations (that of course are normal), the baroreceptor firing rate increases at any given level of MAP. Note also that changes in MAP near the normal value of 100 mm Hg produce the largest changes in baroreceptor discharge rate.

If arterial pressure remains elevated over a period of several days for some reason, the arterial baroreceptor firing rate will gradually return toward normal. Thus, arterial baroreceptors are said to *adapt* to long-term changes in arterial pressure. For this reason, the arterial baroreceptor reflex is not sufficient to serve as a sole mechanism for the long-term regulation of arterial pressure.[1]

Action potentials generated by the carotid sinus baroreceptors travel through the carotid sinus nerves (the Hering's nerves), which join with the glossopharyngeal nerves (IX cranial nerves) before entering the CNS. Afferent fibers from the aortic baroreceptors run to the CNS in the vagus nerves (X cranial nerves). (The vagus nerves contain both afferent and efferent fibers, including, for example, the parasympathetic efferent fibers to the heart.)

CENTRAL INTEGRATION

Much of the central integration involved in reflex regulation of the cardiovascular system occurs in the medulla oblongata in what are traditionally referred to as the *medullary cardiovascular centers*. The neural

---

[1] In the presence of some forms of chronic hypertension, recent work suggests that carotid sinus baroreceptors may continue to fire at a chronically elevated rate but alterations in mechanisms within the central nervous system override the suppressive effects of baroreceptor input on sympathetic neural output to sustain the hypertension.

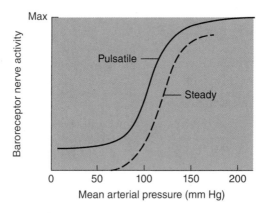

Figure 9-2. The effect of mean arterial pressure on baroreceptor nerve activity.

interconnections between the diffuse structures in this area and higher centers are complex and not completely mapped. Moreover, these structures appear to serve multiple functions including respiratory control, for example. What is known with a fair degree of certainty is where the cardiovascular afferent and efferent pathways enter and leave the medulla. For example, as indicated in Figure 9–1, the afferent sensory information from the arterial baroreceptors enters the medullary *nucleus tractus solitarius*, where it is relayed via polysynaptic pathways to other structures in the medulla (and higher brain centers, such as the hypothalamus, as well). The cell bodies of the efferent vagal parasympathetic cardiac nerves are located primarily in the medullary *nucleus ambiguus*. The sympathetic autonomic efferent information leaves the medulla predominantly from the *rostral ventrolateral medulla* group of neurons (via an excitatory spinal pathway) or the *raphé nucleus* (via an inhibitory spinal pathway). The intermediate processes involved in the actual integration of the sensory information into appropriate sympathetic and parasympathetic responses are not well understood at present. Although much of this integration takes place within the medulla, higher centers such as the hypothalamus are probably involved as well. In the context of this presentation, knowing the details of the integration process is not as important as appreciating the overall effects that changes in arterial baroreceptor activity (input) have on the activities of parasympathetic and sympathetic cardiovascular nerves (output).

Several functionally important points about the central control of the autonomic cardiovascular nerves are illustrated in Figure 9–1. The major external neural influence on the cardiovascular centers comes from the arterial baroreceptors. Because the arterial baroreceptors are active at normal arterial pressures, they supply a tonic input to the central integration centers.

As indicated in Figure 9–1, the integration process is such that increased input from the arterial baroreceptors tends to simultaneously (1) inhibit the activity of the spinal sympathetic excitatory tract, (2) stimulate the activity of the spinal sympathetic inhibitory tract, and (3) stimulate the activity of parasympathetic preganglionic nerves. Thus, an increase in the arterial baroreceptor discharge rate (caused by increased arterial pressure) causes a decrease in the tonic activity of cardiovascular sympathetic nerves and a simultaneous increase in the tonic activity of cardiac parasympathetic nerves. Conversely, decreased arterial pressure causes increased sympathetic and decreased parasympathetic activity.

OPERATION OF THE ARTERIAL BARORECEPTOR REFLEX

The arterial baroreceptor reflex is a continuously operating control system that automatically adjusts to prevent primary disturbances on the heart and/or vessels from causing large changes in MAP. The arterial baroreceptor reflex mechanism acts to regulate arterial pressure in a *negative feedback* manner that is analogous in many ways to the manner in which a thermostatically controlled home heating system operates to regulate inside temperature despite disturbances such as changes in the weather or open windows.[2]

Figure 9–3 shows many events in the arterial baroreceptor reflex pathway that occur in response to a disturbance that decreases MAP. All the events shown in Figure 9–3 have already been discussed, and each should be carefully examined (and reviewed if necessary) at this point because a great many of the interactions that are essential to understanding cardiovascular physiology are summarized in this figure.

Note that in Figure 9–3 the overall response of the arterial baroreceptor reflex to the primary disturbance of *decreased* MAP is a reflex *increase* in MAP (i.e., the response tends to counteract the disturbance). A disturbance of increased MAP would elicit events exactly opposite to those shown in Figure 9–3 and produce the response of decreased MAP; again, the response tends to counteract the disturbance. The homeostatic benefits of the reflex action should be apparent.

One should recall that nervous control of vessels is more important in some areas such as the kidney, the skin, and the splanchnic organs than in the brain and the heart muscle. Thus, the reflex response to a fall in arterial pressure may, for example, include a significant increase in renal vascular resistance and a decrease in renal blood flow without changing the cerebral vascular resistance or blood flow. The peripheral vascular adjustments associated with the arterial baroreceptor reflex take place primarily in organs with strong sympathetic vascular control.

Other Cardiovascular Reflexes and Responses

Seemingly despite the arterial baroreceptor reflex mechanism, large and rapid changes in MAP do occur in certain physiological and pathological situations. These reactions are caused by influences on the medullary

---

[2] In this analogy, arterial pressure is likened to temperature; the heart is the generator of pressure as the furnace is the generator of heat; dilated arterioles dissipate arterial pressure like open windows cause heat loss; the arterial baroreceptors monitor arterial pressure as the sensor of a thermostat monitors temperature; and the electronics of the thermostat controls the furnace as the medullary cardiovascular centers regulate the operation of the heart. Because home thermostats do not usually regulate the operation of the windows, there is no analogy to the reflex medullary control of arterioles. The pressure that the arterial baroreflex strives to maintain is analogous to the temperature setting on the thermostat dial.

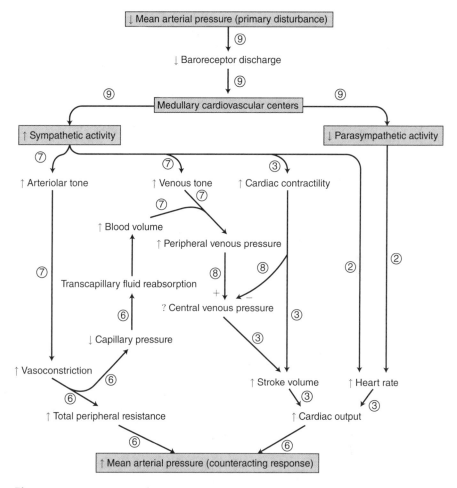

Figure 9–3. Immediate cardiovascular adjustments caused by a decrease in arterial blood pressure. Circled numbers indicate the chapter in which each interaction was previously discussed.

cardiovascular centers *other* than those from the arterial baroreceptors. As outlined in the following sections, these inputs on the medullary cardiovascular centers arise from many types of peripheral and central receptors and from "higher centers" in the CNS such as the hypothalamus and the cortex.

The analogy was made earlier that the arterial baroreceptor reflex operates to control arterial pressure somewhat as a home heating system acts to control inside temperature. Such a system automatically acts to counteract changes in temperature caused by such things as an open window or a dirty furnace. It does not, however, resist changes in indoor temperature caused by someone's resetting of the thermostat dial—in fact, the basic temperature-regulating mechanisms cooperate wholeheartedly in adjusting the temperature to the new desired value.

The temperature setting on a home thermostat's dial has a useful conceptual analogy in cardiovascular physiology often referred to as the *"set point"* for arterial pressure. *Most (but not all) of the influences that are about to be discussed influence arterial pressure as if they changed the arterial baroreceptor reflex's set point for pressure regulation.* Consequently, the arterial baroreceptor reflex does not resist most of these pressure disturbances but assists in producing them.

REFLEXES FROM RECEPTORS IN THE HEART AND LUNGS

A host of mechanoreceptors and chemoreceptors that can elicit reflex cardiovascular responses have been identified in atria, ventricles, coronary vessels, and lungs. The role of these *cardiopulmonary receptors* in neurohumoral control of the cardiovascular system is, in most cases, incompletely understood, but they are likely to be importantly involved in regulating blood volume and body fluid balance.

One general function that the cardiopulmonary receptors perform is sensing the pressure (or volume) in the atria and the central venous pool. Increased central venous pressure and volume cause stretch-activation of these low-pressure receptors, increase afferent activity to the medullary centers, and elicit a reflex decrease in sympathetic activity. Decreased central venous pressure produces the opposite response. In addition to the already described influence of altered sympathetic activity on arterial pressure, these reflexes evoked by changes in low-pressure receptor activity have a great influence on renal function and blood volume regulation as will be discussed in the following sections. Whatever the details, it is clear that cardiopulmonary baroreflexes normally exert a tonic inhibitory influence on sympathetic activity and play an arguably important, but not yet completely defined, role in normal cardiovascular regulation.[3]

CHEMORECEPTOR REFLEXES

Hypoxia (low Po_2), hypercapnia (high Pco_2), and/or acidosis (low pH) levels in the arterial blood cause reflex increases in respiratory rate *and* MAP. These responses appear to be a result of increased activity of *arterial chemoreceptors*, located in the carotid bodies at the bifurcation of the common carotid arteries and the aortic bodies found in the arch of the aorta. *Central chemoreceptors*, located at a variety of sites within the CNS respond to hypercapnia and acidification of the cerebrospinal fluid to regulate respiratory patterns and also influence autonomic output to the heart and vasculature. Chemoreceptors probably play little role in the normal regulation of arterial pressure because arterial blood Po_2 and Pco_2 are normally held very nearly constant by respiratory control mechanisms.

---

[3] Certain other reflexes originating from receptors in the cardiopulmonary region have been described that may be important in specific pathological situations. For example, the *Bezold–Jarisch* reflex that involves marked bradycardia and hypotension is elicited by application of strong stimuli to coronary vessel (or myocardial) chemoreceptors concentrated primarily in the posterior wall of the left ventricle. Activation of this reflex causes certain myocardial infarction patients to present with bradycardia instead of the expected tachycardia.

An extremely strong reaction called the *cerebral ischemic response* is triggered by inadequate brain blood flow (ischemia) and can produce a more intense sympathetic vasoconstriction and cardiac stimulation than is elicited by any other influence on the cardiovascular control centers. Presumably, the cerebral ischemic response is initiated by chemoreceptors located within the CNS. However, if cerebral blood flow is severely inadequate for several minutes, the cerebral ischemic response wanes and is replaced by marked loss of sympathetic activity. Presumably, this situation results when function of the nerve cells in the cardiovascular centers becomes directly depressed by the unfavorable chemical conditions in the cerebrospinal fluid.

Whenever intracranial pressure is increased—for example, by tumor growth or trauma-induced bleeding within the rigid cranium—there is a parallel rise in arterial pressure. This is called the *Cushing reflex* and is a variant of the cerebral ischemic response. It can cause a MAP of more than 200 mm Hg in severe cases of intracranial pressure elevation. The obvious benefit of the Cushing reflex is that it prevents collapse of cranial vessels and thus preserves adequate brain blood flow in the face of large increases in intracranial pressure. The mechanisms responsible for the Cushing reflex are not fully understood but seem to involve central (CNS) chemoreceptors reacting to consequences of reduced cerebral circulation producing very strong sympathetic activation. A major increase in total peripheral vascular resistance occurs. The early phase of the Cushing reflex often includes tachycardia, whereas the late (and more dangerous) phase of this reflex is accompanied by bradycardia (presumably resulting from elevated reflex vagal activity from the arterial baroreceptor input).

REFLEXES FROM RECEPTORS IN EXERCISING SKELETAL MUSCLE

Reflex tachycardia and increased arterial pressure can be elicited by stimulation of certain afferent fibers from the skeletal muscle. These pathways may be activated by chemoreceptors responding to muscle ischemia, which occurs with strong, sustained static (isometric) exercise. This input may contribute to the marked increase in blood pressure that accompanies such isometric efforts. It is uncertain as to what extent this reflex contributes to the cardiovascular responses to dynamic (rhythmic) muscle exercise.

CENTRAL COMMAND

The term *central command* is used to imply an input from the cerebral cortex to lower brain centers during voluntary muscle exercise. The concept is that the same cortical drives that initiate somatomotor (skeletal muscle) activity also simultaneously initiate cardiovascular (and respiratory) adjustments appropriate to support that activity. In the absence of any other obvious causes, central command is at present the best explanation as to why both MAP and respiration increase during voluntary exercise.

THE DIVE REFLEX

Aquatic animals respond to diving with a remarkable bradycardia and intense vasoconstriction in all systemic organs except the brain and the heart.

The response serves to allow prolonged submersion by limiting the rate of oxygen use and by directing blood flow to essential organs. A similar but less dramatic dive reflex can be elicited in humans by simply immersing the face in water. (Note: Cold water enhances the response.) The response involves the unusual combination of bradycardia produced by enhanced cardiac parasympathetic activity and peripheral vasoconstriction caused by enhanced sympathetic activity. This is a rare exception to the general rule that sympathetic and parasympathetic nerves are activated in reciprocal fashion. The dive reflex is sometimes used clinically to reflexively activate cardiac parasympathetic nerves for the purpose of interrupting atrial tachyarrhythmias.

Another, but unrelated, clinical technique for activating parasympathetic nerves to interrupt atrial tachyarrhythmias is called *carotid massage*. In essence, massage of the neck is done to cause physical deformation of the carotid sinuses and "trick" them into sending a "high-pressure" alarm to the medullary control centers.

CARDIOVASCULAR RESPONSES ASSOCIATED WITH EMOTION AND STRESS

Cardiovascular responses are frequently associated with certain acute states of emotion and/or stress. These responses originate in the cerebral cortex and reach the medullary cardiovascular centers through corticohypothalamic pathways. The least complicated of these responses is the *blushing* that is often detectable in individuals with lightly pigmented skin during states of embarrassment. The blushing response involves a loss of sympathetic vasoconstrictor activity *only* to particular cutaneous vessels, and this produces the blushing by allowing engorgement of the cutaneous venous sinuses.

Excitement or a sense of danger often elicits a complex behavioral pattern called the *alerting reaction* (also called the "defense" or "fight or flight" response). The alerting reaction involves a host of responses such as pupillary dilation and increased skeletal muscle tenseness that are generally appropriate preparations for some form of intense physical activity. The cardiovascular component of the alerting reaction is an increase in blood pressure caused by a general increase in cardiovascular sympathetic nervous activity and a decrease in cardiac parasympathetic activity. Centers in the *posterior hypothalamus* are presumed to be involved in the alerting reaction because many of the components of this multifaceted response can be experimentally reproduced by electrical stimulation of this area. The general cardiovascular effects are mediated via hypothalamic communications with the medullary cardiovascular centers.

Some individuals respond to acute situations of extreme stress by fainting, a situation referred to clinically as *vasovagal syncope*. The loss of consciousness is due to decreased cerebral blood flow that is itself produced by a sudden dramatic loss of arterial blood pressure that, in turn, occurs as a result of a sudden loss of sympathetic tone and a simultaneous large increase in parasympathetic tone and decrease in the HR. The influences on the medullary cardiovascular centers that produce vasovagal syncope appear to come from the cortex via depressor centers in the *anterior hypothalamus*. It has been suggested that vasovagal syncope is analogous to the "playing dead" response to peril used by some animals.

Fortunately, unconsciousness (combined with becoming horizontal) seems to quickly remove this serious disturbance to the normal mechanisms of arterial pressure control in humans.

Chronic mental stress (such as may be part of chronic anxiety or depression) can also be associated with altered autonomic and endocrine status and have significant cardiovascular consequences. In these cases, central neural pathways involving the cortex, limbic system, amygdala, and the hypothalamus/pituitary/adrenal axis may be involved.

The extent to which cardiovascular variables, in particular blood pressure, are normally affected by acute or chronic emotional or stressful states is currently a topic of extreme interest and considerable research. As yet, the answer is unclear. However, the therapeutic value of being able to learn to consciously reduce one's blood pressure would be incalculable.

REFLEX RESPONSES TO PAIN

Pain can have either a positive or a negative influence on arterial pressure. Generally, superficial, or cutaneous pain causes a rise in blood pressure in a manner similar to that associated with the alerting response and perhaps over many of the same pathways. Deep pain from receptors in the viscera or joints, however, often causes a cardiovascular response similar to that which accompanies vasovagal syncope, that is, decreased sympathetic tone, increased parasympathetic tone, and a serious decrease in blood pressure. This response may contribute to the state of shock that often accompanies crushing injuries and/or joint displacement.

TEMPERATURE REGULATION REFLEXES

Certain special cardiovascular reflexes that involve the control of skin blood flow have evolved as part of the body temperature regulation mechanisms. Dilation of cutaneous vessels promotes heat loss (as long as the environmental temperature is below the body temperature). Temperature regulation responses are controlled primarily by the hypothalamus, which can operate through the cardiovascular centers to discretely control the sympathetic activity to regulate vasoconstriction of cutaneous vessels and thus skin blood flow. The sympathetic activity of cutaneous vessels is extremely responsive to changes in hypothalamic temperature. Measurable changes in cutaneous blood flow result from changes in hypothalamic temperature of tenths of a degree Celsius.

Cutaneous vessels are influenced by reflexes involved in both arterial pressure regulation and temperature regulation. When the appropriate cutaneous vascular responses for temperature regulation and pressure regulation are contradictory, as they are, for example, during strenuous exercise, then the temperature-regulating influences on cutaneous blood vessels usually prevail.

Summary

Most of the influences on the medullary cardiovascular centers that have been discussed in the preceding sections are summarized in Figure 9–4. This figure is

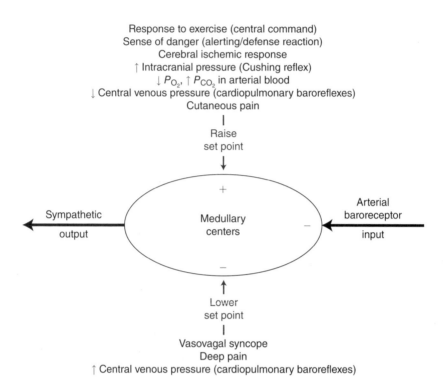

Response to exercise (central command)
Sense of danger (alerting/defense reaction)
Cerebral ischemic response
↑ Intracranial pressure (Cushing reflex)
↓ P_{O_2}, ↑ P_{CO_2} in arterial blood
↓ Central venous pressure (cardiopulmonary baroreflexes)
Cutaneous pain

Raise
set point

+

Sympathetic
output

Medullary
centers

−

Arterial
baroreceptor
input

−

Lower
set point

Vasovagal syncope
Deep pain
↑ Central venous pressure (cardiopulmonary baroreflexes)

Figure 9–4. Summary of the factors that influence the set point of the arterial baroreceptor reflex.

intended first to reemphasize that the arterial baroreceptors normally and continually supply the major input to the medullary centers. The arterial baroreceptor input is shown as inhibitory because an increase in arterial baroreceptor firing rate results in a decrease in sympathetic output. (Decreased sympathetic output should be taken to also imply a simultaneous increase in parasympathetic output that is not shown in this figure.)

As indicated in Figure 9–4, the *nonarterial baroreceptor influences* on the medullary cardiovascular centers fall into two categories: (1) those that *increase* arterial pressure by raising the set point for the arterial baroreceptor reflex and thus cause an increase in sympathetic activity and (2) those that *decrease* arterial pressure by lowering the set point for the arterial baroreceptor reflex and thus cause a decrease in sympathetic activity. Note that certain responses that have been discussed are not included in Figure 9–4. The complex combination of stimuli involved in the dive reflex causes simultaneous sympathetic and parasympathetic activation and cannot be simply classified as either pressure raising or pressure lowering. Also, temperature stimuli that discretely affect cutaneous vessels, but not general cardiovascular sympathetic and parasympathetic activity, have not been included in Figure 9–4.

The nonarterial baroreceptor influences shown in Figure 9–4 may be viewed as disturbances in the cardiovascular system that act on the medullary cardiovascular centers as opposed to disturbances that act on the heart and vessels. These disturbances cause sympathetic activity and arterial pressure to change in the *same direction*. Recall from the discussion of the arterial baroreceptor reflex that cardiovascular disturbances that act on the heart or vessels (such as blood loss or heart failure) produce *reciprocal* changes in arterial pressure and sympathetic activity. These facts are often useful in the clinical diagnoses of blood pressure abnormalities. For example, patients commonly present in the physician's office with high blood pressure in combination with elevated HR (implying elevated sympathetic activity). These same-direction changes in arterial pressure and sympathetic activity suggest that the problem lies not in the periphery but rather with an abnormal pressure-raising input to the medullary cardiovascular centers. The physician should immediately think of those set point–raising influences listed in the top half of Figure 9–4 that would simultaneously raise sympathetic activity and arterial pressure. Often, such a patient does not have chronic hypertension but rather is just experiencing a temporary blood pressure elevation due to the anxiety of undergoing a medical examination (white-coat hypertension).

A more rigorous analysis of the operation of the arterial baroreflex is presented in Appendix E. It is not essential reading, but the serious students may find it enlightening.

LONG-TERM REGULATION OF ARTERIAL PRESSURE

Long-term regulation of arterial pressure is a topic of extreme clinical relevance because of the prevalence of *hypertension* (sustained excessive arterial blood pressure) in our society. The most long-standing and generally accepted theory of long-term pressure regulation is that it crucially involves the kidneys, their sodium handling, and ultimately the regulation of blood volume. This theory is sometimes referred to as the "fluid balance" model of long-term arterial blood pressure control. In essence, this theory asserts that in the long term, MAP is whatever it needs to be to maintain an appropriate blood volume through arterial pressure's direct effects on renal function.

Fluid Balance and Arterial Pressure

Several key factors in the long-term regulation of arterial blood pressure have already been considered. First is the fact that the baroreceptor reflex, however well it counteracts temporary disturbances in arterial pressure, cannot effectively regulate arterial pressure in the long term because the baroreceptor firing rate tends to adapt to prolonged changes in arterial pressure. (In fact, baroreceptor adaptation may be a good thing. Recall that the whole purpose of arterial pressure is *to cause blood to flow through tissues*. Thus, it makes little long-term sense to increase arterial pressure by throttling blood flow to critical organs with reflex arteriolar constriction.)

The second pertinent fact is that circulating blood volume can influence arterial pressure because:

↓ Blood volume
↓
↓ Peripheral venous pressure
↓
Left shift of venous function curve
↓
↓ Central venous pressure
↓
↓ Cardiac output
↓
↓ Arterial pressure

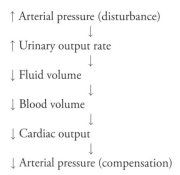 A fact yet to be considered is that arterial pressure has a profound influence on urinary output rate and thus affects total body fluid volume. Because blood volume is one of the components of the total body fluid, blood volume alterations accompany changes in total body fluid volume. The mechanisms are such that an *increase in arterial pressure* causes an increase in urinary output rate and thus a *decrease in blood volume*. But, as outlined in the preceding sequence, decreased blood volume tends to lower arterial pressure. Thus, the complete sequence of events that are initiated by an increase in arterial pressure can be listed as follows:

↑ Arterial pressure (disturbance)
↓
↑ Urinary output rate
↓
↓ Fluid volume
↓
↓ Blood volume
↓
↓ Cardiac output
↓
↓ Arterial pressure (compensation)

Note the negative feedback nature of this sequence of events: increased arterial pressure leads to fluid volume depletion, which tends to lower arterial pressure. Conversely, an initial disturbance of decreased arterial pressure would lead to fluid volume expansion, which would tend to increase arterial pressure. Because of negative feedback, these events constitute a *fluid volume mechanism* for regulating arterial pressure.

As indicated in Figure 9–5, both the arterial baroreceptor reflex and this fluid volume mechanism are negative feedback loops that regulate arterial pressure. Although the arterial baroreceptor reflex is very quick to counteract disturbances in arterial pressure, hours or even days may be required before a change in urinary output rate produces a significant accumulation or loss of total body fluid volume. Whatever this fluid volume mechanism lacks in speed, however, it more than

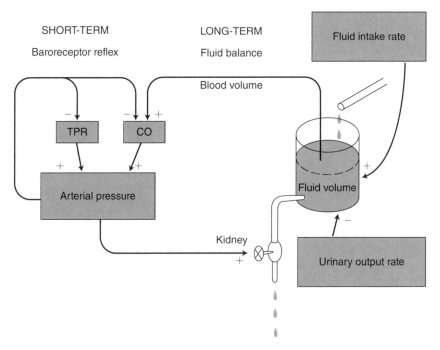

Figure 9–5. Mechanisms of short- and long-term regulations of arterial pressure. TPR, total peripheral resistance; CO, cardiac output.

makes up for that in persistence. As long as there is any inequality between the fluid intake rate and the urinary output rate, fluid volume is changing, and this fluid volume mechanism has not completed its adjustment of arterial pressure. The fluid volume mechanism is in equilibrium only when the urinary output rate exactly equals the fluid intake rate.[4] *In the long term, the arterial pressure can only be that which makes the urinary output rate equal to the fluid intake rate.*[5]

The baroreceptor reflex is, of course, essential for counteracting rapid changes in arterial pressure. The fluid volume mechanism, however, determines the long-term level of arterial pressure because it slowly overwhelms all other influences. Through adaptation, the baroreceptor mechanism adjusts itself so that it operates to prevent acute changes in blood pressure from the prevailing long-term level as determined through fluid balance.

---

[4] In the present discussion, assume that fluid intake rate represents the rate more than the obligatory fluid losses that normally occur in the feces and by transpiration from the skin and structures in the respiratory tract. The processes that regulate voluntary fluid intake (thirst) are not well understood but seem to involve many of the same factors that influence urinary output (e.g., blood volume and osmolality). Angiotensin II may be an important factor in the regulation of thirst.

[5] It is important to comprehend that "fluid balance" implies only that the amount of fluid in the body is in a "steady state" and not changing with time (i.e., input rate = output rate). Being in "fluid balance" does NOT necessarily imply that the *amount* of water in the body is normal.

Effect of Arterial Pressure on Urinary Output Rate

The kidneys play a major role in homeostasis by regulating the electrolyte composition of the plasma and the fluid balance of entire internal environment. One of the major plasma electrolytes regulated by the kidneys is the sodium ion. A key element in the fluid balance mechanism of long-term arterial pressure regulation is the effect that arterial pressure has on sodium excretion and renal urine production rate. The mechanisms responsible for this are briefly described here with emphasis on their cardiovascular implications.

To appreciate how urine formation occurs, we must look at the elegant processes that take place in the kidney. Figure 9–6 represents a schematic view of a single nephron, one of millions, bundled within each kidney. To regulate the plasma electrolyte composition, a large fraction of the plasma fluid that flows into the kidneys is filtered into the nephron across the *glomerular capillaries* so that it enters the *renal tubules*. The fluid that passes from the blood into the renal tubules is called the *glomerular filtrate*, and the rate at which this process occurs is called the *glomerular filtration rate*. Glomerular filtration is a transcapillary fluid movement, the rate of which is influenced by hydrostatic and oncotic pressures, as indicated in Chapter 6. The primary cause of continual glomerular filtration is that glomerular capillary hydrostatic pressure is normally very high ($\simeq 60\,\text{mm Hg}$). The glomerular filtration rate is decreased by factors that decrease glomerular capillary pressure, for example, decreased arterial blood pressure or vasoconstriction of pre-glomerular renal arterioles.

Once fluid is filtered into the renal tubules, it either (1) is *reabsorbed* and reenters the cardiovascular system or (2) is passed along renal tubules and eventually

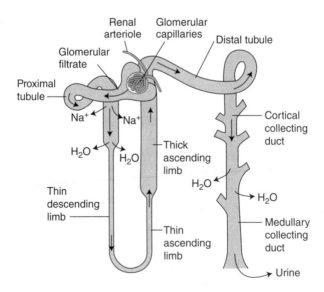

Figure 9–6. Schematic view of a single nephron from the kidney showing how urine is produced.

excreted as urine. Thus, urine production is the net result of glomerular filtration and renal tubular fluid reabsorption:

Urinary output rate = Glomerular filtration rate – Renal fluid reabsorption rate

Most of the reabsorption of fluid that has entered renal tubules as glomerular filtrate occurs because sodium is actively pumped out of the renal tubules by cells in the tubular wall. When sodium leaves the tubules, osmotic forces are produced that cause water to leave with it. Thus, any factor that promotes renal tubular sodium reabsorption (sodium retention) tends to increase the renal fluid reabsorption rate and consequently decrease the urinary output rate. The blood concentration of the hormone *aldosterone*, produced by the adrenal glands, is the primary regulator of the rate of sodium reabsorption by renal tubular cells. Adrenal release of aldosterone is, in turn, regulated largely by the circulating level of another hormone, *angiotensin II*, whose plasma concentration is determined by the plasma concentration of *renin*, an enzyme that is produced in the kidneys. Renin catalyzes the formation of an inactive decapeptide, *angiotensin I*, from *angiotensinogen*, a circulating precursor protein produced by the liver. Angiotensin I then gets quickly converted to angiotensin II (an octapeptide) by the action of *angiotensin-converting enzyme* that is located on the surface of endothelial cells primarily in the lungs. The combination of elements involved in this whole sequence of sodium-regulating events is referred to as the *renin–angiotensin–aldosterone system* and the key controller is the release of renin.

The rate of renin release by the kidneys is influenced by several factors. An increase in the activity of renal sympathetic nerves causes a direct release of renin through a β_1-adrenergic mechanism. Also, renin release is triggered by factors associated with a lowered glomerular filtration rate. The activation of sympathetic vasoconstrictor nerves to renal arterioles thus indirectly causes renin release via lowered glomerular capillary hydrostatic pressure and glomerular filtration rate. The important fact to keep in mind, from a cardiovascular standpoint, is that anything that causes renin release causes a decrease in urinary output rate because increased renin causes increased sodium (and therefore fluid) reabsorption from renal tubules.[6]

In the preceding text, we have emphasized the role of the kidneys in regulating blood volume because of its obvious cardiovascular consequences. But regulating bodily fluid volume is only one of the multiple tasks that the kidneys perform. From a renal perspective, a more immediate concern is the regulation of extracellular osmolarity. In fact, osmolarity is one of the most tightly regulated variables in the internal environment. For example, the ingestion of 8 oz (230 mL) of water will elicit a dramatic renal compensatory response within minutes. That is quite amazing when one considers that adding 230 mL of pure water to 42 L of total body water would only reduce internal osmolarity (i.e., solute concentration) by approximately ½%.

---

[6] Although the renin–angiotensin–aldosterone system is clearly the primary mechanism for the regulation of renal tubular sodium reabsorption, other factors are also involved. A polypeptide natriuretic (salt-losing) factor has been identified in granules of cardiac atrial cells. Atrial distention causes the release of this *atrial natriuretic peptide* into the blood. The possibility that the heart itself may serve as an endocrine organ in the regulation of body fluid volume is stimulating much research interest.

The kidneys regulate extracellular osmolarity primarily by changing the amount of water (not solutes) in the body. They can do this because they have independent mechanisms for controlling their water and solute excretion rates. Renal water excretion rate is controlled by the hormone *vasopressin* (also known as antidiuretic hormone) that is released from the posterior pituitary gland. The primary stimulus for vasopressin release is an increase in internal osmolarity, as detected by osmoreceptors in the hypothalamus. *Inhibition* of vasopressin release occurs with increased afferent input from the cardiopulmonary baroreceptors. Vasopressin increases the water permeability of distal portions of the renal tubules and thus enhances renal water reabsorption and decreases renal water excretion. This is a very rapid and powerful mechanism that essentially keeps internal osmolarity constant in the long term. The bottom line for us is that, given constant internal osmolarity, total extracellular volume must always parallel any changes in total extracellular solute content. Recall that NaCl is by far the most abundant extracellular solute. That is the primary reason that renal sodium handling is of paramount importance in regulating extracellular volume.

Some major mechanisms that influence urinary output rate are summarized in Figure 9–7 with the example of the response to a decrease in arterial pressure. Most important, this figure shows that urinary output rate is linked to arterial pressure by many synergistic pathways. Because of this, modest changes in arterial pressure are associated with large changes in urinary output rate.

The observed relationship between arterial pressure and urinary output for a healthy person is shown in Figure 9–8. Recall that, in the steady state, the urinary output rate must always equal the fluid intake rate and that changes in fluid volume will automatically adjust arterial pressure until this is so. Thus, a healthy person with a normal fluid intake rate will have, as a long-term average, the arterial pressure associated with point A in Figure 9–7. Because of the steepness of the curve shown in Figure 9–7, even rather marked changes in fluid intake rate have minor influences on the arterial pressure of a healthy individual.

PERSPECTIVES

As will be addressed further in Chapter 11, *hypertension* (persistent, excessively high arterial pressure) is a common, serious health issue that all physicians will routinely encounter. Almost always, the primary cause is not evident. So, the standard clinical approach is to try to treat the symptom (high arterial pressure) with drugs logically aimed at decreasing either CO or TPR. An ongoing puzzle is that certain drugs that are effective in some patients are not effective in others. Thus, hypertension treatment often proceeds largely on a trial-and-error basis.

In this text, we have emphasized the role of the kidneys and blood volume control in the long-term regulation of arterial pressure for several reasons. At the core of this hypothesis is the undeniable fact that in the long term (months, years, lifetimes), our urinary fluid output must exactly match our highly variable fluid input. Otherwise, we would gradually either desiccate to cinders or turn into huge water-filled blobs. Any hypothesis about long-term control of arterial pressure

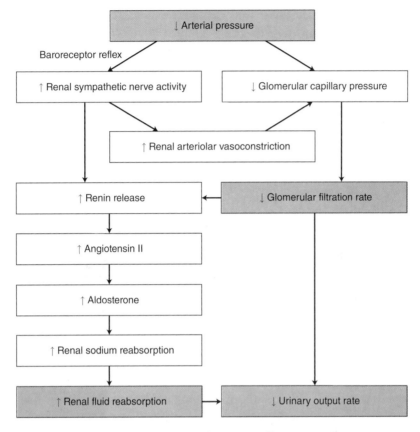

Figure 9-7. Mechanisms by which arterial pressure influences urinary output rate.

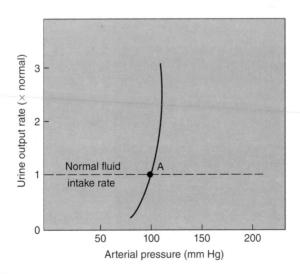

Figure 9-8. The effect of arterial pressure on urinary output rate in a healthy person.

(or any other life variable for that matter) must ultimately work within this constraint. Moreover, the 2 known (but admittedly very rare) definite causes of hypertension (renal artery obstruction or excess aldosterone production from an adrenal gland adenoma) both point to the kidneys.

However, in view of the variable clinical experience in dealing with hypertension, it is well to question whether the kidneys are the sole organ responsible for long-term arterial pressure regulation. Indeed, many argue that the CNS is intimately involved as well. One common hypothesis along these lines is that: *Long-term arterial pressure is regulated to be whatever it needs to be to maintain adequate brain blood flow.* This obviously is somewhat a different mindset than: *Long-term arterial pressure is regulated to be whatever it needs to be to make urine output rate equal to fluid intake rate.* Certainly, the very existence of the "Cushing reflex" lends some credence to the CNS hypothesis. Moreover, even the short-term regulation of arterial pressure is a complex issue that can involve many inputs to the cardiovascular control centers in addition to those from the arterial baroreceptors (see Figure 9–4). It is largely unknown to what extent these "other" influences might be involved in long-term pressure regulation. The bottom line of all this is that the interplay of all the factors involved in the long-term control of arterial pressure is still an active topic of debate.

We remind the student that, whatever the purpose of long-term arterial pressure regulation, changes in MAP can be accomplished only by changing cardiac output and/or TPR. Blood volume is undeniably one important determinant of cardiac output. Thus, we (the authors of this text) conclude that there are elements of truth in both the renal and CNS theories of long-term blood pressure control. It seems that this debate is resulting in some melding of the theories and our understanding of what factors cause chronic hypertension and how individualized treatment strategies can be improved.

KEY CONCEPTS

Arterial pressure is closely regulated to ensure adequate blood flow to the tissues.

The arterial baroreceptor reflex is responsible for regulating arterial pressure in the short term on a second-to-second and moment-to-moment basis.

The arterial baroreceptor reflex involves the following: pressure sensing by stretch-sensitive baroreceptor nerve endings in the walls of arteries; neural integrating centers in the brainstem that adjust autonomic nerve activity in response to the pressure information they receive from the arterial baroreceptors; and responses of the heart and vessels to changes in autonomic nerve activity.

Overall, the arterial baroreflex operates such that an increase in arterial pressure leads to an essentially immediate decrease in sympathetic nerve activity and a simultaneous increase in parasympathetic nerve activity (and vice versa).

The brainstem integrating centers also receive nonarterial baroreceptor inputs that can raise or lower the set point for short-term arterial pressure regulation.

In the long term, arterial pressure is regulated by changes in blood volume that come about because arterial pressure has a strong influence on urinary output rate by the kidney.

STUDY QUESTIONS

9–1. Consider the various components of the arterial baroreceptor reflex and predict whether the following variables will increase or decrease in response to a rise in arterial pressure.

   a. Arterial baroreceptor firing rate
   b. Parasympathetic activity to the heart
   c. Sympathetic activity to the heart
   d. Arteriolar tone
   e. Venous tone
   f. Peripheral venous pressure
   g. Total peripheral resistance
   h. Cardiac output

9–2. Massage of the neck over the carotid sinus area in a person experiencing a bout of paroxysmal atrial tachycardia is often effective in terminating the episode. Why?

9–3. Regarding the baroreceptor reflex and the short-term regulation of arterial pressure, indicate how each of the following stimuli would affect the sympathetic nerve activity at any given arterial pressure.

   a. Low oxygen in arterial blood
   b. Increased intracranial pressure
   c. Increased right atrial pressure
   d. Sense of danger
   e. Visceral pain

9–4. Describe the immediate direct and reflex cardiovascular consequences of giving a healthy person a drug that blocks $\alpha 1$-adrenergic receptors. Describe the possible changes in mean arterial pressure, sympathetic nerve activity, cardiac output, total peripheral resistance, and shifts in the cardiac function and venous return curves.

9–5. What net short-term alterations in mean arterial pressure and sympathetic activity would the following produce?

    a. Blood loss through hemorrhage

    b. Cutaneous pain

    c. Systemic hypoxia

    d. Local metabolic vasodilation in the skeletal muscle

9–6. Your patient has lower-than-normal mean arterial pressure and higher-than-normal pulse rate. Which of the following are possible diagnoses?

    a. Low blood volume

    b. Anxiety

    c. A cardiac valve problem

    d. Elevated intracranial pressure

9–7. In the normal operation of the arterial baroreceptor reflex, a cardiovascular disturbance that lowers mean arterial pressure will evoke a decrease in

    a. baroreceptor firing rate.

    b. sympathetic nerve activity.

    c. heart rate.

    d. total peripheral resistance.

    e. myocardial contractility.

9–8. In general, normal kidneys tend to retain sodium and fluid in the body whenever

    a. arterial pressure is high.

    b. parasympathetic nerve activity is high.

    c. sympathetic nerve activity is high.

    d. plasma aldosterone levels are low.

    e. plasma renin levels are low.

9–9. If your patient's mean systemic arterial pressure changes, it must be because of changes in

    a. the heart rate and/or myocardial contractility.

    b. cardiac output and/or total peripheral resistance.

    c. blood volume and/or venous tone.

    d. sympathetic and/or parasympathetic nerve activity.

    e. arterial compliance and/or stroke volume.

Cardiovascular Responses to Physiological Stresses

10

OBJECTIVES

The student understands the general mechanisms involved in the cardiovascular responses to any given normal homeostatic disturbance in the intact cardiovascular system and can predict the resulting alterations in all important cardiovascular variables:

▶ *Identifies the primary disturbances that the situation places on the cardiovascular system.*

▶ *Lists how the primary disturbances change the influence on the medullary cardiovascular centers from (1) arterial baroreceptors and (2) other sources.*

▶ *States what immediate reflex compensatory changes will occur in sympathetic and parasympathetic nerve activities as a result of the altered influences on the medullary cardiovascular centers.*

▶ *Indicates what immediate reflex compensatory changes will occur in basic cardiovascular variables such as the heart rate, cardiac contractility, stroke volume, arteriolar tone, venous tone, peripheral venous pressure, central venous pressure, total peripheral resistance, resistance in any major organ, and blood flow through any major organ.*

▶ *Predicts what the net effect of the primary disturbance and reflex compensatory influences on the cardiovascular variables listed in the preceding objective will be on mean arterial pressure.*

▶ *States whether mean arterial pressure and sympathetic nerve activity will settle above or below their normal values.*

▶ *Predicts whether and states how cutaneous blood flow will be altered by temperature regulation reflexes.*

▶ *Indicates whether and how transcapillary fluid movements will be involved in the overall cardiovascular response to a given primary disturbance.*

▶ *Indicates whether, why, how, and with what time course renal adjustments of fluid balance will participate in the response.*

▶ *Predicts how each of the basic cardiovascular variables will be influenced by long-term adjustments in blood volume.*

The student understands how respiratory activities influence the cardiovascular system:

▶ *Describes how the "respiratory pump" promotes venous return.*

▶ *Identifies the primary disturbances on cardiovascular variables associated with normal respiratory activity.*

▶ *Describes the reflex compensatory responses to respiratory activity.*

▶ Defines the causes of "normal sinus arrhythmia."

▶ Lists the cardiovascular consequences of the Valsalva maneuver and of positive-pressure artificial ventilation.

The student understands the specific processes associated with the homeostatic adjustments to the effects of gravity:

▶ States how gravity influences arterial, venous, and capillary pressures at any height above or below the heart in a standing individual.

▶ Describes and explains the changes in central venous pressure and the changes in transcapillary fluid balance and venous volume in the lower extremities caused by standing upright.

▶ Describes the operation of the "skeletal muscle pump" and explains how it simultaneously promotes venous return and decreases capillary hydrostatic pressure in the muscle vascular beds.

▶ Identifies the primary disturbances and compensatory responses evoked by acute changes in body position.

▶ Describes the chronic effects of long-term bed rest on cardiovascular variables.

The student understands the specific processes associated with the homeostatic adjustments to exercise:

▶ Identifies the primary disturbances and compensatory responses evoked by acute episodes of dynamic exercise.

▶ Describes the conflict between pressure reflexes and temperature reflexes on cutaneous blood flow.

▶ Indicates how the "skeletal muscle pump" and the "respiratory pump" contribute to cardiovascular adjustments during exercise.

▶ Compares the cardiovascular responses to static exercise with those to dynamic exercise.

▶ Lists the effects of chronic exercise and physical conditioning on cardiovascular variables.

The student understands the cardiovascular alterations that accompany pregnancy, birth, growth, and aging:

▶ Identifies the major maternal cardiovascular adjustments that occur during pregnancy.

▶ Follows the pathway of blood flow through the fetal heart and describes the changes that occur at birth.

▶ Indicates the normal changes that occur in cardiovascular variables during childhood.

▶ Identifies age-dependent changes that occur in cardiovascular variables such as cardiac index, arterial pressure, and cardiac workload.

▶ Describes age-dependent changes in the arterial baroreceptor reflex.

▶ Distinguishes between age- and disease-dependent alterations that occur in cardiovascular function of the aged.

The student understands that sex may influence the cardiovascular system:

▶ Describes sex-dependent differences in cardiovascular variables.

Everything discussed so far has been focused on individual components of the cardiovascular system. In this chapter, we will finally see how these components interact to adjust to a variety of normal everyday situations that tend to disturb normal homeostasis. As had been repeatedly stressed, the primary goal of the cardiovascular system is to provide adequate tissue perfusion throughout the body. However, a key to understanding the cardiovascular adjustments in each of these situations is to recognize that blood flow to the brain and heart muscle is of highest priority and that the arterial baroreceptor reflex and renal fluid balance mechanisms always act to blunt changes in *arterial pressure* to assure adequate perfusion of these critical tissues.

PRIMARY DISTURBANCES AND COMPENSATORY RESPONSES

The cardiovascular alterations in each of the following examples are produced by the combined effects of (1) the direct influences of the *primary disturbance* on the cardiovascular variables and (2) the reflex *compensatory responses* that are triggered by these primary disturbances. In this chapter, all the *primary disturbances* presented represent normal challenges encountered in our everyday lives. In the next chapter, we will consider the effects of *primary disturbances* associated with malfunction of various components of the cardiovascular system. The general pattern of reflex responses is similar in all situations. Rather than trying to memorize the cardiovascular alterations that accompany each situation, the student should strive to understand each response in terms of the primary disturbances and reflex compensatory responses involved. To aid in this process, a list of key cardiovascular variables and their determinants may be found in Appendix C. If the student understands all the relationships indicated in Appendix C, they will have mastered the core of cardiovascular physiology.

A list of important study questions is supplied for this chapter and Chapter 11. These questions are intended to reinforce the student's understanding of complex cardiovascular responses and provide a review of basic cardiovascular principles.

EFFECT OF RESPIRATORY ACTIVITY

The physical processes associated with inhaling air into and exhaling air out of the lungs can have major effects on venous return and cardiac output. During a normal inspiration, intrathoracic pressure falls from approximately negative 2 mm Hg to approximately negative 7 mm Hg (compared to atmospheric pressure) as the diaphragm contracts and the chest wall expands. It rises again by an equal amount during expiration. These periodic pressure fluctuations not only promote air movement into and out of the lungs but also are transmitted through the thin walls of the great veins in the thorax to influence venous return to the heart from the periphery. Because of the unidirectional nature of venous valves, venous return is increased more by inspiration than it is decreased by expiration. The net effect is that venous return from the periphery is generally facilitated by the periodic fluctuations in central venous pressure caused by respiration. This phenomenon is often referred to as the "respiratory pump."

Because of these cyclic changes in intrathoracic pressure, normal breathing is associated with transient changes in heart rate (HR), cardiac output, and arterial pressure. Heart rate in healthy individuals usually fluctuates in synchrony with the respiratory rate. This is referred to as "normal sinus arrhythmia." There are several factors that contribute to this normal arrhythmia.

1. Cyclical alterations in intrathoracic pressure with normal breathing evoke primary disturbances in blood flow and distribution within the cardiovascular system. Some of these disturbances and compensatory responses are illustrated in Figure 10–1. Filling of the right side of the heart is transiently increased during inspiration and, by the Starling law, stroke volume (SV) and thus cardiac output are transiently increased. In addition, the reduction in pulmonary vascular resistance that accompanies inspiration reduces the right

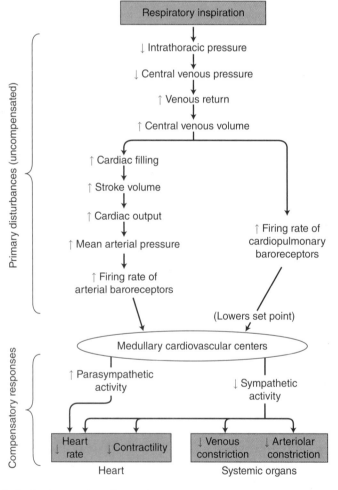

Figure 10–1. Cardiovascular effects of respiratory inspiration.

ventricular afterload, which contributes to a transient increase in right ventricular stroke volume. Because changes in output of the right side of the heart induce changes in output of the left side of the heart within a few beats, the net effect of inspiration will be a transient increase in stroke volume and cardiac output from the left ventricle. This will lead to a transient increase in arterial pressure and a transient increase in firing of the arterial baroreceptors. The output of these high-pressure arterial baroreceptors will act on the medullary cardiovascular centers to produce reflex adjustments to *lower* arterial pressure, by *increasing* cardiac parasympathetic nerve activity, *decreasing* sympathetic nerve activity, and causing a *decrease* in HR.

2. The inspiration-induced decrease in intrathoracic pressure will also stretch low-pressure cardiopulmonary baroreceptors located within the pulmonary vascular bed and cardiac walls and will increase their firing rate. These low-pressure baroreceptor inputs will add to the information from the high-pressure baroreceptors and promote similar pressure-lowering outputs from the medullary cardiovascular centers.

3. Lung mechanoreceptors located primarily within the airways are also stretched during normal inspiration. Unlike the first 2 mechanisms, their input into the medullary centers results in an *inhibition* of the normal tonic vagal activity to the sinoatrial node, causing a transient *increase* in the HR.

Under normal resting conditions, the cyclic change in HR is the most apparent cardiovascular response to respiration. However, because of the complicated and sometimes conflicting mechanisms involved in altering vagal tone to the SA node, specific phase relationships between the respiratory cycle and the cardiovascular effects are hard to predict and are greatly influenced by respiratory rate, depth, and the current average HR. However, total absence of a respiratory arrhythmia is clearly abnormal.

There are a number of instances when the cardiovascular effects of respiratory efforts are exaggerated and extremely important. The following lists several of these situations:

1. During *exercise*, a deep and rapid breathing rate contributes significantly to the venous return by exaggerating the fluctuations in intrathoracic pressure. This is an important example of the *respiratory pump*.

2. *Yawning* is a complex event that includes a significant transient decrease in intrathoracic pressure that is highly effective in increasing venous return (especially when combined with stretching).

3. In contrast to yawning, *coughing* is associated with an *increase* in intrathoracic pressure and, if occurring as a prolonged "fit," can lead to compression of the thoracic vessels, reduced venous return, and such severe reductions in cardiac output as to cause fainting.

4. The *Valsalva maneuver* is a forced expiration against a closed glottis commonly performed by individuals during defecation ("straining at stool") or when attempting to lift a heavy object. There are several phases in this cardiovascular reaction. At the initiation of the Valsalva maneuver, arterial pressure is

abruptly elevated for several beats due to the intrathoracic pressure transmitted to the thoracic aorta. Sustained elevation in intrathoracic pressure then leads to a fall in venous return and a fall in blood pressure, which evokes a compensatory reflex increase in the HR and peripheral vasoconstriction. (During this period, the red face and distended peripheral veins are indicative of high peripheral venous pressures.) At the cessation of the maneuver, there is an abrupt fall in pressure for a couple of beats due to the reduction of intrathoracic pressure. Venous blood then moves rapidly into the central venous pool; stroke volume, cardiac output, and arterial pressure increase rapidly; and a reflex bradycardia occurs. The combination of an episode of high peripheral venous pressure followed by a brief episode of abnormally large stroke volumes, high arterial pressure, and pulse pressure is particularly dangerous for people who are candidates for cerebral vascular accidents (strokes) because this combination may rupture a vessel.

5. Artificial support of respiration with *positive-pressure ventilators* is sometimes necessary for assuring proper gas exchange in the lungs but does have significant adverse cardiovascular consequences. When the lungs are inflated artificially by such ventilators, intrathoracic pressure goes *up* (rather than down, as occurs during normal inspiration). Thus, instead of the normal respiratory pump *increasing* venous return during inspiration, the positive-pressure ventilator *decreases* venous return during lung inflation. In addition, the increase in intrathoracic pressure tends to compress the pulmonary microcirculation and this increases right ventricular afterload. Therefore, when considering the option of putting someone on a respirator, the benefits of improving pulmonary ventilation need to be weighed against the negative effects on the cardiovascular system.

EFFECT OF GRAVITY

Responses to Changes in Body Position

Significant cardiovascular readjustments accompany changes in body position because gravity influences pressures and blood volume distribution within the cardiovascular system. In the preceding chapters, the influence of gravity was ignored, and pressure differences between various points in the systemic circulation were related only to flow and vascular resistance ($\Delta P = \dot{Q} \times R$). As shown in Figure 10–2, this is approximately true only for a recumbent individual. In a standing individual, additional cardiovascular pressure differences exist between the heart and regions of the body that are not at the heart level. This is most important in the lower legs and feet of a standing individual. As indicated in Figure 10–2B, all intravascular pressures in the feet of an upright individual may be increased by 90 mm Hg simply from the weight of the blood in the arteries and veins leading to and from the feet. (On the other hand, the head is higher than the heart while standing and therefore, cerebral arterial pressure will be decreased by about 20 mm Hg.) Note by comparing Figure 10–2A and 10–2B that standing upright does not in itself change the *flow through* the

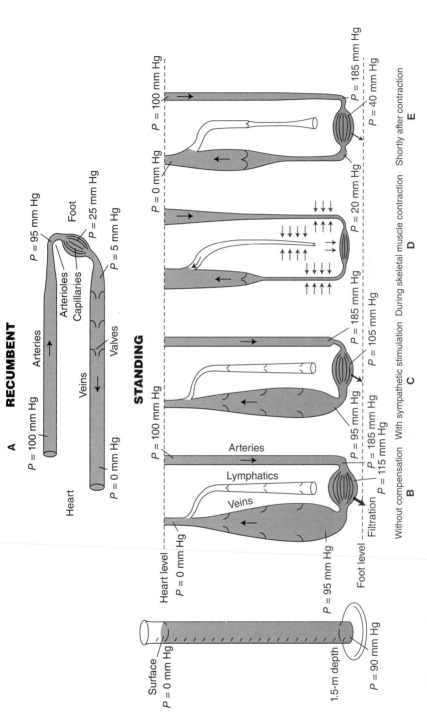

Figure 10–2. The effect of gravity on pressures within a simulated peripheral vascular system. (**A**) System in a recumbent position; (**B–E**) system in an upright position; (**B**) with no compensatory influences; (**C**) with sympathetic stimulation; (**D** and **E**) with the effect of the skeletal muscle pump.

lower extremities, because gravity has the same effect on arterial and venous pressures and thus does not change the *arteriovenous pressure difference* at any one height level.

There are, however, 2 major direct effects of the increased pressure in the lower extremities, which are shown in Figure 10–2B: (1) the increase in venous transmural pressure distends the compliant peripheral veins in the legs and feet and greatly increases the *volume of blood in* these veins by as much as 500 mL in a normal adult and (2) the increase in capillary transmural hydrostatic pressure causes a tremendously high transcapillary filtration rate in the lower legs and feet.

A baroreceptor-induced reflex activation of sympathetic nerves accompanies the transition from a recumbent to an upright position. However, Figure 10–2C shows how vasoconstriction from sympathetic activation is only marginally effective in ameliorating the adverse effects of gravity on the lower extremities. Arteriolar constriction can cause a greater pressure drop across arterioles, but this has only a limited effect on capillary pressure because venous pressure remains extremely high. Filtration will continue at a very high rate. In fact, the normal cardiovascular reflex mechanisms are alone incapable of dealing with upright posture without the aid of the "skeletal muscle pump." A person who remained upright without intermittent contraction of the skeletal muscles in the legs would lose consciousness in 10 to 20 minutes because of the decreased brain blood flow that would stem from sequential steps of diminished central blood volume, leading to reduced stroke volume, depressed cardiac output, and finally lowered arterial pressure.

Effectiveness of the skeletal muscle pump in counteracting venous blood pooling and edema formation in the lower extremities during standing is illustrated in Figure 10–2D and 10–2E. Compression of vessels during skeletal muscle contraction expels both venous blood and lymphatic fluid from the lower extremities (Figure 10–2D). Immediately after a skeletal muscle contraction, both veins and lymphatic vessels are relatively empty because their one-way valves prevent the backflow of previously expelled fluid (Figure 10–2E). Most importantly, the weight of the venous and lymphatic fluid columns is temporarily supported by the closed one-way valve leaflets. Consequently, venous pressure is drastically lowered immediately after skeletal muscle contraction and rises only gradually as veins refill with blood from capillaries. Thus, capillary pressure and transcapillary fluid filtration rate are dramatically reduced for some period after a skeletal muscle contraction. Periodic skeletal muscle contractions can keep the average value of venous pressure at levels that are only moderately above normal. This, in combination with an increased pressure drop across vasoconstricted arterioles, prevents capillary pressures from rising to intolerable levels in the lower extremities. Some transcapillary fluid filtration is still present, but the increased lymphatic flow resulting from the skeletal muscle pump is normally sufficient to prevent noticeable edema formation in the feet.

Actions of the skeletal muscle pump, however beneficial, do not completely prevent a rise in the average venous pressure and blood pooling in the lower extremities on standing. Therefore, assuming an upright position upsets the cardiovascular system and elicits reflex cardiovascular adjustments, as shown in Figure 10–3.

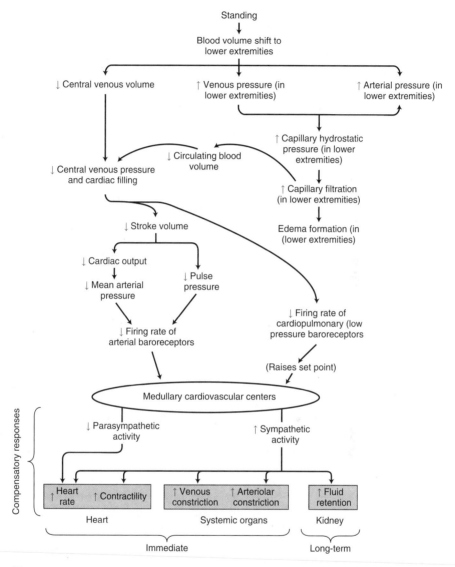

Figure 10–3. Cardiovascular mechanisms involved when changing from a recumbent to a standing position.

As with all cardiovascular responses, the key to understanding the alterations associated with standing is to distinguish the *primary* disturbances from the *compensatory responses*. As shown in the top part of Figure 10–3, the immediate consequence of standing is a shift of blood volume from the central venous pool (i.e., thorax) to the peripheral venous pool (i.e., lower extremities). This results in a decrease in central venous pressure and an increase in both arterial and venous pressures in the lower extremities. By the chain of events shown, the primary disturbances influence the cardiovascular centers by lessening the normal input from both the arterial and the cardiopulmonary baroreceptors.

The consequence of a decreased baroreceptor input to the cardiovascular centers will be reflex adjustments (i.e., the compensatory response) appropriate to increase blood pressure—that is, decreased cardiac parasympathetic nerve activity and increased activity of the cardiovascular sympathetic nerves, as shown in the bottom part of Figure 10–3. The HR and cardiac contractility will increase, as will arteriolar and venous constriction in most systemic organs except the brain and heart.

Heart rate and total peripheral resistance are higher when an individual is standing than when sitting or lying down. Note that these cardiovascular variables are not directly influenced by standing but *are* changed by the compensatory responses. Stroke volume and cardiac output, conversely, are usually decreased below their recumbent values during quiet standing despite the reflex adjustments that tend to increase them. This is because the reflex adjustments do not quite overcome the primary disturbance on these variables caused by standing. This is in keeping with the general dictum that short-term cardiovascular compensations never completely correct the initial disturbance.

Mean arterial pressure (MAP) is often found to increase when a person changes from the recumbent to the standing position. At first glance, this is a violation of many rules of cardiovascular system operation. How can compensation be more than complete? Moreover, how is increased sympathetic activity compatible with higher-than-normal MAP in the first place? In the case of standing, there are many answers to these apparent puzzles. First, the average arterial baroreceptor discharge rate can decrease in spite of a small increase in MAP *if* there is simultaneously a sufficiently large decrease in pulse pressure (which accompanies the smaller stroke volume). Second, the influence on the medullary cardiovascular centers from cardiopulmonary receptors is interpreted as a decrease in blood volume and may raise arterial pressure by mechanisms raising the set point. Third, MAP determined by sphygmomanometry from the arm of a standing individual *overestimates* the MAP being sensed by the baroreceptors in the carotid sinus region of the neck because of gravitational effects.

The kidney is especially susceptible to changes in sympathetic nerve activity (as discussed in the previous chapter and shown in Figure 9–7). Consequently, as shown in Figure 10–3, every reflex alteration in sympathetic activity has influences on fluid balance that become important in the long term. Standing, which is associated with an increase in sympathetic tone, ultimately results in an increase in fluid volume. The ultimate benefit of this is that an increase in circulating blood volume generally reduces the magnitude of the reflex alterations required to tolerate upright posture.

Responses to Long-Term Bed Rest (or to Zero Gravity)

The cardiovascular system of an individual who is subjected to long-term bed rest undergoes a variety of adaptive changes. One of the most significant changes includes a loss in body fluids and circulating blood volume. (This situation is also experienced by people who travel outside the earth's atmosphere at zero gravity.)

One troubling consequence of these adjustments is *orthostatic hypotension*. The steps leading to this disturbing condition can be intuited from Figure 10–3. The most significant immediate change that occurs on assuming a recumbent position (or entering a gravity-free environment) is a shift of fluid from the lower extremities to the upper portions of the body. The consequences of this shift include distention of the head and neck veins, facial edema, nasal stuffiness, and decreases in calf girth and leg volume. In addition, the increase in central blood volume stimulates the cardiopulmonary mechanoreceptors, which influence renal function by neural and hormonal pathways to reduce sympathetic drive and promote fluid loss. The individual begins to lose weight and, within a few days, becomes hypovolemic (by normal earth standards).

When the bedridden patient initially tries to stand up (or when the space traveler reenters the earth's gravitational field), the normal responses to gravity, as described in Figure 10–3, are not as effective, primarily because of the substantial decrease in total circulating blood volume. Upon standing, blood shifts out of the central venous pool into the peripheral veins, stroke volume falls, and the individual often becomes dizzy and may faint because of a dramatic fall in blood pressure. In this case, the normal short-term compensatory mechanisms are not adequate to overcome the loss in blood volume. This phenomenon is referred to as *orthostatic* or *postural hypotension*. Restoration of blood volume involving renal mechanisms and rehydration is required. In addition to the fluid loss, there are other long-term cardiovascular changes (e.g., ventricular remodeling) that may accompany bed rest (or space travel) such that complete reversal of this orthostatic intolerance may take several days or even weeks. (Collectively, these changes are often referred to as *deconditioning* which is a term also used to describe what happens when a person stops exercising, as will be described in the next section.)

Efforts made to diminish the cardiovascular changes for the bedridden patient include intermittent sitting up or tilting the bed to lower the legs and trigger fluid retention mechanisms. Efforts made in space to accomplish the same end may include exercise programs, lower-body negative-pressure devices, and salt and water loading. (To date, these interventions have met with limited success and orthostatic hypotension remains a problem for many astronauts returning to earth.)

EFFECT OF EXERCISE

Responses to Acute Exercise

Physical exercise is one of the most ordinary, yet taxing, situations with which the cardiovascular system must cope. The specific alterations in cardiovascular function that occur during exercise depend on several factors including (1) the type of exercise—that is, whether it is predominantly "dynamic" (rhythmic or isotonic) or "static" (isometric), (2) the intensity and duration of the exercise, (3) the age of the individual, and (4) the level of "fitness" of the individual. The example shown in Figure 10–4 is typical of cardiovascular alterations that might occur in a normal, untrained, middle-aged adult doing a dynamic-type exercise such as running or dancing. Note especially that HR and cardiac output increase greatly during

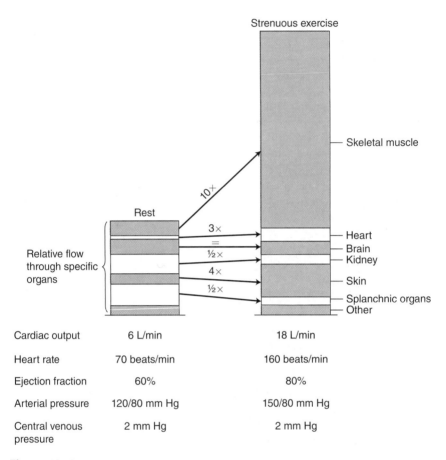

	Rest	Strenuous exercise
Cardiac output	6 L/min	18 L/min
Heart rate	70 beats/min	160 beats/min
Ejection fraction	60%	80%
Arterial pressure	120/80 mm Hg	150/80 mm Hg
Central venous pressure	2 mm Hg	2 mm Hg

Figure 10-4. Changes in cardiovascular variables with strenuous exercise.

exercise and that MAP and pulse pressure also increase significantly. These altera-tions ensure that increased metabolic demands of the exercising skeletal muscle are met by appropriate increases in skeletal muscle blood flow. (Use the data in this figure to answer Study Questions 10–5 to 10–8.)

Many of the adjustments to exercise are due to a large increase in sympa-thetic activity, which results from the mechanisms outlined in Figure 10–5.

One of the primary disturbances associated with the stress and/or antici-pation of exercise originates within the cerebral cortex and exerts an influence on the medullary cardiovascular centers through corticohypothalamic pathways. This set point–raising influence is referred to as *central command* and causes MAP to be regulated to a higher-than-normal level (see Appendix E, Figure E–3A).[1]

---

[1] As was described in Chapter 9, this "non-arterial baroreceptor" input to the medullary CV centers rep-resents a sort of "feedforward" control acting on the cardiovascular system to *initiate* changes by complex neural processes not well understood and is distinguished from the negative feedback control which *reacts* to changes to restore original conditions.

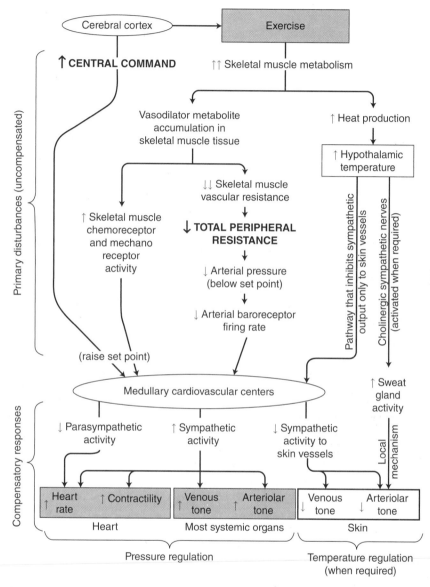

Figure 10–5. Cardiovascular mechanisms involved during exercise.

Also indicated in Figure 10–5 is the possibility that a second set point–raising influence may reach the cardiovascular centers from chemoreceptors and mechanoreceptors in the active skeletal muscles. Such inputs would also contribute to the elevations in sympathetic activity and MAP that accompany exercise.

 A major primary disturbance on the cardiovascular system during dynamic exercise, however, is the decrease in total peripheral resistance (TPR) caused by metabolic vasodilator accumulation and decreased vascular resistance in the active skeletal muscle. As indicated in Figure 10–5, decreased TPR is a pressure-lowering disturbance that elicits a strong increase in sympathetic activity through the arterial baroreceptor reflex.

Although MAP is usually above normal during exercise, the decreased TPR causes it to fall below the elevated level to which it would be regulated by the set point–raising influences on the cardiovascular center alone. The arterial baroreceptor reflex negative feedback pathway responds to this circumstance with a large increase in sympathetic activity. Thus, the arterial baroreceptor reflex is responsible for a large portion of the increase in sympathetic activity that accompanies exercise despite the seemingly contradictory fact that arterial pressure is higher than normal. In fact, were it not for the arterial baroreceptor reflex, the decrease in TPR that occurs during exercise would cause MAP to fall well below normal.

As discussed in Chapter 9 and indicated in Figures 10–4 and 10–5, cutaneous blood flow may increase during exercise despite a generalized increase in sympathetic vasoconstrictor tone. This happens because thermal reflexes involved in keeping body temperature constant can override arterial pressure-regulating reflexes especially as applied to the special case of skin blood flow control. Temperature reflexes, of course, are usually activated during strenuous exercise to dissipate the excess heat being produced by the active skeletal muscles. Cutaneous flow may decrease at the very onset of exercise (as part of the generalized increase in arteriolar tone from increased sympathetic vasoconstrictor activity) and then increase quickly during exercise as body heat builds up.

In addition to the increases in the skeletal muscle and skin blood flow, coronary blood flow increases substantially during strenuous exercise. This is primarily due to local metabolic vasodilation of coronary arterioles as a result of increased cardiac work and myocardial oxygen consumption.

Two important mechanisms that participate in the cardiovascular response to dynamic exercise are not shown in Figure 10–5. The first is the skeletal muscle pump, which was discussed in connection with upright posture. The skeletal muscle pump is a very important factor in promoting venous return during dynamic exercise preventing the reflex-induced increase in cardiac output from drastically lowering central venous pressure. The second factor is the respiratory pump, which also promotes venous return during exercise. Exaggerated respiratory movements that occur during exercise increase the effectiveness of the respiratory pump and thus enhance venous return and cardiac filling.

As indicated in Figure 10–4, the average central venous pressure does not change much, if at all, during strenuous dynamic exercise. This is because the cardiac output and the venous return curves are both shifted upward during exercise. Therefore, cardiac output and venous return will be elevated without a significant change in central venous pressure. Thus, the increase in stroke volume that accompanies exercise (suggested in this figure by the increase in pulse pressure) largely reflects the increased myocardial contractility and increased ejection fraction with decreased end-systolic ventricular volume.

In summary, the profound cardiovascular adjustments to dynamic exercise shown in Figures 10–4 and 10–5 all occur automatically as a consequence of the operation of the normal cardiovascular control mechanisms. The tremendous increase in skeletal muscle blood flow is accomplished largely by increased cardiac output but also in part by diverting flow away from the kidneys and the splanchnic organs.

Static exercise (i.e., isometric) presents a much different disturbance on the cardiovascular system than does dynamic exercise. As discussed in the previous section, dynamic exercise produces large reductions in TPR because of local metabolic vasodilation in exercising muscles. Static efforts, even of moderate intensity, cause a compression of the vessels in the contracting muscles and a reduction in the blood flow through them. Thus, TPR does not usually fall *during* strenuous static exercise and may even increase significantly. The primary disturbances on the cardiovascular system during static exercise seem to be set point–raising inputs to the medullary cardiovascular centers from the cerebral cortex (central command) and from chemoreceptors and mechanoreceptors in the contracting muscle. These inputs result in another example of what is termed the "exercise pressor response."

Cardiovascular effects of static exercise include increases in the HR, cardiac output, and arterial pressure—all of which are the result of increases in sympathetic drive. Static exercise, however, produces less of an increase in the HR and cardiac output and more of an increase in diastolic, systolic, and MAP than does dynamic exercise. Because of the higher afterload on the heart during static exercise, cardiac work is significantly higher than during dynamic exercise.

The time course of recovery of the various cardiovascular variables after a bout of exercise depends on many factors, including the type, duration, intensity of the exercise, and the overall fitness of the individual. Muscle blood flow normally returns to a resting value within a few minutes after dynamic exercise. However, if an abnormal arterial obstruction (such as an atherosclerotic plaque) prevents a normal *active hyperemia* from occurring during dynamic exercise, the recovery will take much longer than normal. After isometric exercise, muscle blood flow often rises to near-maximum levels before returning to normal with a time course that varies with the duration and intensity of the effort. Part of the increase in muscle blood flow that follows isometric exercise might be classified as *reactive hyperemia* in response to the blood flow restriction caused by compressional forces within the muscle during the exercise.

Responses to Chronic Exercise

Physical training or "conditioning" produces substantial beneficial effects on the cardiovascular system. The specific alterations that occur depend on the type of exercise, the intensity and duration of the training period, the age of the individual, and his or her original level of fitness.

In general, however, repeated physical exercise over a period of several weeks is associated with an increase in the individual's work capacity. Cardiovascular alterations seen at rest associated with conditioning may include decreases in HR, increases in cardiac stroke volume, and decreases in arterial blood pressure. During exercise, a trained individual will be able to achieve a given cardiac workload and output with much greater efficiency (lower HR and higher stroke volume) than is possible by an untrained individual. These changes produce a general decrease in myocardial oxygen demand and an increase in the *cardiac reserve* (potential for increasing cardiac output) that can be called on during times of stress.

Much (but not all) of the cardiovascular benefit of exercise conditioning can be attributed to a significant increase in circulating blood volume. This is triggered by the repetitive activation of the sympathetic nervous system during training, which promotes the renal fluid retention mechanisms. Other adaptations to exercise include alterations in arteries, arterioles, and capillaries that adapt in structure and number to maximize perfusion and improve oxygen delivery.

Eccentric cardiac hypertrophy (ventricular chamber enlargement with mild thickening of the ventricular wall) often accompanies dynamic exercise conditioning regimens (endurance training). Concentric cardiac hypertrophy (increases in myocardial mass and ventricular wall thickness) is more pronounced with static exercise conditioning regimens (strength training). These structural alterations improve the pumping capabilities of the myocardium. However, as described in the next chapter, ventricular chamber enlargement and myocardial hypertrophy are not always hallmarks of improved cardiac performance but may be adaptive responses to various pathological states that, if extreme, are not helpful.

Exercise training or "conditioning" with a higher-than-normal blood volume represents the opposite end of a functional spectrum from the "deconditioning" effects of long-term bed rest with lower-than-normal blood volume. "Deconditioning" after cessation of an exercise program occurs rapidly as blood volume returns to resting levels and cardiovascular structural adaptations reverse.

Exercise and physical conditioning can significantly reduce the incidence and mortality of cardiovascular disease. Although studies have not established specific mechanisms for these beneficial effects, there is a positive correlation between physical inactivity and the incidence rate and intensity of coronary heart disease. It is increasingly evident that recovery from a myocardial infarction or cardiac surgery is enhanced by an appropriate increase in physical activity. The benefits of cardiac rehabilitation programs include improvements in various indices of cardiac function and improvements in physical work capacity, percent body fat, serum lipids, psychological sense of well-being, and quality of life.

NORMAL CARDIOVASCULAR ADAPTATIONS

Up to this point, the cardiovascular system of a healthy adult has been described. However, there are some important cardiovascular adaptations that accompany pregnancy, birth, growth, and aging. The material in the following section is a brief overview of these changes.

Maternal Cardiovascular Changes During Pregnancy

Pregnancy causes alterations in vascular structure and blood flow to many maternal organs in order to support growth of the developing fetus. These organs include not only the uterus and developing placenta but also the kidneys and the gastrointestinal organs. However, one of the most striking cardiovascular changes of pregnancy is the nearly 50% increase in circulating blood volume. The placenta, being a low-resistance organ added in parallel with the other systemic organs, reduces the overall systemic TPR by approximately 40%. Without the substantial increase in circulating blood volume to support cardiac filling, the necessary elevation in cardiac output to balance the decrease in TPR would not be possible and pregnancy would result in a substantial decrease in MAP. At birth, the loss of the placenta contributes to the return of maternal TPR back toward normal levels.

Fetal Circulation and Changes at Birth

During fetal development, the exchange of nutrients, gases, and waste products between fetal and maternal blood occurs in the placenta. This exchange occurs by diffusion between separate fetal and maternal capillaries without any direct connection between the fetal and maternal circulations. From a hemodynamic standpoint, the placenta represents a temporary additional large systemic organ for both the fetus and the mother. The fetal component of the placenta has a low vascular resistance and receives a substantial portion of the fetal cardiac output.

Blood circulation in the developing fetus completely bypasses the collapsed fetal lungs. No blood flows into the pulmonary artery because the vascular resistance in the collapsed fetal lungs is essentially infinite (perhaps induced by the hypoxic status of the fetal alveoli). By the special structural arrangements shown in Figure 10–6, the right and left sides of the fetal hearts operate in parallel to pump blood through the systemic organs and the placenta. As shown in Figure 10–6A, fetal blood returning from the systemic organs and placenta fills both the left and right sides of the hearts together because of an opening in the intra-atrial septum called the *foramen ovale*. As indicated in Figure 10–6B, blood that is pumped by the right side of the fetal heart does not enter the occluded pulmonary circulation but is rather diverted into the aorta through a vascular connection between the pulmonary artery and the aorta called the *ductus arteriosis*.

An abrupt decrease in pulmonary vascular resistance occurs at birth with the onset of lung ventilation. The sudden increase in alveolar oxygen causes pulmonary vasodilation. This permits blood to begin flowing into the neonatal lungs from the pulmonary artery and tends to lower pulmonary arterial pressure. Meanwhile, total systemic vascular resistance increases greatly because of separation from the placenta (which is a large organ with low vascular resistance). This causes a rise in neonatal aortic pressure, which retards or even reverses the flow through the ductus arteriosus. Through mechanisms that are incompletely understood but clearly linked to a rise in blood oxygen tension, the ductus arteriosus gradually constricts

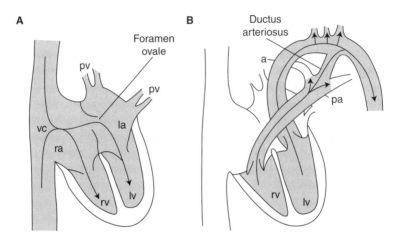

Figure 10-6. Fetal circulation during (**A**) cardiac filling and (**B**) cardiac ejection. pv, pulmonary veins; la, left atrium; lv, left ventricle; rv, right ventricle; ra, right atrium; vc, venae cavae; a, aorta; pa, pulmonary artery.

and completely closes over time, normally ranging from hours to a few days. The circulatory changes that occur at birth tend to simultaneously increase the pressure afterload on the left side of the heart and decrease that on the right. This indirectly causes left atrial pressure to increase above that in the right atrium so that the pressure gradient for flow through the foramen ovale is reversed. Reverse flow through the foramen ovale is, however, prevented by a flap-like valve that covers the opening in the left atrium. Normally, the foramen ovale is eventually closed permanently by the growth of fibrous tissue.

Pediatric Cardiovascular Characteristics

Cardiovascular variables change significantly between birth and adulthood. The healthy neonate has, by adult standards, a high resting HR (average of 140 beats/min) and a low arterial blood pressure (average of 60/35 mm Hg). These average values rapidly change over the first year (to 120 beats/min and 100/65 mm Hg, respectively). By the time the child enters adolescence, these values are near adult levels.

Pulmonary vascular resistance decreases precipitously at birth, as described earlier, and then continues to decline during the first year, at which time pulmonary pressures resemble adult levels. These resistance changes appear to be due to a progressive remodeling of the microvascular arterioles from thick-walled, small-diameter vessels to thin-walled, large-diameter microvessels.

It is noteworthy that distinct differences between right and left ventricular mass and wall thickness develop only after birth. Presumably, they arise because of a hypertrophic response of the left ventricle to the increased afterload it must assume at birth. Accordingly, the electrocardiogram of children shows an early right ventricular dominance (electrical axis orientation) that converts to the normal left ventricular dominance during childhood.

Heart murmurs are also quite common in childhood and have been reported to be present in as many as 50% of healthy children. Most of these murmurs fall in the category of "innocent" murmurs, resulting from normal cardiac tissue vibrations, high flow through valves, and thin chest walls that make noises from the vasculature easy to hear. Less than 1% of them result from various congenital heart defects.

Growth and development of the vascular system parallels growth and development of the body with most of the local and reflex regulatory mechanisms operational shortly after birth.

Cardiovascular Changes with Normal Aging

In general, as persons get older, they get slower, stiffer, and drier. Connective tissue becomes less elastic, capillary density decreases in many tissues, mitotic activity of dividing cells becomes slower, and fixed postmitotic cells (such as nerve and muscle fibers) are lost. Although these changes do not, in general, alter the basic physiological processes, they do have an influence on the rate at which various homeostatic mechanisms operate.

Age-dependent changes that occur in the heart include (1) a decrease in the resting and maximum cardiac index, (2) a decrease in the maximum HR, (3) an increase in the contraction and relaxation time of the heart muscle, (4) an increase in the myocardial stiffness during diastole, (5) a decrease in the number of functioning myocytes, and (6) an accumulation of pigment in the myocardial cells.

Changes that occur in the vascular bed with age may include (1) a decrease in capillary density in some tissues, (2) a decrease in arterial and venous compliance, (3) endothelial dysfunction associated with an increase in total peripheral vascular resistance, (4) an increase in arterial pulse pressure, and (5) an increase in MAP (as discussed in Figure 6–10 in Chapter 6). The increase in arterial pressure may impose a greater afterload on the heart, which may be partially responsible for the age-dependent decreases in cardiac index.

Arterial baroreceptor-induced responses to changes in blood pressure are blunted with age. This is due in part to a decrease in afferent activity from the arterial baroreceptors because of the age-dependent increase in arterial rigidity. In addition, the total amount of norepinephrine contained in the sympathetic nerve endings of the myocardium decreases with age, and the myocardial responsiveness to catecholamines declines. Thus, the efferent component of the reflex is also compromised. These changes may partially account for the apparent age-dependent sluggishness in the responses to postural changes and recovery from exercise.

It is important (although often difficult) to separate true age-dependent alterations from changes due to progressive inactivity or from disease-induced changes in physiological function. Cardiovascular diseases are the major cause of death in an aging population. Atherosclerosis and hypertension are the primary culprits in many populations. These "diseases" lack the universality necessary to be categorized as true aging processes but generally occur with increasing incidence in the older population. Pharmacological interventions and reduction of risk factors (smoking, obesity, inactivity, and high-fat or high-sodium diets) by modification of lifestyle can alter the incidence, intensity, and progression of these cardiovascular diseases. It is also possible that some of the previously mentioned interventions may prevent early expression of some of the normal aging processes and prolong the lifespan of a given individual. No practical intervention, however, is currently available that will increase the maximum potential lifespan of humans.

Sex Differences in Cardiovascular Characteristics

There are an increasing number of well-documented sex-dependent differences in cardiovascular physiology and pathophysiology. While the underlying principles and mechanisms described in the previous chapters apply to all, there are substantial sex-dependent differences in how the system may respond to various challenges. For example, cardiovascular adaptation to endurance training of women is quite different from that of men even with identical training programs. When compared with age-matched men, premenopausal women have a lower left ventricular mass to body mass ratio, which may reflect a lower cardiac afterload in women. This may result from their lower arterial blood pressure, greater aortic compliance, and improved ability to induce vasodilatory mechanisms (such as endothelial-dependent flow-mediated vasodilation). After menopause, some of these sex-based differences tend to disappear. However, older women with ischemic heart disease are more likely than men to have perfusion problems arising from microvascular dysfunction or coronary artery spasm and endothelial dysfunction, whereas men are more likely than women to have occlusive coronary artery disease from atherosclerosis which begins at an earlier age. Older women are also more likely than men to develop heart failure following a myocardial infarction.

Sex-dependent differences in cardiac electrical properties have also been described. Women often have lower intrinsic HRs and longer QT intervals than do men. They are at greater risk of developing long-QT syndrome and torsades de pointes. They are also twice as likely as men to have atrioventricular nodal reentry tachycardias and to develop atrial fibrillation. On the other hand, ischemic sudden death due to arrhythmias is more frequent in men than in women.

Some of the difference between men and women may be a result of cardiovascular protective effects of estrogen but other factors are likely to be involved and specific details are not yet fully understood. It is hoped that tomorrow's practicing physicians will have better understanding of these differences and better strategies for individualizing therapy.

PERSPECTIVES

The ability of the cardiovascular system to adjust to the challenges of the normal life of a healthy individual is very impressive. In all situations, regulation of arterial pressure by changes in cardiac output and vascular resistance assures that blood flow to critical organs is properly regulated and matched to the metabolic needs of the individual cells.

One of the topics missing from this text has to do with maintenance and repair of the cardiovascular components. It is obvious that subcellular mechanisms exist throughout life that are very good at building new structures during growth and development, at adapting existing structures to the demands of everyday life, and mending damaged parts of the cardiovascular system as they are exposed to daily external insults. Major advances in our knowledge of how to care for our cardiovascular system have contributed greatly to the improvement in our longevity and quality of life in the later years. However, we humans seem to have an approximate 100-year maximum limit on our lifespan. Theories of aging suggest that senescence is not totally left to chance or to the accidental accumulation of subcellular errors. Planned obsolescence seems to be a major part of most life forms, and personal longevity is partially controlled by genetics. An age-dependent progressive inability to rebuild and repair our cardiovascular system seems to be a major contributor to overall deterioration of all bodily functions. However, the increasing knowledge about residual stem cell populations found in what has been thought to be tissues made up of fixed postmitotic fully differentiated cells, and about potential use of pluripotent undifferentiated cells for tissue repair suggest that there may be future hope (or concern) that negating age-dependent cardiovascular alterations might prolong human life.

KEY CONCEPTS

 Cardiovascular responses to physiological stresses should be evaluated in terms of the initial effects of the primary disturbance and the subsequent effects of the reflex compensatory responses.

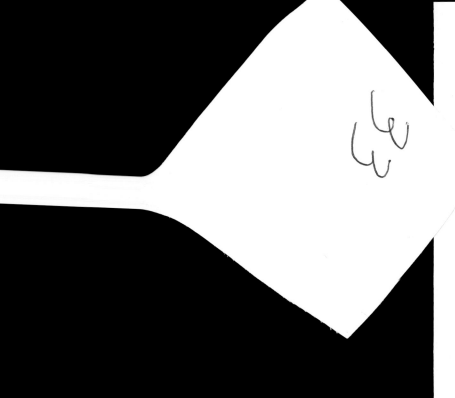 *Cyclical changes in intrathoracic pressure due to respiratory activity have significant effects on the cardiovascular system, partly by influencing venous return and cardiac filling and causing a normal "sinus arrhythmia."*

 Gravity has a significant effect on the cardiovascular system, and various reflex compensatory mechanisms are required to overcome peripheral venous pooling and reduced cardiac filling that accompany changing from a recumbent to an upright position.

 Long-term bed rest causes decreases in circulating blood volume that contribute to orthostatic hypotension.

 The primary cardiovascular disturbances of exercise (central command and skeletal muscle vasodilation) evoke immediate reflex compensatory activity, which permits major changes in muscle blood flow and cardiac output.

 Chronic exercise (training) evokes compensatory adjustments in blood volume and cardiovascular characteristics, permitting greater exercise efficiency achieved by higher stroke volume and lower heart rate.

Pregnancy-induced cardiovascular changes, including a major decrease in total peripheral resistance due to the developing placenta, evoke a significant increase in circulating maternal blood volume.

Circulatory pathways in the fetus are significantly different from those of the newborn and change abruptly at birth with the first breath.

Pediatric cardiovascular characteristics (high resting heart rates and low arterial blood pressures) gradually change to reach the normal adult levels during early adolescence.

Aging results in decreases in the maximal capabilities of cardiovascular responses that are distinct from any disease processes.

Sex-dependent differences influence cardiovascular characteristics and disease susceptibility particularly before the age of menopause in women.

STUDY QUESTIONS

10–1. How are the thin-walled capillaries in the feet able to withstand pressures greater than 100 mm Hg in a standing individual without rupturing?

10–2. Soldiers faint when standing at attention on a very hot day more often than on a cooler day. Why?

10–3. For several days after an extended period of bed rest, patients often become dizzy when they stand upright quickly because of an exaggerated transient fall in arterial pressure (orthostatic hypotension). Why might this be so?

10–4. Vertical immersion to the neck in tepid water produces a diuresis in many individuals. What mechanisms might account for this phenomenon?

10–5. How is the decrease in skeletal muscle vascular resistance evident from the data presented in Figure 10–4?

10–6. Is a decrease in total peripheral resistance implied in Figure 10–4?

10–7. What information in Figure 10–4 implies increased sympathetic activity?

10–8. From the information given in Figure 10–4,

    a. calculate the resting and exercising stroke volumes (SVs).

    b. calculate the resting and exercising end-diastolic volumes (EDVs).

    c. calculate the resting and exercising end-systolic volumes (ESVs).

    d. construct a sketch that indicates, as accurately as possible, how this exercise affects the left ventricular volume–pressure cycle.

10–9. The "iron lung," used to help polio victims breathe in the mid-20th century, applied an external intermittent negative pressure to the patient's thoracic cavity. How might this be better than positive-pressure artificial ventilation of the patient's lungs?

10–10. Blood pressure can rise to extremely high levels during strenuous isometric exercise maneuvers like weight lifting. Why?

10–11. Phenylephrine is a drug that specifically stimulates cardiovascular α-adrenergic receptors. If you gave phenylephrine to a patient, what would you expect would happen to sympathetic nerve activity, to myocardial contractility, to total peripheral resistance, and to heart rate?

10–12. Your 70-year-old 70-~~~~~~~~~~~~~~ ~~ ~iection fraction of 67% at rest. Left ventricular end-dias⁺
these data?

    a. These are normal data for someone this age.

    b. Your patient may be a competitive polka dancer.

    c. Your patient may be suffering from chronic systolic heart failure.

    d. Your patient may be severely hypovolemic.

    e. Stroke volume is $\sim$70 mL.

10–13. All of the following tend to occur when a person lies down. Which one is the primary disturbance that causes all the others to happen?

    a. The heart rate will decrease.

    b. Cardiac contractility will increase.

    c. Sympathetic activity will decrease.

    d. Parasympathetic activity will increase.

    e. Central venous pressure will increase.

10–14. Which of the following represents a normal compensatory response to chronic endurance exercise training?

    a. An increase in circulating blood volume

    b. An increase in the resting heart rate

    c. An increase in resting mean arterial pressure

    d. A decrease in resting stroke volume

    e. A decrease in resting blood flow to the kidneys

10–15. Total peripheral vascular resistance in the systemic circulation of a newborn baby undergoes an abrupt and sustained increase at birth. This is because

    a. circulating blood volume increases.

    b. the high-resistance lungs inflate.

    c. the low-resistance placental circulation is removed.

    d. sympathetic neural stimulation is elevated.

    e. cardiac output rises.

10–16. Aortic stiffness may increase substantially with old age. What is/are the expected consequences of this change?

    a. An increase in total peripheral resistance

    b. An increase in stroke volume

    c. An increase in pulse pressure

    d. An increase in mean arterial pressure

Cardiovascular Function in Pathological Situations

11

OBJECTIVES

The student understands the primary disturbances, compensatory responses, decompensatory processes, and possible therapeutic interventions that pertain to various abnormal cardiovascular situations:

▶ *Defines circulatory shock.*

▶ *Identifies the primary disturbances that can account for cardiogenic, hypovolemic, anaphylactic, septic, and neurogenic shock states.*

▶ *Lists the compensatory processes that may arise during various types of circulatory shock.*

▶ *Identifies the decompensatory processes that may arise during shock and describes how these lead to irreversible shock states.*

▶ *Indicates how coronary artery disease may lead to abnormal cardiac function.*

▶ *Defines the term angina pectoris and describes the mechanisms that promote its development.*

▶ *Indicates the mechanisms by which various therapeutic interventions may alleviate angina and myocardial ischemia in association with coronary artery disease.*

▶ *Defines the term cardiomyopathy and differentiates between dilated and hypertrophied cardiomyopathies.*

▶ *Defines the term heart failure and differentiates between acute and chronic heart failure and between systolic and diastolic failure.*

▶ *Identifies the short-term and long-term compensatory processes that accompany chronic systolic heart failure.*

▶ *Describes the advantages and disadvantages of the fluid accumulation that accompanies systolic heart failure.*

▶ *Defines pulmonary and systemic arterial hypertension.*

▶ *Identifies the various factors that may contribute to the development of systemic hypertension.*

▶ *Describes the role of the kidney in establishing and/or maintaining systemic hypertension.*

Cardiovascular disease represents the number one cause of deaths in most industrialized countries. How and when a person's cardiovascular system breaks down depends upon an increasing number of known risk factors. These include family history and genetic predisposition to various CV system malfunctions, poor diet and/or obesity, inactivity, environmental pollutants, and the acute or chronic effects of various infective agents. In this last chapter, a variety of specific pathologies that may be evoked by these risk factors are introduced. We have already described specific pathologies associated with abnormal cardiac electrical activities and valve function in Chapter 5, so will now focus on the pathologies associated with system-wide abnormalities. It is not intended as an in-depth coverage of cardiovascular diseases but rather as an introductory presentation of how the physiological processes described previously are evoked and/or altered during various abnormal cardiovascular states. In each case, there is generally a *primary disturbance* associated with malfunction of some component of the cardiovascular system that threatens the maintenance of normal arterial pressure. These *primary disturbances* evoke appropriate *compensatory reflex responses* to restore arterial pressure. Often, however, pathological situations also lead to inappropriate "decompensatory processes," which tend to accelerate the deterioration of cardiovascular function. Therapeutic interventions may be required and are often designed to limit or reverse these decompensatory processes. Students are again encouraged to review the summary of cardiovascular variables and their determinants in Appendix C because a thorough knowledge of this material will greatly help understand the physiological consequences of these abnormalities.

CIRCULATORY SHOCK

A state of circulatory "shock" exists whenever there is a generalized, severe reduction in blood supply to the body tissues and the metabolic needs of the tissues are not met. Even with all cardiovascular compensatory mechanisms activated, arterial pressure is usually (though not always) low in shock. In severe shock states of any etiology, inadequate brain blood flow leads to loss of consciousness, often with sudden onset (called *syncope*). The approach to understanding the causes and selecting an appropriate treatment depends on determination of the underlying primary disturbance. Recall that arterial pressure is determined by cardiac output and total peripheral resistance (TPR), so any loss in blood pressure is a result of a decrease in either one or both variables.

Primary Disturbances

In general, the shock state is precipitated by 1 of 3 cardiovascular crises: (1) severely depressed myocardial functional ability; (2) grossly inadequate cardiac filling due to low mean circulatory filling pressure; or (3) profound systemic vasodilation either due to the abnormal presence of powerful vasodilators or due to the absence of neurogenic tone normally supplied by the sympathetic nervous system. The consequences of these primary disturbances are represented in the 5 categories of shock summarized in Figure 11–1.

1. *Cardiogenic shock* occurs whenever cardiac pumping ability is compromised (e.g., as a result of severe arrhythmias, abrupt valve malfunction, coronary occlusions, or myocardial infarction). The direct consequence of any of these abnormalities is a significant fall in cardiac output.

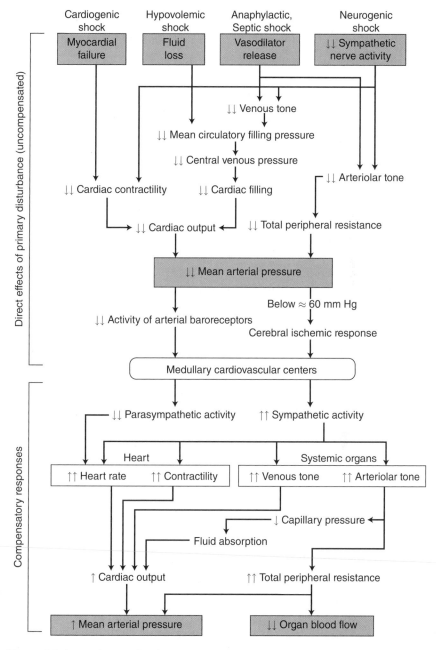

Figure 11–1. Cardiovascular alterations in shock.

2. *Hypovolemic shock* accompanies significant hemorrhage (usually greater than 20% of blood volume), or fluid depletion from lack of adequate fluid intake, severe burns, chronic diarrhea, or prolonged vomiting. These situations induce

shock by depleting body fluids and thus circulating blood volume. The direct consequence of hypovolemia is inadequate cardiac filling and reduced stroke volume.

Note: There are some situations that may result in reduced cardiac filling that is not related to hypovolemia. For example, *cardiac tamponade* associated with fluid accumulation in the pericardial sac (from pericardial infection, coronary vessel rupture, chest wounds, etc.) prevents adequate diastolic filling. Another example of reduced cardiac filling unrelated to hypovolemia is the occurrence of a *pulmonary embolus* (a clot mobilized from systemic veins lodging in a pulmonary vessel). In addition to potential damage to lung tissue, difficulty breathing, and severe discomfort, the disruption of left ventricular cardiac filling may result in a severe systemic shock state.

3. *Anaphylactic shock* occurs as a result of a severe allergic reaction to an antigen to which the patient has developed sensitivity (e.g., insect bites, antibiotics, and certain foods). This immunological event, also called an "immediate hypersensitivity reaction," is mediated by several substances (such as histamine, prostaglandins, leukotrienes, and bradykinin) that, by multiple mechanisms, results in substantial arteriolar vasodilation, increases in microvascular permeability, and loss of peripheral venous tone. These combine to reduce both TPR and cardiac output.

4. *Septic shock* is also caused by profound vasodilation but specifically from substances released into the circulating blood by infective agents. One of the most common is *endotoxin*, a lipopolysaccharide released from bacteria. This substance induces the formation of a nitric oxide synthase (called *inducible* nitric oxide synthase to distinguish it from the normally present *constitutive* nitric oxide synthase) in endothelial cells, vascular smooth muscle, and macrophages that then produce large amounts of the potent vasodilator, nitric oxide. The term *distributive shock* is sometimes used to describe both the anaphylactic and septic shock states.

5. *Neurogenic shock* is produced by loss of vascular tone due to inhibition of the normal tonic activity of the sympathetic vasoconstrictor nerves and often occurs with deep general anesthesia or in reflex response to deep pain associated with traumatic injuries. It may also be accompanied by an increase in vagal activity, which significantly slows the cardiac beating rate. This type of shock is often referred to as a *vasovagal syncope*. The transient syncope evoked by strong emotions is a mild form of neurogenic shock and is usually quickly reversible.

As shown in the top half of Figure 11–1, the common primary disturbances in all forms of shock are decreased cardiac output and/or TPR, leading to decreased mean arterial pressure. Generally, the reduction in arterial pressure is substantial, and so therefore, is the influence on the cardiovascular centers from reduced arterial baroreceptor discharge rate. In addition, in the case of hypovolemic, anaphylactic, and septic shock, diminished activity of the cardiopulmonary baroreceptors due to a decrease in central venous pressure and/or volume acts on the medullary cardiovascular centers to stimulate sympathetic output.[1] If arterial pressure falls below approximately 60 mm Hg, brain blood flow begins to fall, and this elicits the cerebral ischemic response. As indicated in Chapter 9, the cerebral ischemic response causes intense activation of the sympathetic nerves.

Compensatory Mechanisms

In general, the various forms of shock evoke the compensatory responses in the autonomic nervous system that we would expect from a fall in blood pressure.[2] These increases in sympathetic activity and decreases in parasympathetic activity are indicated in the bottom half of Figure 11–1. Cardiac and peripheral vascular compensatory responses to shock, however, may be much more intense than those that accompany more ordinary cardiovascular disturbances. Many of the commonly recognized symptoms of shock (e.g., pallor, cold clammy skin, rapid heart rate, muscle weakness, and venous constriction) are a result of greatly increased sympathetic nerve activity. When the immediate compensatory processes are inadequate, the individual may also show signs of abnormally low arterial pressure and reduced cerebral perfusion, such as dizziness, confusion, or loss of consciousness.

Additional compensatory processes initiated during the shock state may include the following:

1. Rapid and shallow breathing occurs, which promotes venous return to the heart by action of the respiratory pump.
2. Increased renin release from the kidney because of sympathetic stimulation promotes the formation of the hormone, angiotensin II, which is a potent vasoconstrictor and participates in the increase in TPR even in mild shock states.
3. Increased circulating levels of vasopressin (also known as antidiuretic hormone) from the posterior pituitary gland contribute to the increase in TPR. This hormone is released in response to decreased firing of the cardiopulmonary and arterial baroreceptors.
4. Increased circulating levels of epinephrine from the adrenal medulla in response to sympathetic stimulation contribute to systemic vasoconstriction.
5. Reduced capillary hydrostatic pressure resulting from intense arteriolar constriction reduces capillary hydrostatic pressure and promotes fluid movement from the interstitial space into the vascular space.

---

[1] In the case of cardiogenic shock, central venous pressure will increase; and in the case of neurogenic shock, central venous pressure cannot be predicted because both cardiac output and venous return are likely to be depressed. Thus, in these instances, it is not clear how the cardiopulmonary baroreceptors affect autonomic output.

[2] Two primary exceptions to this statement include (1) neurogenic shock, where reflex responses may be absent or lead to further depression of blood pressure and (2) certain instances of cardiogenic shock associated with inferior or posterior wall myocardial infarctions, which elicit a reflex bradycardia, decrease sympathetic drive, and apnea (the Bezold–Jarisch reflex).

6. Increased glycogenolysis in the liver induced by epinephrine and norepinephrine results in a release of glucose and a rise in blood (and interstitial) glucose levels and, more importantly, a rise in extracellular osmolarity by as many as 20 mOsm. This will induce a shift of fluid from the intracellular space into the extracellular (including intravascular) space.

The latter 2 processes result in a sort of "autotransfusion" that can move as much as a liter of fluid into the vascular space in the first hour after the onset of the shock episode. This fluid shift accounts for the reduction in hematocrit that is commonly observed in hemorrhagic shock. The extent of fluid shift may be limited by a reduction in colloid osmotic pressure.

In addition to the immediate compensatory responses shown in Figure 11–1, fluid retention mechanisms are evoked by hypovolemic states that affect the situation in the long term. The production and release of the antidiuretic hormone (vasopressin) from the posterior pituitary promote water retention by the kidneys. Furthermore, activation of the renin–angiotensin–aldosterone pathway promotes renal sodium retention (via aldosterone) and the thirst sensation and drinking behavior (via angiotensin II). These processes contribute to the replenishment of extracellular fluid volume within a few days of the shock episode.

Decompensatory Processes

Often the strong compensatory responses during shock evoked by the intense sympathetic activation can prevent drastic reductions in arterial pressure. However, because the compensatory mechanisms involve overwhelming arteriolar vasoconstriction, perfusion of tissues other than the heart and the brain may be inadequate despite nearly normal arterial pressure. For example, blood flow through vital organs such as the liver, gastrointestinal tract, and kidneys may be reduced nearly to zero by intense sympathetic activation. The possibility of permanent renal, hepatic, or GI tract ischemic damage is a very real concern even in seemingly mild shock situations. Patients who have apparently recovered from a state of shock may die several days later because of renal failure, uremia, or sepsis due to bacterial penetration of the weakened mucosal barrier in the GI tract.

The immediate danger with shock is that it may enter the *progressive stage*, wherein the general cardiovascular situation progressively degenerates, or, worse yet, enter the *irreversible stage*, where no intervention can halt the ultimate collapse of cardiovascular system that results in death.

The mechanisms behind progressive and irreversible shock are not completely understood. However, it is clear from the mechanisms as shown in Figure 11–2 that bodily homeostasis can progressively deteriorate with prolonged reductions in organ blood flow. These homeostatic disturbances, in turn, adversely affect various components of the cardiovascular system so that arterial pressure and organ blood flow are further reduced. Note that the events shown in Figure 11–2 are *decompensatory mechanisms*. Reduced arterial pressure leads to alterations that further reduce arterial pressure rather than correct it (i.e., a *positive feedback process*).

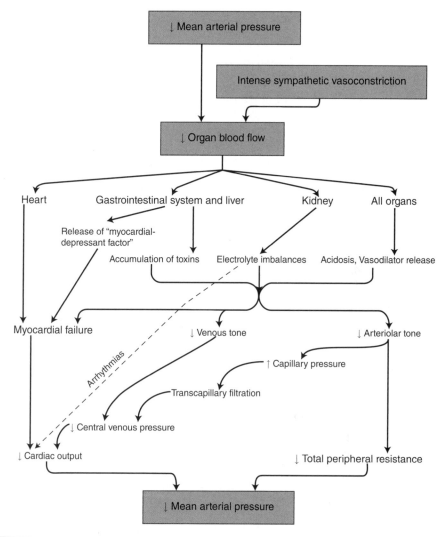

Figure 11-2. Decompensatory mechanisms in shock.

These decompensatory mechanisms that are occurring at the tissue level to lower blood pressure are eventually further compounded by a reduction in sympathetic drive and a change from vasoconstriction to vasodilation with a further lowering of blood pressure. The factors that lead to this unexpected reduction in sympathetic drive from the under-perfused medullary cardiovascular centers are not clearly understood. If the shock state is severe enough and/or has persisted long enough to enter the progressive stage, the self-reinforcing decompensatory mechanisms progressively drive arterial pressure down. Unless corrective measures are taken quickly, death will ultimately result.

CARDIAC DISTURBANCES

Coronary Artery Disease

DEFINITION AND PHYSIOLOGICAL CONSEQUENCES

Whenever coronary blood flow falls below that required to meet the metabolic needs of the heart, the myocardium is said to be *ischemic* and the pumping capability of the heart is impaired. The most common cause of myocardial ischemia is *atherosclerotic disease of the large coronary arteries.* In atherosclerotic disease, localized lipid deposits called *plaques* develop within the arterial walls. With severe disease, these plaques may become calcified and so large that they physically narrow the lumen of arteries (producing a chronic stenosis) and thus greatly and permanently increase the normally low vascular resistance of these large arteries. This extra resistance adds to the resistance of other coronary vascular segments and tends to reduce coronary flow. If the coronary artery stenosis is not too severe, local metabolic vasodilator mechanisms may reduce arteriolar resistance sufficiently to compensate for the abnormally large arterial resistance. Thus, an individual with coronary artery disease may have perfectly normal coronary blood flow when resting. A coronary artery stenosis of any significance will, however, limit the extent to which coronary flow can increase above its resting value by reducing maximum achievable coronary flow. This occurs because, even with very low arteriolar resistance, the overall vascular resistance of the coronary vascular bed is high if resistance in the large arteries is high.

In addition to atherosclerotic disease of large coronary arteries, there is another form of myocardial ischemia caused by abnormalities in the coronary *microvasculature.* Factors involved may include endothelial dysfunction and reduced flow (perhaps due to spasm) in the tiny "resistance" blood vessels of the heart. Because these changes are not characterized by major arterial blockages, they are harder to diagnose. Microvascular abnormalities were previously considered to be rather benign conditions, but studies now suggest that altered microvascular conditions are important pathophysiologic causes of ischemic heart disease especially in women.

Coronary artery disease can jeopardize cardiac function in several ways. Ischemic muscle cells are electrically irritable and unstable, and the danger of developing cardiac arrhythmias and fibrillation is enhanced. During a bout of ischemia, the normal cardiac electrical excitation pathways may be altered, and often ectopic pacemaker foci develop. Electrocardiographic manifestations of myocardial ischemia may be observed in individuals with coronary artery disease during exercise stress tests. In addition, there is evidence that platelet aggregation and clotting function may be abnormal in atherosclerotic coronary arteries and the danger of thrombus or emboli formation is enhanced. It appears that certain platelet suppressants or anticoagulants such as aspirin may be beneficial in the treatment of this consequence of coronary artery disease. (The details of the blood clotting process are included in Appendix D.)

Myocardial ischemia not only impairs the pumping ability of the heart but also may produce chest pain called *angina pectoris*.[3] Anginal pain is often absent in individuals with coronary artery disease when they are resting but is induced during physical exertion or emotional excitement. Both situations elicit an increase in sympathetic tone that increases myocardial oxygen consumption. Myocardial ischemia and chest pain will result if coronary blood flow cannot keep pace with the increase in myocardial metabolism.

DIAGNOSIS

Coronary artery imaging techniques (described in Chapter 4) have proven very useful for determining the extent of coronary artery disease in the large arteries. For example, calcification of plaques (which is a significant indicator of advanced atherosclerosis) can be assessed noninvasively with specialized CT scans or magnetic resonance imaging. Specific information about the site(s) and degree of narrowing of the major coronary vessels can also be obtained invasively by angiography with injection of a radiopaque dye directly into the coronary arteries.

TREATMENTS

Primary treatment of chronic coronary artery disease (and atherosclerosis, in general) should include attempts to lower blood lipids by dietary and pharmacological techniques that prevent (and possibly reverse) further development of the plaques. There are a number of recent strategies proven to be quite helpful. (1) Statins are well-accepted effective lipid-lowering drugs acting by blocking cholesterol production in the liver. (2) Newer drugs that prevent normal inactivation of certain lipid uptake receptors (LDL receptors in the liver) promote lipid removal from the circulation. (3) Because atherosclerotic heart disease is now recognized as a chronic inflammatory vascular disease, new anti-inflammatory drugs are being developed and show promising effects for the treatment of plaque reduction and prevention of infarction. Interested students should consult medical biochemistry and pharmacology texts for a complete discussion of this very important topic.

Treatment of chest pain that is a result of coronary artery disease may involve several different pharmacological approaches. First, quick-acting vasodilator drugs such as nitroglycerin may be used to provide primary relief from an acute anginal attack. In addition to increasing myocardial oxygen delivery by dilating coronary vessels, nitrates reduce myocardial oxygen demand by dilating systemic veins, thereby reducing venous return, central venous filling, and cardiac preload, and by dilating systemic arterioles, which reduces arterial resistance, arterial

---

[3] Definition: "a strangling feeling in the chest." Women are more likely to describe the ischemic episode as intense pressure, squeezing or chest discomfort, and men are more likely to describe it as intense, debilitating pain.

pressure, and cardiac afterload.[4] Second, β-adrenergic blocking agents such as propranolol may be used to block the effects of cardiac sympathetic nerves on the heart rate (HR) and contractility. These agents limit myocardial oxygen consumption and prevent it from increasing above the level that the compromised coronary blood flow can sustain. Third, calcium channel blockers such as verapamil may be used to dilate coronary and systemic blood vessels. These drugs, which block entry of calcium into the vascular smooth muscle cell, interfere with normal excitation–contraction coupling. They have been found to be useful for treating the type of angina caused by vasoconstrictive spasms of large coronary arteries (Prinzmetal angina).

Invasive or surgical interventions are commonly used to eliminate a chronic coronary artery stenosis. X-ray techniques combined with radiopaque dye injections can be used to visualize a balloon-tipped catheter as it is threaded into the coronary artery to the occluded region. Rapid inflation of the balloon squeezes the plaque against the vessel wall and improves the patency of the vessel (*coronary angioplasty*). A small tube-like expandable device called a *stent* is often implanted inside the vessel at the angioplasty site. This rigid implant promotes continued patency of the vessel over a longer period than angioplasty alone. Drug-eluting stents are often used to slowly deliver drugs to the local area that limit the growth of neointimal scar formation that may lead to restenosis. If angioplasty and stent placement are inappropriate or unsuccessful, coronary bypass surgery may be performed. The stenotic coronary artery segments are bypassed by implanting parallel low-resistance pathways formed from either natural (e.g., saphenous vein or mammary artery) or artificial vessels.

Acute Coronary Occlusion—Myocardial Infarction

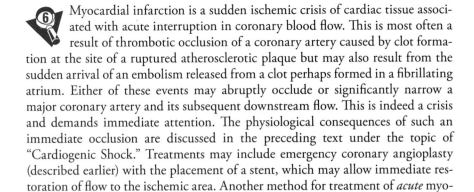

Myocardial infarction is a sudden ischemic crisis of cardiac tissue associated with acute interruption in coronary blood flow. This is most often a result of thrombotic occlusion of a coronary artery caused by clot formation at the site of a ruptured atherosclerotic plaque but may also result from the sudden arrival of an embolism released from a clot perhaps formed in a fibrillating atrium. Either of these events may abruptly occlude or significantly narrow a major coronary artery and its subsequent downstream flow. This is indeed a crisis and demands immediate attention. The physiological consequences of such an immediate occlusion are discussed in the preceding text under the topic of "Cardiogenic Shock." Treatments may include emergency coronary angioplasty (described earlier) with the placement of a stent, which may allow immediate restoration of flow to the ischemic area. Another method for treatment of *acute* myocardial infarction is the intravascular injection of thrombolytic substances (e.g., streptokinase or tissue plasminogen-activating factors) that dissolve blood clots.

---

[4] If blood pressure drops significantly, the beneficial effects of improved coronary circulation and reduced work load may be negated by a reflex increase in heart rate.

This approach is most successful when these "clot busters" are given within a few hours of the infarction.

To emphasize the 2 basic underlying physiological principles for treatment of an acute coronary event: (1) improve coronary blood flow to increase oxygen delivery and (2) minimize cardiac work to lower oxygen demand (by reducing preload, afterload, and contractility).

Cardiomyopathies

 A cardiomyopathy is an abnormality of the cardiac muscle that occurs even though coronary perfusion is usually adequate. They are commonly further classified by specific structural and functional changes as noted below.

Dilated cardiomyopathy (DCM) is characterized by cardiac chamber enlargement with normal ventricular wall thickness. These patients may develop heart failure with a reduced ejection fraction. This type of cardiomyopathy is often a delayed consequence of infections (e.g., herpes, coxsackie, influenza, human immunodeficiency virus), cardiac toxins (e.g., alcohol, cocaine, amphetamine, cancer chemotherapeutics), and other chronic systemic challenges. Familial predisposition has also been noted, and genetic coding for multiple protein abnormalities has been identified including those of the sarcomere, cytoskeleton, ion channels, and extracellular matrix proteins. Abnormalities in the giant protein, titin, that controls sarcomere stiffness, account for about 20% of familial cases of DCM.

Hypertrophic cardiomyopathy (HCM) is the most common genetic heart disease and is characterized by a significant, often asymmetrical, left ventricular wall thickening often leading to ventricular outflow obstruction. This hypertrophy is associated with a disruption of normal muscle cell alignment and various electrical malfunctions. It is often asymptomatic and is a leading cause of ventricular fibrillation and sudden cardiac death in young athletes. Because of its genetic predisposition, echocardiographic prescreening for susceptible populations may be lifesaving.

Takotsubo cardiomyopathy (aka stress cardiomyopathy or broken heart syndrome) is associated with a sudden, temporary, and often localized weakening of the ventricular musculature that is triggered by emotional stress or constant anxiety. Although it is classified as a nonischemic form of cardiomyopathy in that no overt vascular occlusions are identifiable, it may be associated with transient (and reversible) vascular spasm or microcirculatory malfunction. Release of various stress hormones may also produce regional "stunning" of the cardiomyocytes so that pumping is impaired. It differs from an acute myocardial infarction in that it seems to be completely reversible with time and treatment. It is a now well-recognized cause of acute heart failure, lethal arrhythmias, and ventricular rupture.

Chronic Heart Failure

 Heart (or cardiac or myocardial) *failure* is said to exist whenever ventricular function is depressed through myocardial damage, insufficient coronary flow, or any other condition that directly impairs the mechanical performance of the heart muscle. Cardiac failure can be categorized as being associated with systolic abnormalities ("Heart Failure with Reduced Ejection Fraction"—aka HFrEF) or with diastolic filling abnormalities ("Heart Failure with Preserved Ejection Fraction"—aka HFpEF).

Systolic heart failure (HFrEF)—By definition, *systolic* heart failure is associated with a left ventricular ejection fraction of less than 40%. This also implies that the heart is operating on a *lower-than-normal cardiac function curve*, that is, a reduced cardiac output at any given filling pressure. Acute heart failure has already been discussed in the context of sudden coronary artery occlusion, cardiogenic shock, and as part of the decompensatory mechanisms operating in progressive and irreversible shock. Often, however, sustained cardiac "challenges" may induce a chronic state of heart failure. Such challenges might include (1) progressive coronary artery disease, (2) sustained elevation in cardiac afterload as that which accompanies arterial hypertension or aortic valve stenosis, or (3) reduced *functional* muscle mass or contractility as a consequence of various cardiomyopathies or following myocardial infarction. Regardless of the precipitating cause, most forms of systolic failure are associated eventually with a reduced myocyte contractile function. Many specific structural, functional, and biochemical myocyte alterations accompany severe systolic heart failure. Some of the more well-documented abnormalities include (1) reduced calcium sequestration by the sarcoplasmic reticulum and upregulation of the sarcolemmal Na/Ca exchanger (leading to low intracellular calcium levels for excitation–contraction coupling), (2) low affinity of troponin for calcium (leading to reduced cross-bridge formation and contractile ability), (3) altered substrate metabolism from fatty acid to glucose oxidation, and (4) impaired respiratory chain activity (leading to impaired energy production).

The primary disturbance in systolic heart failure (acute or chronic) is depressed cardiac output and thus lowered arterial pressure. Consequently, all the compensatory responses important in shock (Figure 11–1) are also important in heart failure. In chronic heart failure, however, the cardiovascular disturbances may not be sufficient to produce a state of shock. Moreover, long-term compensatory mechanisms are especially important in chronic heart failure.

The circumstances of chronic systolic heart failure are well illustrated by cardiac output and venous function curves such as those shown in Figure 11–3. The normal cardiac output and normal venous function curves intersect at point A in Figure 11–3. A cardiac output of 5 L/min at a central venous pressure of less than 2 mm Hg is indicated by the normal operating point (A). With heart failure, the heart operates on a much lower-than-normal cardiac output curve. Thus, acute heart failure alone (uncompensated) shifts the cardiovascular operation from the normal point (A) to a new position, as illustrated by point B in Figure 11–3—that is, cardiac output falls below normal while central venous pressure rises above normal. The decreased cardiac output leads to decreased arterial pressure and reflex activation of the cardiovascular sympathetic nerves. Increased sympathetic nerve activity tends to (1) increase HR and cardiac contractility to raise the cardiac function curve toward normal and (2) increase peripheral venous pressure

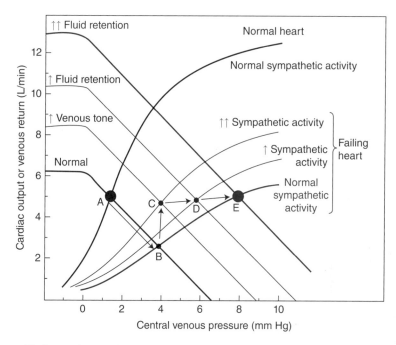

Figure 11–3. Cardiovascular alterations with compensated chronic systolic heart failure.

through venous constriction, and thus raise the venous function curve above normal. Cardiovascular operation will shift from point B to point C in Figure 11–3. Thus, the depressed cardiac output is substantially improved by the immediate consequences of increased sympathetic nerve activity. Note, however, that the cardiac output at point C is still below normal. The arterial pressure associated with cardiovascular operation at point C is likely to be near normal, however, because higher-than-normal TPR will accompany higher-than-normal sympathetic nerve activity.

 In the long term, cardiovascular operation cannot remain at point C in Figure 11–3. Operation at point C involves higher-than-normal sympathetic activity, and this will inevitably cause a gradual increase in blood volume by the mechanisms that are described in Chapter 9. Over several days, there is a progressive rise in the venous function curve as a result of increased blood volume and, consequently, increased mean circulatory filling pressure. Recall that this process involves a sympathetically induced release of renin from the kidney, which activates the renin–angiotensin–aldosterone system that promotes fluid retention. This will progressively shift the cardiovascular operating point from C to D to E, as shown in Figure 11–3.

Note that increased fluid retention (C → D → E in Figure 11–3) causes a progressive increase in cardiac output toward normal and simultaneously allows a *reduction in sympathetic nerve activity toward the normal value.* Reduced sympathetic activity is beneficial for several reasons. First, decreased arteriolar constriction permits renal and splanchnic blood flow to return toward more normal values. Second, myocardial oxygen consumption may fall as sympathetic nerve activity falls, even though cardiac output tends to increase. Recall that the increased HR and increased cardiac contractility caused by sympathetic nerve activation greatly increase myocardial oxygen consumption. Reduced myocardial oxygen consumption is especially beneficial in situations where inadequate coronary blood flow is the cause of heart failure. In any case, once enough fluid has been retained so that a normal cardiac output can be achieved with *normal* sympathetic nerve activity, the individual is said to be in a "compensated" state of chronic heart failure.[5] Note that the primary disturbance (i.e., the depressed cardiac function curve) is still present. Fluid retention did nothing to correct this. However, fluid retention does allow a "normal" cardiac output to now be achieved at the higher-than-normal central venous (i.e., cardiac filling) pressure.

Unfortunately, the consequences of fluid retention in chronic cardiac failure are not *all* beneficial. Note that in Figure 11–3 fluid retention (C → D → E) will cause both peripheral and central venous pressures to be much higher than their normal values. Chronically high central venous pressure causes chronically increased end-diastolic volume (cardiac dilation). Up to a point, cardiac performance is greatly improved by increased cardiac filling volume. Excessive cardiac dilation, however, can impair cardiac function because increased total wall tension is required to generate pressure within an enlarged ventricular chamber ($T = P \times r$; Chapter 2). This increases the myocardial oxygen demand.

The high venous pressure associated with fluid retention also adversely affects organ function because high venous pressure produces transcapillary fluid filtration, edema formation, and congestion (hence the commonly used term *congestive heart failure*). Left-sided heart failure is accompanied by pulmonary edema with dyspnea (shortness of breath) and respiratory crisis.[6] Right-sided heart failure is associated with distended neck veins, ankle edema, and fluid accumulation in the abdomen (ascites) with liver congestion and dysfunction.[7]

In the example shown in Figure 11–3, the depression in the cardiac output curve because of heart failure is only moderately severe. Thus, it is possible, through moderate fluid retention, to achieve a normal cardiac output with essentially normal sympathetic activity (point E). The situation at point E is relatively stable

---

[5] The extracellular fluid volume remains expanded after reaching the compensated state even though sympathetic activity may have returned to near-normal levels. Net fluid loss requires a period of *less-than-normal* sympathetic activity, which does not occur. For reasons not well understood, the cardiopulmonary baroreceptor reflexes apparently become less responsive to the increased central venous pressure and volume associated with heart failure.

[6] Patients often complain of difficulty breathing especially during the night (paroxysmal nocturnal dyspnea). Being recumbent promotes a fluid shift from the extremities into the central venous pool and lungs, making the patient's pulmonary problems worse. Such patients often sleep more comfortably when propped up.

[7] Plasma volume expansion along with abnormal liver function reduces the concentration of plasma proteins by as much as 30%. This reduction in plasma oncotic pressure contributes to the development of interstitial edema that accompanies congestive heart failure.

because the stimulus for further fluid retention (i.e., increased sympathetic drive) has been removed. If, however, the heart failure is more severe, the cardiac output curve may be so depressed that normal cardiac output cannot be achieved by any amount of fluid retention. In these cases, fluid retention is extremely marked, as is the elevation in venous pressure, and the complications of congestion are very serious problems.

Another way of looking at the effects of left ventricular cardiac failure is given in Figure 11–4. The left ventricular pressure–volume loops describing the events of a cardiac cycle from a failing heart are displaced far to the right of those from normal hearts. The untreated patient described in this figure is in serious trouble with a reduced stroke volume and ejection fraction and high filling pressure. Furthermore, the slope of the line describing the end-systolic pressure–volume relationship is shifted downward and is less steep, indicating the reduced contractility of the cardiac muscle. However, because of this flatter relationship, small reductions in cardiac afterload (i.e., arterial blood pressure) will produce substantial increases in stroke volume, as indicated in Figure 11–4, and will significantly help this patient.

As might be expected from the previous discussion, the most common symptoms of patients with congestive heart failure are associated with the inability to increase cardiac output (low exercise tolerance and fatigue) and with the compensatory fluid accumulation (tissue congestion, shortness of breath, and peripheral swelling). In severe cases, the ability of the cardiac cells to respond to increases in sympathetic stimulation is diminished by a reduction in the effective number (downregulation) of the myocyte β_1-adrenergic receptors. This further reduces the ability of the myocytes to increase their contractility and the ability of the heart to increase its beating rate in response to sympathetic stimulation. Thus, low maximal HRs contribute to the reduced exercise tolerance.

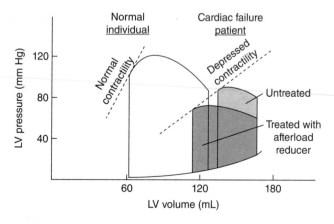

Figure 11–4. Left ventricular pressure–volume loops showing systolic heart failure (loops to the right) characterized by depressed contractility, increased end-diastolic volume, and reduced ejection fraction.

Treatment of the patient with congestive systolic heart failure is a difficult challenge. Treatment of the precipitating condition is of course the ideal approach, but often this cannot be done effectively. Cardiac glycosides (e.g., digitalis)[8] have been used to improve cardiac contractility (i.e., to increase the ejection fraction, shift the cardiac function curve upward, increasing contractile force of the myocyte at any given starting length).[9] These drugs are unfortunately quite toxic and often have undesirable side effects.

Treatment of the congestive symptoms involves balancing the need for enhanced cardiac filling with the problems of too much extracellular fluid. Drugs that promote renal fluid loss (diuretics such as furosemide or thiazides) are extremely helpful as are the angiotensin-converting enzyme (ACE) inhibitors and the angiotensin II receptor blockers (ARBs).[10] A potent diuretic can quickly save a patient from drowning in the pulmonary exudate and reduce diastolic volume of the dilated heart to acceptable levels, but it can also lower blood pressure to dangerous levels.

Chronic heart failure patients often have elevated sympathetic drive if they have not completely compensated for the depressed cardiac function by fluid retention and increased blood volume. Although high sympathetic drive is an important initial compensatory mechanism, the energy cost of a chronically elevated HR and contractility can put the heart with diminished coronary circulation at a disadvantage. Therefore, treatment with β-adrenergic receptor blockers can reduce metabolic demand to a level more easily met by a compromised vascular supply. Again, if elimination of the effect of elevated sympathetic drive on the heart is too aggressive, cardiac output may fall and worsen a failure state.

Diastolic heart failure (HFpEF)—Up to one-half of patients with heart failure have normal or near normal (i.e., "preserved") ejection fraction (>50%). In these cases, the problem is not with the systolic pressure-developing processes but rather with the diastolic relaxation and passive distension processes. As shown in Figure 11–5, diastolic dysfunction implies a stiffened heart during diastole such that increases in cardiac filling pressure do not produce normal increases in end-diastolic volume.

Some individuals (primarily elderly patients with hypertension and cardiac hypertrophy) who have some symptoms of cardiac failure (exertional dyspnea,

---

[8] A "tea" made from the leaves of the foxglove plant (*Digitalis purpurea*) was used for centuries as a common folk remedy for the treatment of "dropsy" (congestive heart failure with significant peripheral edema). With the formal recognition of its medicinal benefits in the late 18th century by the English physician Sir William Withering, digitalis became a valuable official pharmacological tool.

[9] The mechanism of cardiac glycoside action is thought to involve the inhibition of the sodium/potassium adenosine triphosphatase (Na^+/K^+-ATPase) leading to increases in intracellular Na^+, which is then exchanged for extracellular calcium via the Na^+/Ca^{2+} exchanger. This results in "loading" of the sarcoplasmic reticulum during diastole and increased calcium release for subsequent excitation–contraction coupling.

[10] ACE inhibitors can be helpful to the congestive heart failure patient for several reasons. By inhibiting the conversion of angiotensin I into its more active form, angiotensin II, peripheral vasoconstriction is reduced (which improves cardiac pumping by afterload reduction) and aldosterone levels are reduced (which promotes diuresis). In addition, ACE inhibitors and the ARBs seem to prevent some of the apparently inappropriate myocyte and collagen growth (i.e., remodeling) that occurs with cardiac overload and failure.

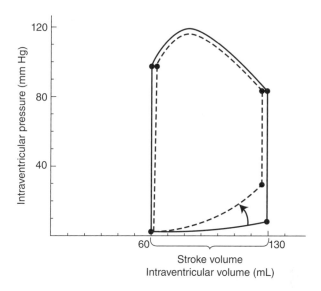

Figure 11–5. Left ventricular pressure–volume loops showing diastolic heart failure (*dashed lines*) characterized by increased diastolic stiffness, increased end-diastolic pressure, and normal ejection fraction.

fluid retention, pulmonary edema, and high end-diastolic pressures) seem to have normal systolic function (ejection fractions >50%), and normal or even reduced ventricular end-diastolic volumes despite increased cardiac filling pressure. Thus, the terms *diastolic heart failure* and *heart failure with preserved systolic function* have been used to describe this situation.

This condition is associated with many common risk factors (hypertension, atrial fibrillation, diabetes or metabolic syndrome, older age, female sex, inactivity, renal dysfunction, and/or obesity). Most of the time, angiographic evaluation of the coronary circulation does not show significant large vessel disease. The symptoms mimic those of systolic heart failure (i.e., with reduced ejection fraction) (e.g., exertional dyspnea, fatigue, congestion, chest pain). Some degree of diastolic dysfunction is also commonly present in patients with reduced ejection fraction and may precede systolic problems.

Potential causes of altered diastolic properties in heart failure include: (1) decreased cardiac tissue passive compliance due to extracellular remodeling, collagen cross-linking, and other extracellular matrix protein alterations often associated with left ventricular hypertrophy resulting from hypertension; (2) loss of myocardial elastic recoil that is partly responsible for early ventricular filling after systole; (3) increased myofibrillar passive stiffness due to alterations in the myofibrillar giant protein, titin; (4) delayed myocyte relaxation early in diastole due to slow cytosolic calcium removal processes; (5) inadequate adenosine triphosphate levels required to disconnect the myofilament cross-bridges rapidly; and (6) residual, low-grade cross-bridge cycling during diastole due to calcium leaking from the sarcoplasmic reticulum. Metabolic comorbidities (diabetes, obesity) may trigger a systemic inflammatory state that leads to microvascular endothelial dysfunction, allowing inflammatory cells to enter the myocardium. These trigger various paracrine signals that initiate various processes that lead to the passive compliance changes.

At this point, therapeutic strategies that directly influence diastolic properties are not well developed. Attempts to reduce interstitial fibrosis (with ACE inhibitors and/or angiotensin receptor antagonists) and to reduce diastolic calcium leak from the sarcoplasmic reticulum (with β-adrenergic blockers) have had limited success. Correcting underlying comorbidities and treatment with anti-inflammatory therapies are possibilities. Reduction of afterload seems to be most helpful, especially if it reduces left ventricular hypertrophy. In any case, "heart failure with preserved ejection fraction" is currently difficult to diagnose and to effectively treat.

HYPERTENSION

Hypertension is defined as a chronic elevation in arterial blood pressure and can exist in either the pulmonary or the systemic vascular system.

Pulmonary hypertension is less common than systemic hypertension and less is known about its causes, progression, and treatments. Pulmonary hypertension is designated when mean pulmonary artery pressure is greater than 25 mm Hg. It can be caused by either structural alterations in the lung vasculature (associated with smoking, environmental toxins, left heart failure with pulmonary congestion) or by altered vascular smooth muscle reactivity. Right-sided heart failure resulting from chronic pulmonary hypertension is called *cor pulmonale*. Although there is a genetic component to its incidence, it seems to be highly correlated with conditions involving chronic hypoxia (e.g., chronic obstructive pulmonary disease, cystic fibrosis, and pneumoconiosis).[11] The increased prevalence of obesity with accompanying obstructive sleep apnea may account for a recent increase in reported incidence of this disease. It is relatively hard to diagnose until symptoms appear as the consequences of elevated pulmonary arterial pressures. These symptoms may include systemic edema, pulmonary congestion, shortness of breath, chest pain, and fatigue.

There is no cure for pulmonary hypertension at present, and strategies used for the treatment of systemic hypertension have had little or no effect on the pulmonary bed. However, several pharmacological approaches are proving to be useful: (1) endothelin receptor antagonists block the biological activities of the vasoconstrictor, endothelin; (2) phosphodiesterase-5 inhibitors prevent the breakdown of cyclic guanosine monophosphate, thus promoting the vasorelaxant effects of nitric oxide; and (3) prostacyclin derivatives provide an exogenous supply of the vasodilator, prostacyclin, or drugs that activate a prostacyclin receptor.

---

[11] It is noteworthy that *acute* pulmonary hypertension and pulmonary edema are recognized risks of mountain climbing to extreme altitudes without the aid of supplemental oxygen.

Systemic hypertension is defined as an elevation of mean systemic arterial pressure above 140/90 mm Hg. It is an extremely common cardiovascular problem, affecting more than 20% of the adult population in the western world. It has been established beyond doubt that hypertension increases the risk of coronary artery disease, myocardial infarction, heart failure, stroke, and many other serious cardiovascular problems. Moreover, it has been clearly demonstrated that the risk of serious cardiovascular incidents is reduced by proper treatment of hypertension.[12]

In approximately 90% of cases, the primary abnormality that produces high blood pressure is unknown. This condition is sometimes referred to as primary or essential hypertension because the elevated level is thought to be "essential" to drive the blood through the systemic circulation. In the remaining 10% of hypertensive patients, the cause can be traced to a variety of sources, including epinephrine-producing tumors (pheochromocytomas), aldosterone-producing tumors (in primary hyperaldosteronism), certain forms of renal disease (e.g., renal artery stenosis, glomerular nephritis, and toxemia of pregnancy), certain neurological disorders (e.g., brain tumors that increase intracranial pressure), certain thyroid and parathyroid disorders, aortic coarctation, lead poisoning, drug side effects, abuse of certain drugs, obstructive sleep apnea, or even unusual dietary habits. The high blood pressure that accompanies such known causes is referred to as secondary hypertension. Most often, however, the true cause of the hypertension remains a mystery, and it is only the symptom of high blood pressure that is treated.

Facts about Systemic Hypertension

Amid an enormous amount of information about systemic hypertension, a few universally accepted facts stand out:

1. Genetic factors contribute importantly to the development of hypertension. Familial tendencies for high blood pressure are well documented. In addition, hypertension is generally more common in men than in women and racial differences in incidence have been identified.
2. Chronic conditions such as obesity, diabetes, kidney disease, and sleep disorders are strongly associated with systemic hypertension.
3. Environmental factors or behaviors can greatly influence the development of hypertension. Physical inactivity, use of tobacco, excess alcohol consumption, high-sodium or low-potassium diets, and/or certain forms of psychological stress may either aggravate or precipitate hypertension in genetically susceptible individuals.
4. Structural changes in the left side of the heart and arterial vessels occur in *response* to systemic hypertension. Early alterations include hypertrophy of muscle cells and thickening of the walls of the ventricle and systemic resistance vessels.

---

[12] Because an increased risk of cardiovascular complications with even mildly elevated blood pressure has been identified, a category designated *prehypertension* has been added to include blood pressures ranging from 120 to 139 mm Hg systolic and 80 to 89 mm Hg diastolic.

Late changes associated with the deterioration of function include increases in connective tissue and loss of elasticity.

5. The established phase of hypertension is associated with an increase in TPR. Cardiac output and/or blood volume may be elevated during the early developmental phase, but these variables are usually normal after the hypertension is established.

6. The increased TPR associated with established hypertension may be due to (a) *rarefaction* (decrease in density) of microvessels, (b) pronounced structural adaptations that occur in the peripheral vascular bed, (c) continuously increased activity of the vascular smooth muscle cells,[13] (d) increased sensitivity and reactivity of the vascular smooth muscle cells to external vasoconstrictor stimuli, and/or (e) diminished production and/or effect of endogenous vasodilator substances (e.g., nitric oxide).

7. The chronic elevation in blood pressure does not appear to be due to a sustained elevation in sympathetic vasoconstrictor neural discharge nor is it due to a sustained elevation of any blood-borne vasoconstrictive factor. (Both neural and hormonal influences, however, may help initiate primary hypertension.)

8. Blood pressure–regulating reflexes (both the short-term arterial and cardiopulmonary baroreceptor reflexes and the long-term, renal-dependent, pressure-regulating reflexes) become adapted or "reset" to regulate blood pressure at a higher-than-normal level.

9. Disturbances in renal function contribute importantly to the development and maintenance of primary hypertension. Recall that the urinary output rate is influenced by arterial pressure, and, in the long term, arterial pressure can stabilize only at the level that makes urinary output rate equal to fluid intake rate. As shown by point N in Figure 11–6, this pressure is approximately 100 mm Hg in a normal individual.

All forms of hypertension involve an alteration somewhere in the chain of events by which changes in arterial pressure produce changes in urinary output rate (see Figure 9–6) such that the renal function curve is shifted rightward, as indicated in Figure 11–6. The important feature to note is that *higher-than-normal arterial pressure is required to produce a normal urinary output rate in a hypertensive individual.* Although this condition is always present with hypertension, it is not clear whether it could be the common cause of hypertension or simply another one of the many adaptations to it.

Consider that the untreated hypertensive individual in Figure 11–6 would have a very low urinary output rate at the normal mean arterial pressure of 100 mm Hg. Recall from Figure 9–5 that whenever the fluid intake rate exceeds

---

[13] Continuous activation of vascular smooth muscle might be evoked by autoregulatory responses to increased blood pressure, as discussed in Chapter 6. A *total body autoregulation* could produce an increase in total peripheral resistance so that total systemic flow (i.e., cardiac output) would remain nearly normal in the presence of increased mean arterial pressure.

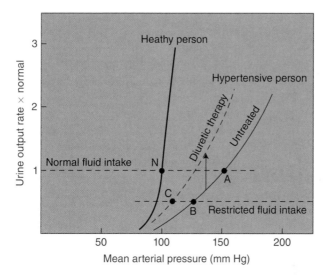

Figure 11–6. Renal function curves in healthy and hypertensive people.

the urinary output rate, fluid volume must rise and consequently so will cardiac output and mean arterial pressure. With a normal fluid intake rate, this untreated hypertensive patient will ultimately stabilize at point A (mean arterial pressure 150 mm Hg). Recall from Chapter 9 that the baroreceptors adapt within days so that they have a normal discharge rate at the *prevailing* average arterial pressure. Thus, once the hypertensive individual has been at point A for a week or more, even the baroreceptor mechanism will begin resisting acute changes from the 150-mm Hg pressure level.

A most important fact to realize is that, although either high cardiac output or high TPR must always ultimately sustain high blood pressure, neither needs to be the *primary* cause of the hypertension. A shift in the relationship between arterial pressure and urinary output rate, as illustrated in Figure 11–6, however, will always produce hypertension. The possibility that the kidneys actually "set" the blood pressure is supported by evidence accumulating from kidney transplant studies. In these studies, the blood pressure is shown to "follow" the kidney (i.e., putting a hypertensive kidney in a normotensive individual produces a hypertensive individual, whereas putting a normotensive kidney in a hypertensive individual produces a normotensive individual). Further support for an essential role of the kidney comes from recent studies showing that catheter-based, high-frequency radiowave ablation of renal sympathetic nerves effectively reduces hypertension in drug-resistant patients.

Therapeutic Strategies for Treatment of Systemic Hypertension

In certain hypertensive individuals, restricting salt intake produces a substantial reduction in blood pressure because of the reduced requirement for water retention to osmotically balance the salt load. In the example in Figure 11–6, this effect is illustrated by a shift from point A to point B. The efficacy of lowering salt intake to lower arterial pressure depends heavily on the slope of the renal function curve in the hypertensive individual. The arterial pressure of a healthy individual, for example, is affected only slightly by changes in salt intake because the normal renal function curve is so steep.

A second common treatment for hypertension is diuretic therapy. Many diuretic drugs are available, but most have the effect of inhibiting renal tubular salt (and therefore fluid) reabsorption. The net effect of diuretic therapy, as shown in Figure 11–6, is that the urinary output rate for a given arterial pressure is increased; that is, diuretic therapy raises the renal function curve. The combined result of restricted fluid intake and diuretic therapy for the hypertensive individual in Figure 11–6 is illustrated by point C.

A third therapeutic intervention is treatment with β-adrenergic blockers that inhibit sympathetic influences on the heart and renal renin release. This approach is most successful in hypertensive patients who have high circulating renin levels.

A fourth antihypertensive strategy is to block the effects of the renin–angiotensin system either with ACE inhibitors blocking the formation of the vasoconstrictor angiotensin II or with ARBs. Other pharmacological interventions may include use of α-adrenergic receptor blockers, which prevent the vasoconstrictive effects of catecholamines, and calcium channel blockers, which act directly to decrease vascular smooth muscle tone.

Alterations in lifestyle, including reduction of stress, decrease in caloric intake, limitation of the amount of saturated fats in the diet, and establishment of a regular exercise program, may help reduce blood pressure in certain individuals.

The possibility of catheter-based renal sympathetic denervation for the treatment of refractory hypertension is quite intriguing and may become another approach to handling this condition in the future.

PERSPECTIVES

Medical knowledge is constantly expanding and it is difficult, if not impossible, to keep up. However, we hope that this chapter's overview of some common cardiovascular diseases will reassure the student that *memorizing* everything is not necessary. *Understanding* the basic principles of normal cardiovascular operation should provide a firm foundation for identifying the underlying abnormalities, distinguishing the primary disturbances from the compensatory responses, understanding the mechanisms responsible for the symptoms, and appropriately treating the condition. What the future brings with new mechanistic insights, new diagnostic techniques, and new strategies for the treatment (or better yet, for prevention) of these diseases will most assuredly be built on these basic underlying principles.

KEY CONCEPTS

 Circulatory shock is defined as a generalized, severe reduction in tissue blood flow so that metabolic needs are not met.

 The primary disturbances that can lead to shock can be categorized as those that directly interfere with pump function, those that interfere with ventricular filling, or those that cause sustained vascular dilation.

 Shock is usually accompanied by a compensatory increase in sympathetic activity aimed at maintaining arterial pressure via augmented cardiac output and vascular resistance.

 Decompensatory processes precipitated by the shock state are generally caused by inadequate tissue blood flow, loss of local homeostasis, and tissue damage leading to a progressive and irreversible fall in arterial pressure.

 Coronary artery disease, usually associated with development of atherosclerotic plaques, results in a progressive compromise in coronary blood flow that becomes inadequate to meet the tissue's metabolic needs.

 Acute heart failure due to an abrupt blockage of a major coronary artery is a form of cardiogenic shock.

 Cardiomyopathies are primarily associated with deficits in myocyte function rather than inadequate coronary blood flow.

 Systolic heart failure is defined as a reduction of cardiac muscle contractility that results in a depressed cardiac output at all preloads with reduced ejection fraction.

 Compensatory fluid retention mechanisms are evoked in heart failure to improve cardiac filling, but when fluid retention is excessive, congestive complications arise (e.g., pulmonary edema and abdominal ascites).

 Diastolic dysfunction resulting from reduced cardiac compliance and impaired diastolic filling may precipitate heart failure even though ejection fraction is preserved.

 Pulmonary hypertension that accompanies acute or chronic conditions of hypoxia is relatively uncommon but can lead to right-sided heart failure (cor pulmonale).

 Systemic hypertension is a common and serious condition influenced by multiple genetic and environmental factors and is usually associated with chronic elevation in total peripheral resistance.

11–1. *Clinical signs of hypovolemic shock often include pale and cold skin, dry mucous membranes, weak but rapid pulse, muscle weakness, and mental disorientation or unconsciousness. What are the physiological conditions that account for these signs?*

11–2. *Which of the following would be helpful to hemorrhagic shock victims?*

    a. Keep them on their feet

    b. Warm them up

    c. Give them fluids to drink

    d. Maintain their blood pressure with catecholamine-type drugs.

11–3. *What happens to hematocrit?*

    a. During hypovolemic shock resulting from prolonged diarrhea

    b. During acute cardiogenic shock

    c. During septic shock

    d. With chronic bleeding

11–4. *Left ventricular chamber enlargement with congestive heart failure increases the wall tension required to generate a given systolic pressure. True or false?*

11–5. *Why are diuretic drugs often helpful in treating patients with congestive heart failure?*

11–6. *What is the potential danger of vigorous diuretic therapy for patients with heart failure?*

11–7. *Why does renal artery stenosis produce hypertension?*

11–8. *Your 70-year-old, 70-kg patient has an ejection fraction of 70%. Left ventricular end-diastolic volume is 100 mL. Which of the following statements best fits these data?*

    a. Stroke volume is approximately 30 mL

    b. Left ventricular end-systolic volume is approximately 70 mL

    c. Your patient may be dehydrated

    d. Your patient may be suffering from chronic systolic heart failure

    e. These are normal values for someone this age

11–9. *All the following are compensatory processes that help maintain circulation during states of hypovolemic shock except*

    a. hepatic glycogenolysis to increase extracellular glucose concentration.

    b. rapid respiratory effort to promote venous return of blood to the heart.

    c. vasoconstrictive contributions from increases in circulating epinephrine.

    d. autotransfusion of interstitial fluid into capillary beds.

    e. increased blood flow to the kidney.

11–10. Predict the status of each of the following variables in most individuals with chronic systemic hypertension.

    a. Cardiac output

    b. Heart rate

    c. Arterial pulse pressure

    d. Total peripheral resistance

    e. Renal urinary output

11–11. Compression stockings are often used by people with congestive heart failure. Why?

11–12. Would compression stockings be helpful for someone who suffers from leg pain after walking a short distance?

11–13. Would compression stockings be helpful for someone with a large clot in a major vein (deep vein thrombosis).

Answers to Study Questions

CHAPTER 1

1–1. The lungs always receive more blood flow than any other organ because 100% of the cardiac output passes through the lungs.

1–2. False. Flow through any vascular bed depends on its resistance to flow and the arterial pressure. As long as this pressure is maintained constant (a critical point that is dependent on adjustments in cardiac output), alterations in flow through any individual bed will have no influence on flow through other beds in parallel with it.

1–3. A leaky aortic valve will cause a diastolic murmur. Normally, the aortic valve is closed during diastole when there is a large reverse pressure difference between the aorta and left ventricle.

1–4. False. Slowing conduction through the AV node will have no effect on the heart rate but will increase the interval between atrial and ventricular excitation. The heart rate is normally slowed by decreases in the rate of action potential initiation by pacemaker cells in the SA node.

1–5. a. Saying that the diameter of a vessel increases by 10% is equivalent to saying that its radius increases by 10%; that is, the radius after the change is 1.1 times the radius before the change. The Poiseuille equation says that other factors equal, resistance is proportional to 1 over radius to the fourth power:

$$R \propto 1/r^4$$

Thus,

$$R_{before} \propto 1/(r_{before})^4$$

$$R_{after} \propto 1/(1.1r_{before})^4 = [1/(1.1)^4][1/(r_{before})^4]$$

$$= (1/1.46)R_{before} = 0.68R_{before}$$

Therefore, a 10% increase in vessel radius will reduce its resistance by 32%.

b. Because $\dot{Q} = \Delta P / R$, and $R_{after} = 0.68\ R_{before}$

$$\dot{Q}_{after} = \Delta P / 0.68 R_{before}$$

... and for a given ΔP ...

$$\dot{Q}_{after} = 1 / 0.68 R_{before} = 1.46 \dot{Q}_{before}$$

Therefore, for a given ΔP, a 10% increase in vessel diameter will increase flow by 46%.

[*Note:* One must always use change *factors* NOT *percentage* changes in these equations.]

1–6. a. Wrong! The pulmonary and systemic circuits are arranged in series and therefore must have the same output flow in the steady state.
   b. Wrong! The right and left hearts are served by a common electrical excitation system and therefore beat at the same rate.
   c. Wrong! Although it is true that the right ventricle is less muscular than the left, that fact does not explain why pulmonary pressure is so low. Actually, it is the other way around because pulmonary arterial pressure is low, the right ventricle does not have to be very muscular to pump blood into the lungs.
   d. Right! $\Delta P = \dot{Q} \times R$. Because $\dot{Q}$ is the same (= CO) through the lungs and the systemic circulation, the only way pulmonary arterial pressure could be relatively low is for pulmonary vascular resistance to be relatively low.
   e. Wrong! CO = HR × SV. CO and HR are the same for both the right and left pumps. Therefore, the SV of the right ventricle must be equal to that of the left.
   f. This is a complete cop-out for a reasoned explanation!

1–7. Significant blood loss has a profound negative effect on cardiac pumping because there is not enough blood left to fill the heart properly. This results in decreased cardiac output because of the Starling law of the heart. The consequence of decreased cardiac pumping ability is a lessened pressure difference between arteries and veins. Because of the basic flow equation, less ΔP causes less flow through the systemic organs. Interstitial homeostasis is compromised when there is abnormally low blood flow through capillaries. Improper interstitial conditions impair nerve function and cognitive ability in the brain and cause weakness in skeletal muscles.

1–8. Norepinephrine is the normal sympathetic neurotransmitter substance, so the same cardiovascular effects that normally accompany activation of sympathetic nerves should be predicted. These include increased heart rate, increased forcefulness of cardiac contraction, arteriolar constriction, and venous constriction. (Not all of these things may actually happen in the intact individual for complex reflex reasons presented in Chapter 9.)

1–9. Arteriolar and venous constriction would be expected because the sympathetic nerve effects on these vessels are normally mediated via α-receptors.

No direct effects on the heart would be expected because the sympathetic effects on the heart are mediated by β-receptors.

1–10. Among other effects, β-adrenergic receptor blockade tends to reduce heart rate and the forcefulness of ventricular contraction. Both these results tend to decrease cardiac output. The β-receptor blockade does not directly influence the arteriolar smooth muscle and thus does not directly change the resistance to flow through the systemic vasculature. According to the basic flow equation, less flow through a constant resistance implies a smaller pressure difference exists $(\Delta P = \dot{Q} / R)$. Because the venous pressure is normally 0 mm Hg, and ΔP is arterial minus venous pressure, this translates to a lowered arterial pressure.

1–11. Plasma sodium concentration will be 140 mEq/L because serum is just plasma minus a few clotting proteins. Interstitial sodium ion concentration will also be 140 mEq/L because sodium ions are in diffusional equilibrium across capillary walls. Intracellular sodium ion concentration cannot be predicted because sodium is actively pumped out of all cells.

1–12. $\dot{Q} = \Delta P / R$. The ΔP across your kitchen faucet is the pressure in the water supply pipes in your house minus the atmospheric pressure at the end of its waterspout. Turning the faucet handle does not change either of these pressures; that is, ΔP is constant. Therefore, changes in outflow must be caused by changes in the resistance to flow through the faucet mechanism. What the faucet handle does is control the degree of opening of a valve within the mechanism. When the handle is in the "off" position, this valve is completely closed and has an infinite resistance to flow, in which case $\dot{Q}$ is 0 regardless of ΔP. As this valve is progressively opened, its resistance to flow progressively decreases and consequently $\dot{Q}$ progressively increases.

1–13. Physical exercise requires an increase in CO. Normally, this is accomplished in large part by an increase in HR. The presence of β-blocker interferes with the normal ability to increase HR via sympathetic nerve activation.

1–14. e. 20 L. Extracellular volume is interstitial volume plus plasma volume. As indicated in Figure 1–1, this amounts to approximately 15 L in a "standard person" weighing 70 kg (154 lb). The rule of thumb is that body weight is approximately 60% water with the intracellular volume at approximately 40% of body weight and the extracellular volume at approximately 20% of body weight. Thus, a 100-kg person would be expected to have approximately 20 L of extracellular fluid.

1–15. The Fick principle states that

$$\dot{G}_{m} = \dot{Q} \times ([G]_{a} - [G]_{v})$$

Thus,

$$\dot{G}_{m} = 60\,\text{mL/min} \times (50 - 30)\,\text{mg/100 mL} = 12\,\text{mg/min}$$

1–16. False. Normally, the rate at which an organ removes a substance from the blood is determined by the organ's use rate of the substance, which is normally determined by the metabolic activity within the tissue. The Fick principle implies that when an organ's metabolism of a substance is constant, an increase in blood flow will result in an increase in the venous blood concentration of the substance. One way of looking at the Fick principle is that the first term $(\dot{Q} \times [X]_a)$ indicates at what rate a substance is offered to an organ. From this, the organ takes whatever it has an appetite for $(\dot{X})$ and leaves the excess in the venous blood $(\dot{Q} \times [X]_v)$. Obviously, an organ can never continuously "consume" more than it receives, so the first term $(\dot{Q} \times [X]_a)$ indicates the maximum sustained tissue metabolic rate $(\dot{X})$ that is possible in a given situation. Thus, in abnormal circumstances, low blood flow $(\dot{Q})$ and/or arterial concentration $([X]_a)$ could adversely affect tissue metabolism of X.

1–17. 1. An electrical arrhythmia would obviously influence heart rate. Depending on the nature of the arrhythmia, HR might be high or low. Because CO = HR × (EDV – ESV), a low HR would tend to reduce CO, whereas a high HR, in and of itself, would do the opposite. In some cases where the HR is extremely high, a counteracting influence of decreased EDV volume may develop because of decreased diastolic filling time. Certain arrhythmias cause the individual ventricular muscle cells not to contract in unison. To develop high pressure in the ventricular chamber, the cells in the ventricular wall must be contracting at the same time. When they do not do so, ventricular ejection is impaired and ESV increases as a result.

2. A "stenotic" valve has an abnormally high resistance to flow when it is supposed to be fully open. A stenotic input valve impedes diastolic filling and reduces EDV. A stenotic output valve impedes ventricular ejection and tends to increase ESV.

3. An "insufficient" valve allows backward flow when it is supposed to be closed. An insufficient inlet valve adversely affects effective SV because some of the volume that the ventricle "pumps" during systole goes backwards into the atria. An insufficient outlet valve adversely affects effective stroke volume because some of the volume that the ventricle pumps out during systole leaks back into the ventricle during diastole.

4. When the heart muscle cells themselves are "failing," they have diminished ability to generate pressure within the ventricle during systole. This ultimately results in increased ESV.

5. "Inadequate diastolic filling" is just another way of saying, "decreased EDV." One commonly encountered situation where this occurs is with extreme blood loss.

CHAPTER 2

2–1. a. The potassium equilibrium potential will become less negative because a lower electrical potential is required to balance the decreased tendency for net K^+ diffusion out of the cell $[E_{eqK^+} = (-61.5 \text{ mV}) \log ([K^+]_i / [K^+]_o)]$.

  b. Because the resting membrane is most permeable to K^+, the resting membrane potential is always close to the K^+ equilibrium potential. Lowering the absolute value of the K^+ equilibrium potential will undoubtedly also lower the absolute resting membrane potential (i.e., depolarize the cells).

  c. Two things can happen when the resting membrane potential is decreased: (1) the potential is closer to the threshold potential, which should increase excitability; and (2) the fast sodium channels become inactivated, making the cell less excitable. Thus, small increases in $[K^+]_o$ may increase excitability, whereas large increases in $[K^+]_o$ decrease excitability.

2–2. Elevations in extracellular potassium depolarize cardiac muscle cell membranes, as can be ascertained from the Nernst equation (see study question 2–1). A large depolarization that will accompany 20 mM KCl will inactivate all sodium and calcium channels, making the cells unexcitable and thus stopping the heart in a relaxed state (diastole). This cessation of contractile activity significantly reduces oxygen demands and helps protect the heart tissue against hypoxic injury.

2–3. a. Sodium channel blockers delay the opening of the fast sodium channels in cardiac myocytes. This will slow the rate of depolarization during the action potential (phase 0), which will in turn slow conduction velocity. This results in a prolongation of the PR interval and a widening of the QRS complex.

  b. Calcium channel blockers slow the firing rate of SA nodal cells by blocking the calcium component of the diastolic depolarization. They will reduce the rate of rise of the AV nodal cell action potential (which is largely due to calcium entry into the cells) and slow the rate of conduction through the AV node. In addition, calcium channel blockers will decrease the amount of calcium made available to the contractile machinery during excitation–contraction coupling and thus will decrease the tension-producing capabilities of the cardiac muscle cell.

  c. Potassium channel blockers inhibit the delayed increase in potassium permeability that contributes importantly to the initiation and rate of repolarization of the cardiac myocyte. This prolongs the duration of the plateau phase of the action potential, prolongs the QT interval of the ECG, and prolongs the effective refractory period of the cell.

2–4. False. It is true that increase in sympathetic activity will increase the heart rate (a positive chronotropic effect). However, the electrical refractory period of cardiac cells extends throughout the duration of the cell's contraction. This prevents individual twitches from ever occurring so closely together that they could summate into a tetanic state.

2–5. The correct answers are a and c. Increase in preload increases the amount of shortening by increasing the starting length of the muscle, whereas increase in contractility increases the amount of shortening from a given starting length. Increase in afterload limits the amount of shortening because of increase in tension requirement. (See Figures 2–9 and 2–10.)

2–6. b, because activation of this channel initiates repolarization (phase 3 of the action potential).

2–7. e, because changes in the configuration of the action potential at any given time after the initial rising phase have no influence on the conduction from cell to cell.

2–8. c, because normally about 80% of the transient increase in cytoplasmic calcium during a contraction is sequestered back into the SR.

CHAPTER 3

3–1. The ventricular systolic pressure is also 24 mm Hg because the normal pulmonic valve provides negligible resistance to flow during ejection. The right ventricular diastolic pressure, however, cannot be determined from the pulmonary artery pressure. It is determined by systemic venous pressure and normally will be close to 0 mm Hg.

3–2. All of them are correct answers: a, by increasing preload; b, by decreasing afterload; and c and d by augmenting contractility.

3–3. One cannot tell from the information given because the two alterations would have opposite effects on cardiac output (i.e., although decreased filling will reduce stroke volume, increased sympathetic tone will increase both stroke volume and heart rate). A complete set of ventricular function curves and quantitative information about the changes in filling pressure and sympathetic tone would be necessary to answer the question. (See Figure 3–8.)

3–4. True. (See Figure 3–6.) Increased sympathetic activity will increase contractility and ejection fraction.

3–5. b, because the ST segment of the ECG occurs during systole, whereas all the other events occur during diastole.

3–6. a, because the isovolumic contraction phase is the most energetically costly part of the cardiac cycle and increases in heart rate multiply this effect. Note, increases in end-diastolic volume (choice c) will also increase myocardial oxygen demands (because wall tension is proportional to pressure and radius, $T \sim Pr$) but to a much lesser extent than do increases in heart rate.

3–7. b, because sympathetic activation will increase action potential conduction through the AV node and thereby *decrease* the PR interval. All of the other choices will be increased by activation of cardiac sympathetic nerves. (The increase in metabolic demands will increase coronary blood flow by mechanisms described in more detail in Chapter 7.)

3–8. False. Recall that changes in TPR are caused by peripheral vascular responses and that the heart normally responds by adjustments in its cardiac output to keep arterial pressure constant. At constant arterial pressure, an increase in TPR implies a reduction in CO. According to the cardiac external work rate equation (WR = MAP × CO), a decrease in CO at constant MAP will cause a decrease in the work rate of the heart. *This is the main reason that your heart is working less hard when you are at rest than when you are exercising.*

3–9. False. Whereas basic thermodynamics says that to produce any given amount of external work, the heart must expend at least an equal amount of chemical energy. But the heart muscle is only about 30% efficient in converting chemical energy into mechanical work. Thus for openers, to produce any given external work, the heart consumes roughly 3 times that amount of chemical energy. Moreover, because of the peculiarities of cardiac muscle, the heart is somewhat more efficient in producing a given CO with higher SV and lower HR than the other way around. *So, metabolic requirements depend on how a given CO is accomplished.*

CHAPTER 4

4–1.
$$\dot{Q} = \frac{\dot{V}_{O_2}}{[O_2]_{SA} - [O_2]_{PA}}$$
$$= \frac{600 \, \text{mL/min}}{(200 - 140) \, \text{mL/L}}$$
$$= 10 \, \text{L/min}$$

This is a high resting cardiac output but may be normal during exercise.

4–2. Ejection fraction is 0.66 or 66%, which is within a normal range.

4–3. The correct answer is c.

4–4. The correct answer is b. According to the standard ECG polarity conventions, the P, R, and T waves will normally all be downward deflections on lead aVR.

4–5. According to the electrocardiographic conventions, the electrical axis is at 45 degrees and falls within the normal range (in the patient's lower-left quadrant). The smallest amplitude deflection will occur on the lead to which the electrical axis is most perpendicular. Lead III and lead aVL are both within 15 degrees of being perpendicular to 45 degrees and therefore will have equally small deflections.

4–6. d.

4–7. e.

4–8. c.

CHAPTER 5

5–1. a. Pulmonic valve stenosis or tricuspid valve regurgitation will both cause systolic murmurs.

   b. Pulmonic valve stenosis will increase the right ventricular pressure development during systole, which will promote right ventricular hypertrophy. The increased muscle mass on the right will be reflected as a shift in the net electrical dipole to the right during ventricular depolarization. Tricuspid valve regurgitation does not increase right ventricular pressures or stimulate cardiac muscle hypertrophy.

   c. No. Neither pulmonic stenosis nor tricuspid regurgitation will cause elevation in pulmonary vascular pressures or pulmonary edema. If anything, congestion from malfunction of either of these valves on the right side will appear upstream in the systemic system as swollen ankles or as ascites (fluid in the abdominal space).

5–2. a and b, because filling time is reduced; c, if ventricular rate is rapid; d, for obvious reasons; but not e, because ventricular pacemakers produce a lower heart rate, which is associated with a longer filling time and therefore, a larger stroke volume.

5–3. a. Aortic stenosis produces a significant pressure difference between the left ventricle and the aorta during systolic ejection (a time when this valve normally should be widely open and create little resistance to flow).

   b. Mitral stenosis produces a significant pressure difference between the left atrium and the left ventricle during diastole (a time when *this* valve normally should be widely open).

5–4. Tricuspid insufficiency. With proper positioning of the patient, pulsations in the neck veins can be observed. Regurgitant flow of blood through a leaky tricuspid valve during systole produces this large abnormal wave.

5–5. Irregular giant *a* waves (called cannon waves) are observed in the jugular veins whenever the atrium contracts against a closed tricuspid valve (i.e., during ventricular systole). Because in third-degree heart block the atria and ventricles are beating independently, this situation may occur at irregular intervals.

5–6. Given the abnormal pressure gradient (30 mm Hg) across the mitral valve during diastole, we conclude it is stenotic. This would be associated with a diastolic murmur and, because of the elevated left atrial and pulmonary venous pressure, could be associated with shortness of breath and/or pulmonary congestion. The resistance across this valve is calculated as the abnormal pressure difference divided by the flow.

$R = \Delta P/CO$
$R = 30/\text{mm Hg}/3 \text{ L/min}$
$R = 10 \text{ mm Hg per L/min}$

5–7. Aortic insufficiency.

5–8. d. The total dissociation of atrial and ventricular rates indicates lack of AV communication.

5–9. Although atrial fibrillation is the most likely diagnosis, without ECG validation, paroxysmal supraventricular tachycardia, atrial flutter, AV nodal block, and even ventricular flutter cannot be ruled out. Subsequent steps should include chronic cardiac monitoring over a week or more (Holter monitor), followed by pharmacological interventions to subdue the arrhythmia and, if atrial fibrillation, an anticoagulant to suppress clot formation in the atria and potential stroke.

CHAPTER 6

6–1. Since

$$\dot{F} = K[(P_c - P_i) - (\pi_c - \pi_i)]$$

then

$$\dot{F} = K[28 - (-4) - 24 + 0]\text{mm Hg} = K \times 8 \text{ mm Hg}$$

The result is positive, indicating net movement of fluid out of the capillaries.

6–2. All do: a and d, by allowing interstitial protein buildup; b, by raising P_c; and c for decreasing plasma oncotic pressure.

6–3. a. By the parallel resistance equation, the equivalent resistance (R_p) for the parallel pair is $R_p = R_e/2$.

Then by the series resistance equation,

$$R_n = R_e + R_p = 3R_e / 2$$

b. Since more resistance precedes the junction (R_e) than follows it $(R_e/2)$, P_j will be closer to P_o than to P_i.

6–4. Since

$$\dot{Q} = \frac{\Delta P}{R}$$

then

$$R = \frac{\Delta P}{\dot{Q}}$$

and

$$\text{TPR} = \frac{\bar{P}_A - P_{CV}}{CO}$$

Therefore,

$$\text{TPR} = \frac{100 - 0\,\text{mm Hg}}{6\,\text{L/min}}$$

$$= 16.7\,\text{mm Hg} \times \text{min/L}$$

6–5. False. TPR is less than the resistance to flow through any of the organs. Each organ, in effect, provides an additional pathway through which blood may flow. Thus, the individual organ resistances must be greater than the total resistance and

$$\frac{1}{\text{TPR}} = \frac{1}{R_1} + \frac{1}{R_2} + \dots + \frac{1}{R_n}$$

6–6. True.

6–7. True. Because arteriolar constriction tends to reduce the hydrostatic pressure in the capillaries, reabsorptive forces will exceed filtration forces, and net reabsorption of interstitial fluid into the vascular bed will occur.

6–8. True. $\bar{P}_A = CO \times TPR$.

6–9. False. Increases in cardiac output are often accompanied by decreases in total peripheral resistance. Depending on the relative magnitude of these changes, mean arterial pressure could rise, fall, or remain constant.

6–10. True. $P_p \simeq SV / C_A$. Acute rapid changes in arterial compliance usually do not occur.

6–11. False. An increase in TPR (with CO constant) will produce approximately equal increases in P_S and P_D and increase $\bar{P}_A$ with little influence on pulse pressure.

6–12. $\bar{P}_A \approx P_D + \dfrac{1}{3}(P_S - P_D)$

$\bar{P}_A \approx 70 + \dfrac{1}{3}(110 - 70)\,\text{mm Hg}$

$\bar{P}_A \approx 83\,\text{mm Hg}$

6–13. a. Recall that $SV \simeq P_p \times C_A$. P_p increased by a factor of 1.15 (from 39 to 45 mm Hg) during exercise. Because C_A is a relatively fixed parameter in the short term, the increase in P_p must have been produced by an increase in stroke volume of approximately 15%.

b. Recall that $CO = HR \times SV$. HR increased by a factor of 2 (from 70 to 140 beats/min) during exercise, and because SV increased by a factor of about 1.15, cardiac output must have increased by approximately 130%. [2.0 (1.15) = 2.3 times the original level.]

c. Recall that $TPR = \bar{P}_A / CO$. P_A increased by a factor of 1.13 (from 93 to 105 mm Hg) during exercise, whereas CO increased by approximately 2.3 times. Thus, total peripheral resistance must have decreased by approximately 55% (1.13/2.3 = 0.45 of the original level).

6–14. d.

CHAPTER 7

7–1. The correct answers are a, b, and c.

7–2. False. Autoregulation of blood flow implies that vascular resistance is adjusted to maintain constant flow in spite of changes in arterial pressure.

7–3. All, because they all increase myocardial oxygen consumption. Myocardial blood flow is controlled primarily by local metabolic mechanisms.

7–4. False. Sympathectomy will cause some dilation of skeletal muscle arterioles but not a maximal dilation because skeletal muscle arterioles have a strong inherent basal tone.

7–5. Hyperventilation decreases the blood P_{CO_2} level. This, in turn, causes cerebral arterioles to constrict (recall that cerebral vascular tone is highly sensitive to changes in P_{CO_2}). The increased cerebral vascular resistance causes a decrease in cerebral blood flow, which produces dizziness and disorientation.

7–6. It is likely that the increased metabolic demands evoked by the exercising skeletal muscle cannot be met by an appropriate increase in blood flow to the muscle. This patient may have some sort of arterial disease (atherosclerosis) that provides a high resistance to flow that cannot be overcome by local metabolic vasodilator mechanisms.

7–7. High left ventricular pressures must be developed to eject blood through the stenotic valve (Figure 5–4A). This increases myocardial oxygen consumption, which tends to increase coronary flow. At the same time, however, high intraventricular pressure development enhances the systolic compression of coronary vessels and tends to decrease flow. The local metabolic mechanisms may be adequate to compensate for the increased compressional forces and meet the increased myocardial metabolic needs in a resting individual. However, there may not be enough "reserve" to meet additional needs such as those that accompany exercise. Coronary perfusion pressure may also be decreased if the systemic arterial pressure is lower than normal.

7–8. b.

7–9. c.

7–10. a.

7–11. a. Hypoxic arteriolar vasoconstriction is a phenomenon that is known to occur only in the lungs.

7–12. True. During systole, coronary vessels are collapsed by external compression forces.

CHAPTER 8

8–1. None of the choices are correct. (The tiny change in vascular volume that accompanies a decrease in arteriolar tone is not sufficient to have a significant effect on mean circulatory filling pressure.)

8–2. Central venous pressure always settles at the value that makes cardiac output and venous return equal. Therefore, anything that shifts the cardiac function curve or the venous return curve affects central venous pressure (see the list of influences on P_{CV} in Appendix C).

8–3. False. Starling's law of the heart says that, *if other influences on the heart are constant,* cardiac output decreases when central venous pressure decreases (e.g., A → B in Figure 8–7). In the intact cardiovascular system, where many things may happen simultaneously, cardiac output and central venous pressure may change in opposite directions (e.g., B → C in Figure 8–7).

8–4. None. Venous return must always equal cardiac output in the steady-state situation.

8–5. Because cardiac preload *is* central venous pressure, the physician will try to lower central venous pressure. This requires a left shift of the venous return curve. The two ways that can be done are decreasing circulating volume or decreasing venous tone. The former is often accomplished with diuretic drugs, and the latter can be achieved with certain vasodilator drugs that specifically influence venous tone (i.e., venodilators).

8–6. e. Dehydration directly tends to lower blood volume, mean circulatory filling pressure, cardiac filling pressure, end-diastolic volume, and stroke volume. Heart rate will increase as a compensatory response to maintain cardiac output and arterial pressure.

8–7. b.

8–8. a.

CHAPTER 9

9–1. a and b will increase; the rest will decrease.

9–2. Carotid sinus massage causes arterial baroreceptors to fire, which in turn increases parasympathetic activity from the medullary cardiovascular centers. This can either slow the pacemaker activity or interrupt a reentry tachycardia and allow a more normal rhythm to be established.

9–3. a, b, and d would increase sympathetic nerve activity; c and e would decrease it.

9–4. Step 1. The influence of sympathetic nerve activity on arteriolar tone will be blocked. Arteriolar tone will fall and so will TPR. This will directly lower mean arterial pressure.

Step 2. The arterial baroreceptor firing rate will decrease, which will increase sympathetic nerve activity from the medullary CV centers.

Step 3. The heart rate and cardiac output will reflexively increase because of the cardiac effects of the increased sympathetic activity on β_1-adrenergic receptors. Total peripheral resistance will not be improved by the increase in sympathetic drive because the drug has blocked the α_1-adrenergic receptors.

Step 4. The cardiac function curve will shift upward, but the venous return curve will not shift, because the α-receptor blockade blocks the effect of increased sympathetic activity on the veins. Consequently, central venous pressure will be lower than normal (see Figure 8–6).

9–5. a and d are primary disturbances to the cardiovascular system. These will directly reduce the mean arterial pressure. Reflex adjustments largely mediated by the arterial baroreceptors will result in a higher-than-normal sympathetic activity.

b and c elicit set point–increasing inputs to the medullary cardiovascular system that result in a higher-than-normal sympathetic output for any given level of input from the arterial baroreceptors. Thus, in the presence of these disturbances, the system will operate at higher-than-normal mean arterial pressure *and* sympathetic activity.

9–6. a and c. These disturbances would tend to directly lower blood pressure, which would then lead to a reflex increase in the heart rate. Disturbances b and d have no direct effect on the heart or vessels. Rather, they act on the medullary cardiovascular centers to raise the set point and cause an increase in sympathetic activity. Consequently, one would expect b (and d in early phases) to cause increases in *both* the heart rate and the mean arterial pressure. In the case of prolonged and severely elevated intracranial pressure, the increased sympathetic activity does indeed raise arterial pressure to very high levels, but the arterial baroreceptors can fight this by simultaneously increasing parasympathetic drive to decrease the heart rate (second phase of Cushing reflex).

9–7. a.

9–8. c.

9–9. b.

CHAPTER 10

10–1. Because capillaries have such a small radius, according to the law of Laplace ($T = P \times r$), the tension in the capillary wall is rather modest despite very high internal pressures.

10–2. Fainting occurs because of decreased cerebral blood flow when mean arterial pressure falls below approximately 60 mm Hg. On a hot day, temperature reflexes override pressure reflexes to produce the increased skin blood flow required for thermal regulation. Thus, TPR may be lower when standing on a hot day than on a cool one. This vasodilation combined with the absence of the skeletal muscle pump during standing motionless at attention makes it quite likely that brain blood flow will be compromised.

10–3. The cardiovascular response to lying down is just the opposite of that shown in Figure 10–3. Therefore, during extended bed rest, patients tend to lose rather than retain fluid and end up with lower-than-normal blood volumes. Because of low blood volume, central venous pressure and cardiac filling are significantly reduced when the patient assumes an upright posture. Short-term compensatory actions (increased sympathetic drive, skeletal muscle pump, and respiratory pump) may be inadequate and blood pressure may fall. This may lead to a decrease in brain blood flow and dizziness ensues. Such patients are less able to cope with standing until blood volume is restored to normal values.

10–4. The pressure produced by the water on the lower part of the body enhances reabsorption of fluid into the capillaries, compresses peripheral veins, reduces the peripheral venous volume, and increases the volume of blood in the central venous pool. This stimulates the low-pressure cardiopulmonary mechanoreceptors and evokes a diuresis by way of the various neural and hormonal pathways discussed in Chapter 9.

10–5. $R = \bar{P}_A / \dot{Q}$. Skeletal muscle resistance must have decreased considerably during exercise because skeletal muscle flow increased 10-fold (100%), whereas mean arterial pressure increased much less (from 93 to 103 mm Hg or $\simeq 11\%$).

10–6. TPR $= \bar{P}_A / CO$. Total peripheral resistance must have decreased during exercise because cardiac output increased 3-fold (300%), which is relatively much larger than the 11% increase in mean arterial pressure.

10–7. 1. The heart rate during exercise is well above the intrinsic rate ($\simeq 100$ beats/min). This indicates activation of the cardiac sympathetic nerves because withdrawal of cardiac parasympathetic activity cannot increase the heart rate above the intrinsic rate (Chapter 2).

2. Increased arterial pulse pressure and ejection fraction at constant central venous pressure indicate increased stroke volume and cardiac contractility and thus increased activity of cardiac sympathetic nerves (Chapter 3).

3. Decreased renal and splanchnic blood flows despite increased mean arterial pressure indicate sympathetic vasoconstriction in these organs (Chapter 6).

10–8. a. SV = CO/HR
   SV = 6000/70 = 86 mL/beat at rest
   SV = 18,000/160 = 113 mL/beat during exercise
   [You may recall that, in the absence of other information, changes in SV can be estimated from changes in arterial pulse pressure, P_p. The information in Figure 10–4 indicates that P_p increased 1.75 times (from 40 to 70 mm Hg) as a result of exercise, whereas SV actually increased only 1.32 times (from 86 to 113 mL), as calculated earlier. This discrepancy emphasizes that although SV is a major determinant of P_p, changes in other factors, such as the compliance of arteries (C_A), can influence P_p as well (see Appendix C). Part of the increase in P_p that accompanies exercise is due to a decrease in effective arterial compliance. The latter is due to (1) an increase in mean arterial pressure with exercise and (2) the nonlinear nature of the arterial volume–pressure relationship (see Figures 6–8 and 6–10).]

   b. Ejection fraction = SV/EDV, therefore EDV = SV/ejection fraction
   EDV = 86/0.60 = 143 mL at rest
   EDV = 113/0.80 = 141 mL during exercise

[Recall that central venous pressure, P_{CV}, is the cardiac filling pressure or preload and is therefore the primary determinant of EDV. The EDV changed little with exercise because exercise caused little or no change in P_{CV}.]

c. SV = EDV − ESV, therefore ESV = EDV − SV

ESV = 143 − 86 = 57 mL at rest

ESV = 141 − 113 = 28 mL during exercise

[Recall that the primary determinants of ESV are cardiac afterload (mean arterial pressure) and myocardial contractility (see Appendix C). Cardiac afterload increases during exercise and thus goes in the wrong direction to account for a decrease in ESV. Therefore, an increased myocardial contractility, secondary to increased cardiac sympathetic nerve activity, must be primarily responsible for the decrease in ESV that accompanies exercise.]

d.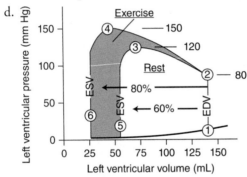

Key features on this figure:

Point 1. End-diastolic volume during both rest and exercise is approximately 140 mL.

Point 2. Ventricular ejection (decreasing ventricular volume) begins when intraventricular pressure reaches the diastolic aortic pressure and the aortic valve opens. Figure 10−4 indicates an arterial diastolic pressure of 80 mm Hg both at rest and during exercise. Thus, ventricular ejection will begin at an intraventricular pressure of 80 mm Hg in both situations.

Points 3 and 4. Peak intraventricular pressure normally equals peak (systolic) arterial pressure. Hence, the systolic arterial pressure values in Figure 10−4 indicate peak intraventricular pressures of 120 and 150 mm Hg during rest and exercise, respectively.

Points 5 and 6. As calculated in section c above, end-systolic volume is 57 mL at rest and decreases to 28 mL during exercise. This reduction in end-systolic volume accounts for the increase in stroke volume during exercise.

10–9. The external negative pressure served to expand the thorax and "pull" air into the lungs through the patient's airways in much the same way that the thoracic muscle and diaphragm expand the thorax in normal breathing. This method of ventilating the lungs did not have the adverse cardiovascular consequences that positive-pressure artificial ventilation has.

10–10. Blood flow through muscles is reduced or stopped by compressive forces on skeletal muscle vessels during an isometric muscle contraction. Thus, during an isometric maneuver, total peripheral resistance (TPR) may be higher than normal rather than much lower than normal as it is during phasic exercises such as running. In the absence of decreased TPR but the presence of especially strong set point–raising influences (central command) from the cortex on the medullary cardiovascular centers, mean arterial pressure may be regulated to very high values (see point 2 in Figure E-3A of Appendix E). The other process that often accompanies strenuous isometric exercise is the use of a Valsalva maneuver. This forced attempt to exhale with a closed glottis has several cardiovascular consequences (described in Chapter 10). However, one of the beneficial effects for weight lifters is the high intrathoracic and intraabdominal pressures achieved when the air cannot escape from the highly inflated lungs. These pressure-filled cavities "insulate," and therefore provide core support for the lumbar and thoracic spine.

10–11. By acting specifically on α-adrenergic receptors, the *primary* disturbance of phenylephrine will be to increase total peripheral resistance. (Recall that almost all cardiac effects of catecholamines are all mediated via *beta* receptors.) The resulting increase in arterial blood pressure and increased firing of the arterial baroreceptors will cause a *compensatory reflex* decrease in sympathetic nerve activity (and increase in parasympathetic activity), which will reflexly decrease both myocardial contractility and heart rate. (Withdrawal of sympathetic tone to arterioles will not reduce the vasoconstriction because the direct effect of the drug overrides the neural signal.)

10–12. b. Stroke volume is ~140 mL, which is higher-than-normal at rest. High stroke volumes (coupled with low resting heart rates) are typical for trained athletes.

10–13. e. All other choices are part of the reflex compensatory responses to the increase in central venous pressure.

10–14. a.

10–15. c.

10–16. c. Although aging is often associated with an increase in mean arterial pressure, that is not a consequence of changes in aortic stiffness but rather changes in TPR, as described in Chapter 6.

CHAPTER 11

11–1. Intense sympathetic activation drastically reduces skin blood flow, promotes transcapillary reabsorption of fluids, increases the heart rate and contractility (but may not restore stroke volume because of low central venous pressure), and reduces skeletal muscle blood flow. Cerebral blood flow falls if the compensatory mechanisms do not prevent mean arterial pressure from falling below 60 mm Hg.

11–2. a. Not helpful because gravity tends to promote peripheral venous blood pooling and cause a further fall in arterial pressure.
  b. Not helpful if carried to an extreme. Cutaneous vasodilation produced by warming adds to the cardiovascular stresses.
  c. Helpful if the victim is conscious and can drink because fluid will be rapidly absorbed from the gut to increase circulating blood volume.
  d. Might be helpful as an initial emergency measure to prevent brain damage due to severely reduced blood pressure, but prolonged treatment will promote the decompensatory mechanisms associated with decreased organ blood flow.

11–3. a. In hypovolemic shock from diarrhea, the hematocrit will probably increase because, even though the compensatory processes will evoke a substantial "autotransfusion" by shifting fluid from the intracellular and interstitial space into the vascular space, this amount of fluid is limited to a liter or less. Therefore, a substantial loss of fluid (without red blood cells) will *raise* the hematocrit significantly.
  b. In cardiogenic shock, the hematocrit may decrease because compensatory actions evoked to maintain blood pressure may promote a fluid shift into the vascular space. However, because central venous pressure (and perhaps peripheral venous pressures) may also be elevated, capillary hydrostatic pressures (and thus fluid shifts) are difficult to predict.
  c. In septic shock, peripheral vasodilation and peripheral venous pooling may actually promote filtration of fluid out of the vasculature in some beds (which would lead to an increased hematocrit), but the low arterial and central venous pressures may counteract this shift, so changes in hematocrits are difficult to predict in this situation.
  d. Chronic bleeding disorders are usually associated with low hematocrit and anemia because red blood cell production may not keep pace with red cell losses, whereas the volume-regulating mechanisms may be able to maintain a normal blood volume.

11–4. True. The law of Laplace states that when the radius (r) of a cylinder (or in this case, the irregularly shaped ventricular chamber) increases, the wall tension (T) for a given internal pressure (P) must also increase: $T = P \times r$.

11–5. Excessive fluid retention can induce decompensatory mechanisms that further compromise an already-weakened heart (e.g., inadequate oxygenation of the blood as it passes through edematous lungs, marked cardiac dilation and increased myocardial metabolic needs, and liver dysfunction due to congestion). Diuretic therapy reduces fluid volume and the high venous pressures that are the cause of these problems.

11–6. If blood volume and central venous pressure are reduced too far with diuretic therapy, stroke volume may fall to unacceptably low levels according to Starling's law of the heart and blood pressure may fall. Subsequent compensatory increases in heart rate may not be tolerable by those in heart failure.

11–7. Because of the high resistance of the stenosis and the pressure drop across it, glomerular capillary pressure and therefore glomerular filtration rate are lower than normal when arterial pressure is normal. Thus, a renal artery stenosis reduces the urinary output rate caused by a given level of arterial pressure. The renal function curve is shifted to the right, and hypertension follows.

11–8. c.

11–9. e.

11–10. All variables will be normal except for d which will be above normal.

11–11. Applying external pressure with elastic stockings on the lower limbs and feet counteracts the tendency for high peripheral venous pressures to cause edema in the lower extremities. Because congestive failure is associated with high central venous and therefore peripheral venous pressures, this strategy will aid in keeping fluid within the vascular circulation.

11–12. Probably not. This condition (called intermittent claudication) is usually a result of "poor circulation" not able to increase blood flow in response to increase oxygen demand in exercising leg muscles. It is most often caused by severe atherosclerotic narrowing of major arteries (peripheral artery disease) providing a fixed high resistance that cannot be overcome by vasodilation in the microvasculature. Compression stocking will not be helpful (unless there is some other complication resulting in high peripheral venous pressures).

11–13. Yes. A clot in a large vein can increase upstream venous pressure and lead to significant edema, swelling, pressure, and pain. A compression stocking can be used to minimize these symptoms but will not correct the primary problem. Note that deep vein thrombosis (DVT) is a dangerous condition. If a piece of the clot breaks off, passes through the right ventricle, and lodges in the lung (pulmonary embolis), it can significantly interfere with gas exchange and cardiac filling. There is some evidence that these stockings can help *prevent the formation* of these clots in people who will be experiencing long periods of inactivity (e.g., plane trip, bed rest, paralysis) or have other situations that may promote formation of DVT (pregnancy, vascular surgery, obesity).

Appendix A

Normal Values of Erythrocytes, Leukocytes, and Platelets in Adult Human Blood*

Erythrocytes	Male: 4.3–5.7 million/μL blood Female: 3.9–5.1 million/μL blood
Hemoglobin	Male: 13.5–17.5 g/dL Female: 12.0–15.5 g/dL
Hematocrit	Male: 38.8%–50% Female: 34.9%–44.5%
Platelets	150,000–450,000/μL of blood
White blood cells	4000–11,000/μL of blood

Types of leukocytes	Percentage of total leukocytes	Primary role
Polymorphonuclear granulocytes		
Neutrophils	40–80	Phagocytosis
Eosinophils	1–6	Allergic hypersensitivity reactions
Basophils	<1–2	Allergic hypersensitivity reactions
Monocytes	1–6	Phagocytosis and antibody production
Lymphocytes	20–40	Antibody production and cell-mediated immunity

*Normal reference ranges vary somewhat with age and race. They may also vary from laboratory to laboratory. To confuse the issue further, various unit measurements are used to report blood data, and so caution must be used in examining data.

Appendix B

Some Normal Constituents of Adult Human Plasma

Class	Constituent	Amount/normal concentration range
Electrolytes (inorganic)		
Cations	Sodium (Na^+)	136–145 meq/L
	Potassium (K^+)	3.5–5.0 meq/L
	Calcium (Ca^{2+})	2.1–3.7 meq/L
	Magnesium (Mg^{2+})	1.2–1.8 meq/L
	Iron (Fe^{3+})	60–160 μg/dL
	Copper (Cu^{2+})	70–155 μg/dL
	Hydrogen (H^+)	35–45 nmol/L (pH = 7.35–7.45)
Anions	Chloride (Cl^-)	95–105 meq/L
	Bicarbonate (HCO_3^-)	23–28 meq/L
	Sulfate (SO_4^{2-})	0.9–1.1 meq/L
	Phosphate (HPO_4^{2-} mostly)	2.5–4.5 mg/dL
Proteins	Total (7% of plasma weight)	6–8 g/dL
	Albumin	3.4–5.0 g/dL
	Globulins	2.2–4.0 g/dL
	Fibrinogen	150–400 mg/dL
Lipids	Cholesterol—Total	<200 mg/dL
	LDL cholesterol	<100 mg/dL
	HDL cholesterol	>60 mg/dL
	Triglycerides	<150 mg/dL
Carbohydrates	Glucose	80–120 mg/dL
	Lactate	0.67–1.8 meq/L
Waste products	Uric acid (from nucleic acids)	2.6–7.0 mg/dL
	Blood urea nitrogen (from protein)	7–20 mg/dL
	Creatinine (from creatine)	0.5–1.1 mg/dL
	Bilirubin (from heme)	0.3–1.0 mg/dL

Appendix C

Key Cardiovascular Variables and Their Normal Determinants[1]

$$\bar{P}_A = CO \times TPR$$

$$CO = SV \times HR$$

$$SV = EDV - ESV$$

Ejection fraction $= SV/EDV$

$$SV \xleftarrow{\text{ventricular pump}} \begin{cases} (+) \uparrow \text{ cardiac preload (via effect on EDV)} \\ (+) \uparrow \text{ cardiac contractility (via effect on ESV)} \\ (-) \uparrow \text{ cardiac afterload (via effect on ESV)} \end{cases}$$

Cardiac preload $\propto P_{CV}$ ("$\propto$" means "is proportional to")

$$P_{CV} \xleftarrow{\text{central blood volume}} \begin{cases} (+) \uparrow \text{ total blood volume} \\ (+) \uparrow \text{ peripheral venous tone} \\ (+) \text{ skeletal muscle pump} \\ (+) \text{ respiratory pump} \\ (-) \text{ standing} \\ (-) \uparrow \text{ cardiac output} \end{cases}$$

Venous tone $\leftarrow \{(+) \uparrow$ sympathetic activity (via NE, α-receptors)

Contractility $\xleftarrow{\text{ventricular cells}} \{(+) \uparrow$ sympathetic activity (via NE, β-receptors)

Cardiac afterload $\propto \bar{P}_A$

$$HR \xleftarrow{\text{SA node cell firing rate}} \begin{cases} (+) \uparrow \text{ sympathetic activity (via NE, } \beta\text{-receptors)} \\ (-) \uparrow \text{ parasympathetic activity (via ACh)} \end{cases}$$

$$TPR \xleftarrow{\text{arteriolar tone}} \begin{cases} (+) \uparrow \text{ sympathetic activity (via NE, } \alpha\text{-receptors)} \\ (-) \uparrow \text{ local metabolites (} \uparrow \text{ local metabolic rate)} \end{cases}$$

$$P_p \propto SV / C_A$$

---

[1] $\bar{P}_A$, mean arterial pressure; CO, cardiac output; TPR, total peripheral resistance; SV, stroke volume; HR, heart rate; ESV, end-systolic volume; EDV, end-diastolic volume; P_{CV}, central venous pressure; NE, norepinephrine; ACh, acetylcholine; P_p, arterial pulse pressure; C_A, arterial compliance; SA, sinoatrial.

Appendix D

Hemostasis

Whenever damage occurs to a blood vessel, a variety of processes are evoked that are aimed at preventing or stopping blood from exiting the vascular space. The 3 primary processes are summarized in the following list:

I. **Platelet aggregation and plug formation:** Occur as a result of the following steps:
   A. Vessel injury with endothelial damage and collagen exposure.
   B. Platelet adherence to collagen (mediated by the plasma protein, von Willebrand factor).
   C. Platelet shape change (from disks to spiny spheres) and degranulation with release of the following:
      1. Adenosine diphosphate, which causes platelet aggregation and "plugs" the hole.
      2. Thromboxane, which causes vasoconstriction and potentiates platelet adhesion and aggregation.
II. **Local vasoconstriction:** Mediated largely by thromboxane but may also be induced by local release of other chemical signals that constrict local vessels and reduce blood flow.
III. **Blood clotting:** The formation of a solid gel made up of the protein, fibrin, platelets, and trapped blood cells.

The critical step in blood clotting is the formation of thrombin from prothrombin, which then catalyzes the conversion of fibrinogen to fibrin. The final clot is stabilized by covalent cross-linkages between fibrin strands catalyzed by factor XIIIa (the formation of which is catalyzed by thrombin).

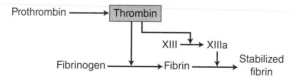

The cascade of reactions that leads from vessel injury to the formation of thrombin is shown in the figure below and is described as follows:

A. Vessel injury or tissue damage with blood exposure to subendothelial cells that release thromboplastin ("tissue factor").

B. The plasma protein factor VII binds to the tissue factor, which converts it to an activated form, factor VIIa.

C. VIIa catalyzes the conversion of both factors IX and X to activated forms IXa and Xa, respectively.

D. IXa also helps convert factor X to Xa (Stuart factor).

E. Xa converts prothrombin to thrombin.

F. Thrombin.

    1. Activates platelets (makes them sticky, induces degranulation, and promotes attachment of various factors that participate in clotting).

    2. Converts fibrinogen to fibrin.

    3. Recruits the "intrinsic pathway," which amplifies further formation of factor Xa and facilitates the conversion of prothrombin to thrombin by promoting the following reactions:

        a. Conversion of factor XI to its activated form, XIa, which then converts factor IX to IXa, which then attaches to activated platelets and converts factor X to Xa.

        b. Conversion of factor VIII (missing in hemophiliacs) to its activated form, VIIIa, which attaches to activated platelets and accelerates conversion of factor X to Xa.

        c. Conversion of factor V to its activated form, Va, which attaches to activated platelets and accelerates conversion of prothrombin to thrombin.

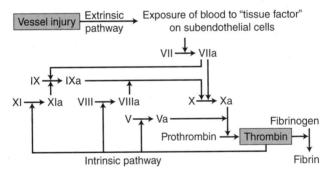

Several agents clinically used as *anticoagulants* interfere with various steps in this clotting process. *Aspirin* and other *cyclooxygenase inhibitors* are anticoagulants because they prevent the formation of thromboxane. *Dicoumarol* and *coumadin* block the activity of vitamin K, which is necessary for synthesis of many of the clotting factors by the liver. Specific inhibitors of the actions of various clotting factors are also now available. *Heparin* activates a plasma protein called *antithrombin III*, which, in turn, inactivates thrombin and several of the other clotting factors. In addition, a separate class of drugs that focus on preventing platelet aggregation are also useful in preventing clot formation. Because calcium is an important clotting cofactor, calcium chelators such as *EDTA*, *oxalate*, and *citrate* are used to prevent stored blood from clotting. Various *thrombolytic agents* modeled after the endogenous *tissue plasminogen activator* (*tPA*) are also available that promote dissolution of the fibrin clot after it is formed. These agents promote the formation of plasmin from plasminogen, which enzymatically attacks the clot, turning it into soluble peptides.

Appendix E

Analysis of the Arterial Baroreflex

For most purposes, the simple "thermostat analogy" provides a sufficient understanding of how the arterial baroreflex operates. However, in certain situations—especially when there are multiple disturbances in the cardiovascular system—a more detailed understanding is helpful. Consequently, the operation of the arterial baroreflex is presented in this appendix with a more formal control system approach.

The complete arterial baroreceptor reflex pathway is a control system made up of two distinct portions, as shown in Figure E–1: (1) an *effector portion*, including the heart and peripheral blood vessels; and (2) a *neural portion*, including the arterial baroreceptors, their afferent nerve fibers, the medullary cardiovascular centers, and the efferent sympathetic and parasympathetic fibers. Mean arterial pressure is the *output* of the effector portion and simultaneously the *input* to the neural portion. Similarly, the activity of the sympathetic (and parasympathetic) cardiovascular nerves is the *output* of the neural portion of the arterial baroreceptor control system and, at the same time, the *input* to the effector portion. For convenience, we omit continual reference to parasympathetic nerve activity in the following discussion. Throughout, however, an indicated change in sympathetic nerve activity should usually be taken to imply a reciprocal change in the activity of the cardiac parasympathetic nerves.

A host of reasons why mean arterial pressure *increases* when the heart and peripheral vessels receive *increased* sympathetic nerve activity were discussed in this textbook. All this information is summarized by the curve shown in the lower graph in Figure E–1, which describes the operation of the effector portion of the arterial baroreceptor system alone. In Chapter 9, how *increased* mean arterial pressure acts through the arterial baroreceptors and medullary cardiovascular centers to *decrease* the sympathetic activity has also been discussed. This information is summarized by the curve shown in the upper graph in Figure E–1, which describes the operation of the neural portion of the arterial baroreceptor system *alone*.

When the arterial baroreceptor system is intact and operating as a closed loop, the effector portion and neural portion retain their individual rules of operation, as described by their individual function curves in Figure E–1. Yet in the closed loop, the two portions of the system must interact until they come into balance with each other at some operating point with a mutually compatible combination of mean arterial pressure and sympathetic activity. The analysis of the complete

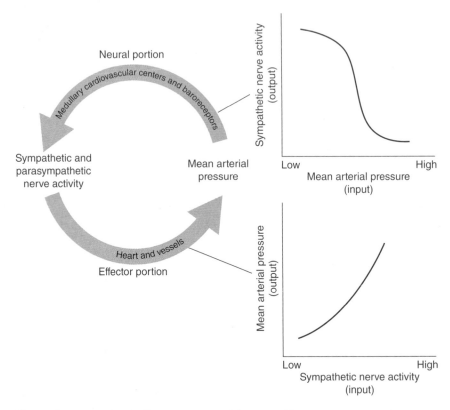

Figure E-1. Neural and effector portions of the arterial baroreceptor control system.

system begins by plotting the operating curves for the neural and effector portions of the systems together on the same graph, as shown in Figure E–2A. To accomplish this superimposition, the graph for the neural portion (the upper graph in Figure E–1) was flipped to interchange its vertical and horizontal axes. Consequently, the neural curve (but not the effector curve) in Figure E–2A must be read in the unusual sense that its independent variable, arterial pressure, is on the vertical axis and its dependent variable, sympathetic nerve activity, is on the horizontal axis.

Whenever there is any outside disturbance on the cardiovascular system, the operating point of the arterial baroreceptor system shifts. This happens because *all* cardiovascular disturbances cause a shift in one or the other of the two curves in Figure E–2A. For example, Figure E–2B shows how the operating point for the arterial baroreceptor system is shifted by a cardiovascular disturbance that lowers the operating curve of the effector portion. The disturbance in this case could be anything that reduces the arterial pressure produced by the heart and vessels *at each given level of sympathetic activity.* Blood loss, for example, is such a disturbance because it lowers central venous pressure and, through the Starling's law, lowers cardiac output and thus mean arterial pressure at any given level of

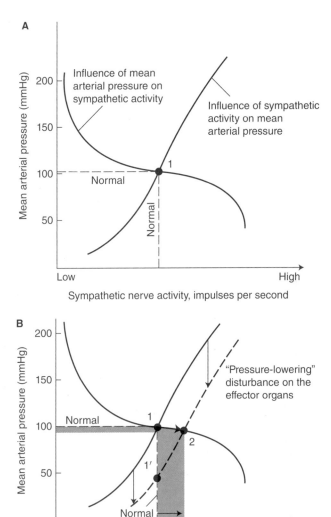

Figure E–2. Operation of the arterial baroreceptor control system: (**A**) normal balance and (**B**) operating point shift with disturbance on the effector portion.

cardiac sympathetic nerve activity. Metabolic vasodilation of arterioles in exercising skeletal muscle is another example of a pressure-lowering disturbance on the effector portion of the system because it lowers the total peripheral resistance and thus the arterial pressure that the heart and vessels produce at any given level of sympathetic nerve activity.

As shown by point 2 in Figure E–2B, any pressure-lowering disturbance on the heart or vessels causes a new balance to be reached within the baroreceptor system at a slightly lower-than-normal mean arterial pressure and a higher-than-normal sympathetic activity level. Note that the point 1' in Figure E–2B indicates how far the mean arterial pressure would have fallen as a consequence of the disturbance, had not the sympathetic activity been automatically increased above normal by the arterial baroreceptor system.

As indicated previously in Chapter 9 and in this appendix, many disturbances act on the neural portion of the arterial baroreceptor system rather than directly on the heart or vessels. These disturbances shift the operating point of the cardiovascular system because they alter the operating curve of the neural portion

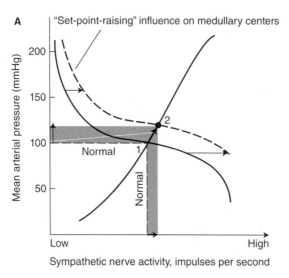

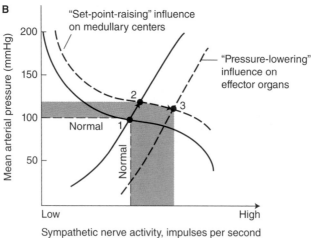

Figure E–3. The effect of neural influences on the arterial baroreceptor control system: (**A**) operating point shift with disturbance on the neural portion and (**B**) operating point shift with disturbances on both neural and effector portions.

of the system. For example, the influences listed in Figure 9–4 that raise the set point for arterial pressure do so by shifting the operating curve for the neural portion of the arterial baroreceptor system to the right, as shown in Figure E–3A, because they increase the level of sympathetic output from the medullary cardio-vascular centers *at each and every level of arterial pressure* (i.e., at each and every level of input from the arterial baroreceptors). For example, a sense of danger will cause the components of the arterial baroreceptor system to come into bal-ance at a higher-than-normal arterial pressure and a higher-than-normal sympa-thetic activity, as shown by point 2 in Figure E–3A. Conversely, but not shown in Figure E–3, any of the set-point-lowering influences listed in Figure 9–4 acting on the medullary cardiovascular centers will shift the operating curve for the neural portion of the arterial baroreceptor system to the left, and a new balance will be reached at lower-than-normal arterial pressure and sympathetic activity.

Many physiological and pathological situations involve simultaneous dis-turbances on both the neural and effector portions of the arterial baroreceptor system. Figure E–3A illustrates this type of situation. The set-point-increasing disturbance on the neural portion of the system alone causes the equilibrium to shift from point 1 to point 2. Superimposing a pressure-lowering disturbance on the heart or vessels further shifts the equilibrium from point 2 to point 3. Note that, although the response to the pressure-lowering disturbance in Figure E–3B (point 2 to point 3) starts from a higher-than-normal arterial pressure, it is essentially identical to that which occurs in the absence of a set-point-increasing influence on the cardiovascular center (see Figure E–2B). Thus, the response is an attempt to prevent the arterial pressure from falling below that at point 2. The overall implication is that any of the set-point-increasing influences on the med-ullary cardiovascular centers listed in Figure 9–4 cause the arterial baroreceptor system to regulate arterial pressure to a higher-than-normal value. Conversely, the set-point-lowering influences on the medullary cardiovascular centers listed in Figure 9–4 would cause the arterial baroreceptor system to regulate arterial pres-sure to a lower-than-normal value.

Several situations that involve a higher-than-normal sympathetic activity at a time when arterial pressure is itself higher-than-normal are discussed in Chapters 10 and 11. It should be noted that higher-than-normal sympathetic activity and higher-than-normal arterial pressure can exist together only when there is a set-point-raising influence on the *neural* portion of the arterial baroreceptor system.

Index

Page numbers followed by *f, t, and n* indicate figures, tables, and notes, respectively.